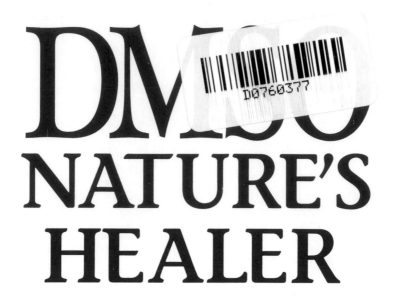

DMSO
NATURE'S
HEALER

Dr. Morton Walker

A DR. MORTON WALKER HEALTH BOOK

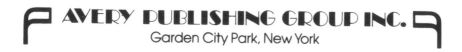

AVERY PUBLISHING GROUP INC.
Garden City Park, New York

The medical information and procedures contained in this book are not intended as a substitute for consulting your physician. All matters regarding your physical health should be supervised by a medical professional.

Cover Design: Rudy Shur and Ann Vestal
In-House Editors: Bonnie Freid
Typesetter: Bonnie Freid
Printer: Paragon Press, Honesdale, PA

Library of Congress Cataloging-in-Publication Data

Walker, Morton
    DMSO : nature's healer / Morton Walker.
      p. cm.
    Includes bibliographical references and index.
    ISBN 0-89529-548-2
    1. Dimethyl sulphoxide—Therapeutic use. I. Title.
RM666.D56W337   1993
615'.783—dc20   92-34981
                                                CIP

Copyright © 1993 by Dr. Morton Walker

All rights reserved. No part of this publication may be reproduced, stored in a retrieval system, or transmitted, in any form or by any means, electronic, mechanical, photocopying, recording or otherwise, without the prior written permission of the copyright owner.

Printed in the United States of America

10 9 8 7 6 5 4 3 2

Contents

To that singular humanitarian who loves people,
Chrystyne M. Jackson, publisher of Explore magazine,
who has saved more people's lives
with counseling, lectures, referrals, and publications
than have most individual physicians
who use conventional medical practices.

Acknowledgments

My appreciation is extended to the medical consultant for a first edition of this book. Ten years ago, William Campbell Douglass, M.D., then of Sarasota, Florida, put together a three-day medical conference comprised of experts on dimethyl sulfoxide. They came to Sarasota from around the United States and six foreign countries and brought specialty knowledge of DMSO with them. They shared this knowledge with each other, and I was the medical journalist who recorded their information, produced magazine and clinical journal articles, and eventually the first edition of this book. The present second edition is an update and then rewrite of that initial published effort.

Preface

The American Medical Association (AMA) held a leadership conference the weekend of February 14, 1981, and one of its speakers was Otis
R. Bowen, M.D. Dr. Bowen is former governor of Indiana, a leader in
medicine, management, and politics. In his presentation to the AMA,
he shocked the assembly by admitting that he took the law into his own
hands and used an illegal drug to ease his wife's pain while she was
dying. Beth Bowen died January 1, 1981, after months of agony from
multiple myeloma, a type of bone cancer.

Dr. Bowen, who was preparing to step down from the governorship
at the time, turned to dimethyl sulfoxide, or DMSO, to ease his wife's
intense pain. He had obtained the liquid solvent from a veterinarian
and found that it relieved his wife's suffering "in minutes," he said.

The Food and Drug Administration (FDA) forbids the use of DMSO
in humans except in treating a rare urinary bladder condition. Even in
the face of the government ban, Dr. Bowen did what he knew was right
for his wife by administering intravenous DMSO. "Why can't dying
persons, with severe pain, have easy prescription access to it?" he asked
in his speech. "The only excuse I could find was that, after prolonged
use and heavy dosage, it caused an occasional cataract in dogs only."

Before you've read very far into this book, you'll probably be asking
questions similar to Dr. Bowen's. It won't be difficult to identify with
the patients involved here, some of whom have been forced to take
treatment into their own hands by turning to DMSO.

In fact, DMSO has *not* been found unsafe for humans. Any side
effects are merely minor irritations. DMSO stops bacterial growth. It
relieves pain. As a vasodilator, the drug enlarges small blood vessels,
increasing the circulation to an area. It softens scar tissue and soothes
burns. DMSO's anti-inflammatory activity relieves the swelling and

inflammation of arthritis, bursitis, tendinitis, and other musculoskeletal injuries. And it does many more good things of a therapeutic nature
for anyone who is injured or ill.

I recommend that you use DMSO strictly under the supervision of a
doctor who is skilled in its application. Only the pure pharmaceutical
grade should be employed, not the crude industrial grade.

DMSO is both a drug and a good solvent. Industry values it for
removing paints and varnishes, and dissolving certain plastics such as
rayon, polyvinyl chloride, polyurethane, methacrylate, and acrylic. It
doesn't affect cotton, wool, nylon, leather, or polyesters.

More important, it benefits human body cells, tissues, and organs in
unique ways. DMSO is the twenty-first century's newest healing principle with a very wide range of usefulness. It represents an entirely
different means of treating diseases—not as an ordinary drug that
works for a given disease, but as a holistic ingredient that brings
whole-body cellular function back to normal.

Dimethyl sulfoxide has had a battered thirty-year history. But because of the general public outcry about its ban, DMSO has become a
household word and a medical-political cause célèbre. Those of us who
have been using the drug for twenty-six to twenty-eight years never
dreamed that it would become a focal point in the continuing battle
between individual freedom and the power of government.

My colleagues and I have been criticized, ridiculed, and even perse-
cuted in some medical circles for promoting and using DMSO. But I, and
others like me, came to the conclusion, having observed establishment
medical thinking for forty years, that the only way a truly revolutionary
treatment principle can be brought to the patient is by appealing to the
general population through the information media. That is the purpose
of this book.

Much of my material will appear anecdotal to the scientist, but such
language is what the public understands best. And sometimes a hundred patient stories, heard by a sensitive and intelligent physician, are
as good as or better than a double-blind research project. Double-blind
studies are often just that—everyone involved is blind and stays that
way until, many years and thousands of patients later, it is discovered
that the particular drug doesn't work or is too toxic to warrant its use.

Good current examples of toxic drugs are the arthritis agents Motrin,
Tolectin, Nalfon, and Naprosyn. They all underwent extensive double-
blind testing. All are weak organic acids and prostaglandin inhibitors—
like aspirin. About as effective as aspirin, these four drugs have two

distinct differences: they are more toxic than aspirin and cost ten to thirty times more money. So much for double-blind studies.

Whether you agree or disagree with current claims, it's likely you'll affirm that if a drug has been proven safe, doctors should be free to use this agent when they believe it will help their patients. With all the extremely potent and dangerous drugs on the market, it is absurd to keep such an effective product as DMSO from pharmacy shelves.

Certainly not all of the claims for DMSO will prove to be valid, but in my opinion, many of them have already shown themselves to be true. And the most dramatic use of the medication is likely yet to be discovered.

Another purpose for my book is to point out the myriad applications of this unique substance. Once DMSO is legalized for use in all states and ethically produced for topical, parenteral, and oral administration, people won't have to smuggle the feed-store grade and the crude industrial grade into their homes to paint on their arthritic joints.

DMSO will eventually find its place in the armamentarium of American medicine. We who believe in the substance want to see it happen sooner than later. The clinical evaluation of DMSO began in the United States in 1963 and now, in 1992, the FDA still has not approved the drug for more than one use. This situation gives rise to some underlying questions you may find running throughout this book. How do we get the FDA to see beyond its blind spot? How can we either bring DMSO to the people or declare the substance useless once and for all?

You will find lots of answers in these pages. DMSO needs even more public pressure than has been leveled at the regulatory process already. We want doctors to be able to prescribe DMSO without fear of censure from the medical world or the hospitals that employ them. If this doesn't happen, it appears that little will be done to ensure that a pure, medical grade of DMSO will be made available for patients.

In writing this book, I have found a distinct reticence by doctors to have their names mentioned in connection with DMSO. Often they provided me with glowing case reports of successes with the drug treatment, but their fear of colleague criticism prevented my revealing their identities. I had to discard such reports, and there were hundreds of them.

DMSO has the largest potential number of uses ever documented for a single chemical. My wish is that this book will bring more of them into the public domain than has been allowed to this point. It should be well understood by everyone at the outset that I don't say the substance is some kind of miracle cure. More properly, DMSO is a very effective and versatile compound that has been successfully adapted for a number of health problems. I want to get it into the hands of more people so that they may be relieved of discomforts and diseases for which DMSO is appropriate. I hope you will agree that mine is a worthy goal.

Morton Walker, D.P.M.
Stamford, Connecticut

CHAPTER 1
The Painkiller
With a Problem

In the late spring of 1980, Eva Lee Snead, M.D., then a family practice specialist in San Antonio, Texas, learned that her friend, thirty-two-year-old psychologist Marjorie Saloman, was supposed to undergo a hysterectomy, the removal of her uterus. Mrs. Saloman's genital system problem arose from a stenosis of the cervical os. This condition is a narrowing or stricture at the mouth of the neck-like opening to the uterus where it extends into the vagina.

The psychologist described to Dr. Snead how several unsuccessful attempts at cervical dilatation had been attempted by her gynecologist. He tried to relax the cervix by injecting local anesthesia at its lower quadrant. Such an anesthetic technique usually is simple and effective, but this particular block had been no help to the woman even after many tries. Mrs. Saloman's gynecologist admitted that for her the attempted cervical dilatation was a complete failure.

The pain had been so great for this patient that when the dilatation instrument was inserted she had fainted. Her gynecologist quickly removed the instrument because the anesthetic was not allaying the pain. None of his attempts to relieve the problem worked; surgical removal of the uterus was the next procedure of choice.

Dr. Snead asked her friend to wait a week before having the hysterectomy, if delay was agreeable to the gynecologist. Complying with this request, Marjorie Saloman had her physician telephone Dr. Snead to learn the medical reasoning behind it.

Having some prior experiences with DMSO (dimethyl sulfoxide) treatment, Dr. Snead persuaded him to combine the substance with vitamin E and apply it topically to the patient's cervical area. Dr. Snead wanted to try to reduce the woman's scar tissue and adhesions, which DMSO is able to do.

"I was lucky enough to run into the gynecologist on the day that we were going to apply the DMSO," Dr. Snead wrote me, "and he inserted the substance himself with the vitamin E. Before five minutes were over, his instrument slipped into the cervix without any sensation felt by the patient."

A month later, the gynecologist rechecked the woman's constricted cervix and found it was still overly narrow. He repeated the application of DMSO and vitamin E, and after a few minutes was able to insert the instrument to stretch the opening without any problem. This time it was a highly successful procedure, and the hospital appointment for surgery was cancelled.

The patient wore a device that was inserted to keep the cervical canal's wall stretched. In the meantime, Dr. Snead placed her friend on megavitamin therapy using high doses of nutrient substances to restore health to surrounding tissues.

One month after the device had been inserted, the woman was again checked by her gynecologist who found the cervical os perfectly expanded. He was able to insert probes without first applying DMSO or anesthesia and without the patient feeling any discomfort. Marjorie Saloman had definitely been saved from having a hysterectomy.

Yet Dr. Eva Lee Snead had her medical license revoked for repeatedly employing DMSO and other forms of complementary medicine— what some have labelled "quackery" but that rightly may be considered alternative methods of healing. The state of Texas is not predisposed to allowing deviations from the medical mainstream. And, as you will see, use of dimethyl sulfoxide by forward-looking physicians is out of the medical mainstream.

*   *   *

Lorae Avery, Ph.D., director of The Health Center, Inc., an acupuncture and nutrition clinic in Auburndale, Florida, expressed her amazement to me at the effectiveness of DMSO in eliminating pain. She saw excellent results when physicians working for The Health Center applied the substance externally to patients. One of them was sixty-five-year-old Anna Goldeman, who had been suffering for years with bursitis of the right shoulder. She went to The Health Center for relief of the bursitis in November, 1980, and was gratified by the results of DMSO treatment.

More dramatic than the patient's alleviation of her shoulder pain was the easing of a discomfort that had begun four years previously. Mrs. Goldeman had undergone amputation of the left hip high in the groin, which resulted in "phantom limb pain." After amputation of a limb, or a portion of it, the amputee may experience strange sensations as though the part were still there. This feeling of phantom pain is generally considered to be a stump hallucination. It arises from various types of nerve stimuli, resulting in burning, tingling, pricking, tickling, or really severe pain. Such sensations are not uncommon for an amputee and are not readily treatable.

With application of DMSO to her right shoulder, phantom limb pain with its constant twitching went out of Mrs. Goldeman's left groin. She no longer sensed that she still had an extremity. Now she could feel more at peace with her situation.

Dr. Avery said, "We did not attempt to treat the phantom limb pain; our physicians were concerned with the bursitis. Yet, the phantom pain disappeared coincidentally from application of DMSO to the woman's shoulder. Thus, what happened is, DMSO applied to one part of the body caused phantom pain to go away in another part of the body. And it's permanently stayed away."

Checking back with Dr. Avery over ten years later, I learned that Mrs. Goldeman continues in comfort knowing that DMSO is available to cease her pain whenever needed.

* * *

Murray Franklin, M.D., of Chicago, is a Clinical Associate Professor of Medicine at the University of Illinois College of Medicine, as well as the medical director of the Union Health Service, the largest pre-paid medical plan in the state of Illinois. He received a supply of DMSO in the fall of 1980 and decided to try it for the benefit of some patients for whom nothing else had worked. One of the people receiving topical therapeutic applications was Lucas Sheinholtz, fifty-two, who had been troubled with rheumatoid-osteoarthritis of both knees for more than a decade. Mr. Sheinholtz, hobbling with the assistance of two canes, arrived at Dr. Franklin's office complex to visit another physician. The patient had previously received many injections of cortisone, which his regular physician administered routinely. But no appreciable improvement in his arthritis had been observed by either the patient or his doctor.

"I suggested to the man's physician that we might paint some DMSO on both of his painful knees," Dr. Franklin said. "His right knee was swollen; the left knee was not. The right knee was warm to the touch. The patient's doctor agreed to a therapeutic trial, and I applied DMSO in three applications. Since I was not fully acquainted with how to use the solution, I allowed an application to dry and then put it on again and again. Within fifteen to twenty minutes the patient said he felt no pain and was able to walk practically without the use of a cane.

"He returned in one week and described his pain in the left knee as having disappeared completely," said Dr. Franklin. "There just wasn't any. The pain in the swollen right knee had returned just a little. I applied the DMSO again and the man got a similar result within a quarter of an hour. No more pain! I haven't seen him since and presume he is feeling fine."

THE NEW MEDICAL BREAKTHROUGH FOR PAIN

The people have a new medical breakthrough for pain: dimethyl sulfoxide, called DMSO. By itself or in combination with other medical ingredients, dimethyl sulfoxide should be useful in treating almost every disease known to mankind. The substance, a byproduct of pulp and paper manufacturing, has been employed safely and successfully by millions of people around the world to control swelling; reduce discomfort; take away inflammation; slow the growth of, and in many instances kill, bacteria, viruses, and fungi. It heals burns and relieves sprains, strains, and arthritic joints. It has worked effectively against cataracts, sports injuries, scleroderma, myasthenia gravis, tuberculosis, and even lessened mental retardation in people with Down's syndrome.

Cancer seems to respond well to DMSO. At Mount Sinai Hospital in New York City, Charlotte Friend, M.D., has turned cancerous cells into harmless normal ones in the test tube by putting them in touch with the DMSO solutions. Thus, DMSO cancer research is in progress.

Reported in the *Journal of Clinical Oncology,* in November 1988, twenty cancer patients with extravasation of anthracycline (destructive secretions from tissues of the toxic chemotherapeutic agent anthracycline onto the recipient's skin with the potential to form cancerous ulcers) were treated on a single-arm pilot study with topically-applied 99 percent dimethyl sulfoxide and observed for three months with regular examinations and photographs. DMSO was applied to approximately twice the area affected by the extravasation and allowed to air dry. This was repeated every six hours for fourteen days. The initial signs of extravasation included swelling, redness, and pain. The median area of damage on the skin of these patients was 8.25 square centimeters (cm^2) and a median of twenty-five minutes elapsed between extravasation and application of DMSO.

In no patient did extravasation progress to ulceration or require surgical intervention, as is usual with this toxic chemotherapeutic agent for cancer. The authors of this report suggest with 95 percent confidence that ulceration was likely to have occurred in at least 17 percent of these patients. They go on to say that at three months there was no sign of residual damage in half the patients, while a pigmented indurated area remained in ten. The only side effects of DMSO included a burning feeling on applications, subsequently associated with itch, redness, and mild scaling. Slight blisters occurred in four patients, and six reported a characteristic breath odor associated with oysters. The oncologists stated that topical DMSO appears to be a safe and effective treatment for the cancer-related condition, anthracycline extravasation.[1]

DMSO tends to prevent the formation of scar tissue, or to dissolve it once present. The contracture (drawing together) of scar tissue ordinarily left after a burn doesn't take place.

Chilean physicians have published their results of using the substance, which indicate that it reduces the incidence of heart attacks or angina pain. It has been credited with preventing damage to heart muscle when tested in animal experiments. As with its use in stroke, DMSO may be lifesaving if employed early in heart attacks. Investigation is continuing.

Studies in Chile also show DMSO to be a penetrant across the blood-brain barrier. It carries drugs effective against certain forms of mental illness directly into the brain.

Placed into the nostrils, DMSO can open blocked sinuses within a few minutes.

It transports antibiotics right into the middle ear to lessen infections. It does the same against viruses and reduces the symptoms of herpes zoster (shingles) and herpes simplex (fever blisters). The viruses are hit with antiviral drugs by the DMSO transport. Furthermore, the herpes II venereal disease is greatly relieved by application of DMSO directly to the genitalia.

Periodontists in Poland have cleared up gum disease and reduced tooth decay and their associated pain by painting DMSO on the involved areas. Some pioneering dentists are dropping it into empty tooth sockets after extractions, especially those for wisdom teeth. It stops post-extraction swelling.

A 1987 paper coming out of Russia described the treatment of patients having generalized periodontitis with indomethacin in a suspension of dimethyl sulfoxide. Periodontitis is disease of the structures supporting the teeth such as the gums, periodontal membrane, and alveolar bone. The action of bacteria on food debris accumulated around the margins of the gums causes the formation of plaque, which eventually forms a hard deposit, tartar (or calculus). This accumulates in the gingival crevices (the spaces between the gums and the surface of the teeth), which become abnormally enlarged to form gingival pockets. It's an early stage of periodontal disease.

In chronic gingivitis, the gums are marked by chronic inflammation, and they become swollen and bleed easily. Calculus accumulates in the gingival pockets, causing bleeding and ulceration. Untreated, the plaque spreads to the underlying periodontal membrane and alveolar bone, which are destroyed. In this stage of chronic periodontitis, the teeth become loosened and eventually fall out.

Periodontal disease is the major cause of tooth loss in middle-aged and elderly people. It is brought on by poor oral hygiene and also by ill-fitting dentures and badly made artificial crowns and fillings. The early stages of periodontitis are treated by scaling to remove the calculus and polishing to remove the plaque, combined with careful oral hygiene. In advanced disease the gingival pockets are surgically removed by gingivectomy (gum excision).

Now periodontal disease is being treated with indomethacin and DMSO, in combination. Indomethacin is a drug with anti-inflammatory, antifever, and pain-killing properties, but containing no corticosteroids. Its mode of action, like that of certain other anti-inflammatory drugs, is not known.[2]

Before this Russian publication, clinical results from the treatment of a hemorrhagic form of periodontosis were reported from Bulgaria. The clinicians used a complex herb extract and 15 percent DMSO to rid their patients of periodontal disease.[3]

American podiatrists have found DMSO effective for the treatment of painful corns, calluses, ingrown toenails, bunions, hammertoes, heel spurs, and even the inflammation of gouty big toes. DMSO appears to control gout pain after just seven days of application.

Inflammations such as pink eye from viral invasion go away after a few applications of DMSO.

All this happens in a way that medical scientists have yet to fully understand. They don't know how DMSO actually works. For this reason primarily, DMSO is not approved by the United States Food and Drug Administration (FDA) for any other human medicinal use except as a treatment for interstitial cystitis, a condition that causes scarring and gradual shrinkage of the bladder.

Bruce H. Stewart, M.D., of the Cleveland Clinic Foundation, and Sheridan Shirley, M.D., of the University of Alabama, administered DMSO to 213 patients and found it quickly healed the bladder condition despite the fact that the patients had not responded to traditional treatment. Before the success of DMSO, people suffering with interstitial cystitis faced either major surgery of the bladder, or even its complete removal. They suffered from the urge to urinate as frequently as every ten minutes.

Unlike criteria laid down for studying the use of DMSO for other conditions, the study on interstitial cystitis was done following an elementary protocol. The patients were ill, didn't improve spontaneously, and all forms of treatment were ineffective. They then received DMSO and improved markedly. DMSO had eliminated the patients' health problems and won approval by the FDA for use in bladder treatment—but only for interstitial cystitis.

THE FDA OBJECTION TO OTHER DMSO USES

"The fundamental problem from the point of view of the FDA is the quality of the scientific information that is available to support the various claims that are made for DMSO," said J. Richard Crout, M.D., Director of the Bureau of Drugs with the Food and Drug Administration. Dr. Crout made his statement at a hearing before the House Select Committee on Aging, 96th Congress, held March 24, 1980.

Dr. Crout continued, "I want to make it clear that the Food and Drug Administration has approved DMSO for the indication for which there is evidence that meets the statutory standard. We are prepared to approve it for any other indications when the evidence comes along that it does meet that statutory standard."

In brief, the drug can be approved if clinical researchers show substantial evidence of its effectiveness by providing the FDA with well-controlled trials. The "possibility" that DMSO is effective, according to the present statute, is simply not enough. For this reason, the only thing holding up FDA approval of DMSO for any of the substance's indications is the availability of well-controlled trials that meet statutory standards, said Dr. Crout. There is a basic conflict between the quality of the scientific evidence available and the statutory standard for approval.

This fundamental confrontation is best illustrated by a new drug application (NDA) submitted in 1978 by Research Industries Corporation of Salt Lake City, Utah, the major producer of a human medicinal grade of DMSO in 50 percent concentration called Rimso-50. Research Industries Corporation wanted to extend the use of its product and market it for the symptomatic relief of pain and ulceration in the fingers of patients with scleroderma. Scleroderma is a rare collagen disorder that results in thickening of the skin from the swelling of fibrous tissue. It most often involves the hands, especially causing ulcers on the fingers, and less frequently on other tissues in the body. After detailed review by the FDA's Bureau of Drugs staff and its Arthritis Advisory Committee, the NDA was refused on the grounds that the available clinical trials did not yet demonstrate that DMSO was effective for scleroderma. Medical science's current investigative techniques using double- or single-blind studies seemed inadequate for evaluating the effectiveness of DMSO in this instance.

Research Industries Corporation relied principally on one particular study to demonstrate DMSO's effectiveness against scleroderma. This study had each patient dip only one hand into a solution of DMSO. The untreated hand was observed as a control. Both hands had ulcerations of the skin of the fingers, and investigators thought that DMSO's effectiveness in healing sclerodermatous ulcers would clearly be shown by what happened to the two hands.

Dr. Crout described what happened. "There was a general improvement trend in the healing of ulcers of the fingers in many patients, and in a few this was quite striking. Interestingly, however, this improvement occurred in both hands in these patients with scleroderma; that is, both the treated and untreated hands tended to heal."

Now, DMSO is different from any other known medical substance in that it is easily absorbed into the body. Paint an amount the size of a silver dollar anywhere on your upper body and in thirty seconds you'll taste it on the tip of your tongue. It penetrates the skin and travels through the blood stream that fast.

The officials of the Research Industries Corporation argued that both hands of the affected patients healed because DMSO worked equally well on the hand in touch with the liquid and on the control hand. Simply, DMSO healed the control hand by traveling through the blood stream to the ulcer site. Absorption of the substance into the body from the treated hand was inevitable because of its unique power of penetrability. Current techniques utilizing the scientific method as it is understood today cannot be applied to the study of DMSO.

Dr. Crout said, "Our staff and advisory committee felt, to the contrary, that improvement of the untreated hand raised the strong possibility that the general improvement trend in the whole trial was attributable to a nonspecific effect of DMSO. Everyone agreed that the trial showed that DMSO may be effective, but few felt that the trial proved the point.

"Because the statutory standard for approval of a drug is substantial evidence of effectiveness as shown by well-controlled trials, not simply the possibility of effectiveness," continued the FDA chief, "we are unable to approve DMSO for this indication at this time."

In order for a new drug to be recognized by the FDA it must conform to section 505 of the Food, Drug, and Cosmetic Act, which holds that the standard for effectiveness is "substantial evidence" of effectiveness. This means evidence must come from controlled clinical investigations conducted by experts qualified by scientific training and experience to evaluate the effectiveness of drugs.

Dr. Crout declared that applications for an investigational new drug (IND) submitted for DMSO during the previous eighteen years were faulty. They had not been assembled into scientifically designed studies. They had not followed that certain discipline required by research. All INDs must go through a standard FDA procedure to win approval. The prior investigational new drug applications submitted by three pharmaceutical companies of national repute were poorly prepared, said Dr. Crout, and the companies did not know how to present an IND application to the FDA to show proper evidence of value in the use of DMSO. He made this statement despite the fact that these same pharmaceutical firms had previously won approval for other drugs.

FLAWS IN FDA PROCEDURE

Of course, the pharmaceutical companies disagreed. The codiscoverer of the therapeutic properties of DMSO, Stanley W. Jacob, M.D., Associate Professor of Surgery at the University of Oregon Medical School, certainly disagreed. He believed the advisory committee that made recommendations against FDA approval of DMSO was biased against DMSO. Dr. Jacob told the House Committee on Aging: "I am not at all satisfied that the FDA is giving DMSO a fair shake."

The DMSO researchers who worked with patients on a case-by-case basis pointed out that the FDA advisory committee was negatively disposed. The committee members had never themselves used DMSO as a therapeutic tool. And this was admitted by Dr. Crout.

The Honorable Claude Pepper, former Chairman of the House Select Committee on Aging, was inclined to agree with the analysis made by Dr. Jacob. Congressman Pepper told Dr. Crout, "If there is a drug for which there was an enormous amount of prospect of good that was being pressed upon you by three drug companies who apparently thought the drug had enormous potential, in a case like that, I would think that you would be eager to see if the claims that were made could be justified. You would be looking for satisfactory proof that would square with your conscience and your judgment that that product might give relief to a lot of people and could be put on the market.

"Now, the public—and I must say up to now I share the opinion—has the impression that your agency in its desire to be careful and its desire not to let anybody be hurt, has denied perhaps a lot of people relief in fear that if they allowed the thing to be approved as it was presented, that they might be hurt by it; that yours is a negative attitude, that you don't tell them what is wrong with the application in an informal way so they can attempt to correct it and the like; that you are not eager to see the users of the country that might profit from it get the advantage of it," said the Congressman.

"You say, 'It is no skin off my back,' as the old saying goes, 'if these folks cannot comply with the technicalities. That is the law, it is none of our responsibility. Let them get a better lawyer or somebody else. We are not running it. We are just sitting up here trying to protect the public interest.'

"Are you sure that there is no justification for the public or even members of Congress having that impression of our regard of your duties?" asked Congressman Pepper. "Are you sure there is no foundation for that fear?"

Dr. Crout discounted such a possibility and implied that DMSO was having difficulties because it was so unorthodox. He said it would be far easier for a new drug to have its application approved if it was closer to something already in the marketplace, such as a new antibiotic or tranquilizer that duplicates an existing one.

DMSO is a substance totally strange to medical science. It has a novel mode of action not understood within the context of our current healing concepts. It is an altogether new principle that will possibly revolutionize therapeutics once it is studied in a more exacting way. For now, however, DMSO is not being studied in accordance with the standard double- or single-blind procedures commonly used in the scientific method. This is the present problem. And it is one that has perplexed the medical community ever since DMSO was first discovered to have therapeutic value to counter human injury and heal human disease.

The existence of this new anti-inflammatory painkiller raises the questions: How can it be established with certainty the degree to which DMSO does or does not work for the numerous and varied conditions reported in the medical literature by clinicians using it successfully? Are we able to break the logjam that enables a federal agency to keep this drug from general use because its research studies don't conform to the regulations laid down by that same federal government for its citizens' protection? Does DMSO have a history of controversy among pioneering health professionals and bureaucratic medical conservatives alike, because neither group truly comprehends how radically this substance departs from known principles of healing? Must DMSO remain controversial?

CHAPTER 2
DMSO's
Controversial History

On November 10, 1980, United States Food and Drug Administration officials entered the office of Dr. Stanley Jacob at the University of Oregon Health Sciences Center. They were looking for research reports on possible damage to human eyes from the use of DMSO. They had an administrative search warrant issued by a federal judge and were prepared to rifle through and seize the files kept by Dr. Jacob.

William Zuber and Dr. Alan B. Lisook of the FDA were refused access to any documents by Jacob even in the face of the federal warrant. Instead, Jacob's attorney, Jay Geller, answered the warrant point-by-point in federal court. Mr. Geller said such reports or documents didn't exist or, if they did, were not in Jacob's possession.

Geller added that certain documents requested were privileged patient information and not available even under court order except in cases where patients give permission. Zuber and Lisook walked away with only one paper that Jacob provided, a two-page memo on DMSO and its legal use in treating interstitial cystitis. Otherwise, they got no response to questions they asked. Zuber admitted he did not have any authority to question the physician, since the Food, Drug, and Cosmetic Act does not give the FDA "access to people, just things."

When Lisook asked Geller whether the reports had ever been in Jacob's possession in the past, Geller assured the investigators that they had not and that no documents had been removed from the doctor's office since the warrant was issued. Zuber and Lisook then terminated the meeting, saying they didn't believe they could obtain any information "central to this warrant."

Geller accused the FDA of harassing Jacob. He said much of the information requested in this federal warrant was on record from previous hearings.

Jacob said there was no evidence of damage to the human eye caused by DMSO. "Allegations of hidden toxicity are false," he stated.[1]

Such controversy, with legal actions and reactions, has commonly surrounded the puzzling painkiller dimethyl sulfoxide. Its exciting biological and medical uses have made the substance one of the stormiest and most disputed drugs of our day. It lay dormant for nearly one hundred years after its discovery; now it had burst on the medical scene amidst contention, discord, charges and countercharges—literally a war of words intended to convince others of the truth.

The loser in all this intraprofessional argument is the medical consumer. Patient advocacy doesn't seem to exist when it relates to DMSO. Welfare for the people has been abandoned. The facts remain undetermined with certainty; guidance to help victims of illness make the wisest health decisions for themselves has been ignored. Health professionals and medical bureaucrats apparently are failing to fulfill their responsibilities to the public.

THE SOURCE AND ORIGIN OF DIMETHYL SULFOXIDE

DMSO was first synthesized in 1866 by Russian scientist Alexander Saytzeff in Kazan, on the Volga River in Central Russia. He saw that the substance was colorless, had a garlic-like odor, felt oily to the touch, looked like mineral oil when poured from the test tube, and left an aftertaste similar to clams or oysters. It had laboratory curiosity value for Dr. Saytzeff and his fellow chemists because dimethyl sulfoxide combined with almost any chemical he dropped into the liquid. It was an excellent solvent, useful as a degreaser, paint thinner, and antifreeze. For about eighty years, the only publication advising scientists about the stuff was a paper Dr. Saytzeff had submitted to an obscure German chemistry journal that printed his article in 1867.

After World War II, chemists started to show active interest in the substance. A number of papers appeared in chemical literature in 1948, showing DMSO to be an excellent solvent. In 1959, a group in Great Britain demonstrated that the solvent would protect red blood cells and other tissues against freezing conditions.

Dr. H. Harry Szmant, Chairman of the University of Detroit's chemistry department, explained that the liquid has a tremendous capacity to dissolve substances. It is a reagent that can speed up some chemical reactions a "billionfold."

"The unique capability of DMSO to penetrate living tissues without causing significant damage is most probably related to its relatively polar nature, its capacity to accept hydrogen bonds, and its relatively small and compact structure," he said. "This combination of properties results in the ability of DMSO to associate with water, proteins, carbohydrates, nucleic acid, ionic substances, and other constituents of living systems. Of foremost importance to our understanding of the possible functions of DMSO in biological systems is its ability to replace some of the water molecules associated with the cellular constituents, or to affect the structure of the omnipresent water."[2]

Controversy began to surround DMSO in 1962 when Dr. Jacob first became interested in how to safely freeze human kidneys and considered the solvent for this purpose. He asked Robert Herschler, a chemical applications supervisor at the Crown Zellerbach Paper Company, for some of the chemical. Crown Zellerbach had plenty to spare, since DMSO is a byproduct of its paper-making process. For five dollars a quart it can be produced commercially in crude form for refining into human medicinal application.

At their first meeting, Robert Herschler mentioned that he had difficulty washing the stain off his hands when both DMSO and dye got on them. Dr. Jacob recalls: "We painted DMSO on our skin and within fifteen minutes noticed an oyster and garlic taste. The skin where the chemical had been was dry."

The drying effect of dimethyl sulfoxide set off the DMSO explosion. Dryness of a therapeutic agent makes it valuable in the treatment of burns, since moisture tends to promote infection. Jacob and Herschler tried it on burned rats and found those treated were quieter in behavior than the untreated. The drug relieved burn pain. "From that point on, DMSO usage just spread like wildfire," Dr. Jacob said in an interview.

In the United States DMSO is derived from *lignin,* the cement substance of trees. In Europe and other places it is synthesized from coal, petroleum, or other organic substances.

Collaborative efforts between Jacob's staff representing the University of Oregon Medical School and Herschler representing Crown Zellerbach Corporation demonstrated in laboratory tests that DMSO would not only pass through the skin and mucous membranes, but during passage would carry with it a certain number of other substances. For instance, penicillin can be dissolved in DMSO and be carried through the skin without a needle. Local anesthetic can be carried the same way.

In these early studies, DMSO was shown to relieve pain, reduce swelling, slow the growth of bacteria, improve blood supply, soften scar tissue, enhance the effectiveness of other pharmacologic agents, act as a diuretic, and function as a muscle relaxant. It eliminated the pain of sprains, strains, and arthritis, and even the pain of broken bones.

Veterinarians used the substance, by prescription, for arthritic conditions or injuries in animals. In arthritic greyhounds, an injection of either DMSO or corticoid (a substance that has an action like a hormone of the adrenal cortex) will enable the animal to race again. In six months 60 percent of the corticoid-treated dogs will have a recurrence, but less than 20 percent of the dogs treated with DMSO show such recurrence.

THE FDA ENTERS THE PICTURE
AND CONTROVERSY STARTS

The first report on the use of DMSO as a pharmacologic agent was written by Jacob in 1963 and published February 1, 1964. It caused a flood of trials and wild enthusiasm over the new "miracle" drug that carried other substances through the skin and into all organs of the body. It was soon obvious that the chemical could relieve inflammation and pain in many conditions, some heretofore untreatable any other way.

The first investigational new drug (IND) application for the clinical study of DMSO in humans was submitted to the FDA on October 25, 1963, and subsequently approved. Enormous interest in the drug developed rapidly, to the point where it began to be used very extensively, especially for the treatment of sprains, bruises, and minor burns. The drug was supplied at no charge to great numbers of investigators in general medicine, specialty medicine, and to paramedical professionals, including physiotherapists, a few dentists, nurses, and the author of this book, a former practicing podiatrist.

By 1965 an estimated 100,000 patients had received the medication. Studies were being conducted but the FDA did not consider them to be well enough controlled to document clearly that the observed benefits were actually due to the drug. *The New York Times,* in a lead editorial on April 3, 1965, called DMSO "the closest thing to a wonder drug produced in the 1960s." An international symposium of medical scientists in Berlin, West Germany, in July 1965, was held to exchange information on the effects of DMSO.

Still, when three new drug applications (NDAs) on DMSO were submitted to the FDA in 1965, all three were turned down. The pharmaceutical companies Merck, Syntex, and Gibb submitted their NDAs with the statement that DMSO was ready to be a prescriptive agent. The FDA denied their statement and applications, and in fact published its own statement in the *Federal Register* terminating all clinical use of DMSO. The agency cited toxicological studies showing that high doses of the drug changed the refractive index of the eye lens in experimental animals. That is, a change occurred in their focusing power and a certain cloudiness came over the lenses.

The agency's concern was that visual damage might occur in humans exposed to DMSO. Researchers and bureaucrats didn't know at that time that the eye changes were limited to particular species. Nothing happens to monkeys or, most important, to human beings.

A year later this prohibitive policy was relaxed somewhat. The FDA permitted new investigations for the clinical evaluation of DMSO in serious conditions, such as scleroderma, persistent herpes zoster, and severe rheumatoid arthritis, for which no satisfactory therapy is available.

In September 1968 the FDA published a further revision, a relaxation of its DMSO policy that allowed topical application to the skin for not more than fourteen days for less serious disabilities such as acute musculoskeletal conditions—for example, sprains, bursitis, and tend-initis. This relaxation of rules was based on a toxicological study of people that provided a reassuring result: no evidence of human eye toxicity due to DMSO was present.

Yet, again, another NDA submitted by Gibb Pharmaceutical Company in 1971, stating that DMSO was ready to be prescribed in the United States, was denied.

An NDA, on the use of DMSO for scleroderma, was submitted by Research Industries Corporation in 1978. The study was planned by Arthur L. Scherbel, M.D., then Chief of Rheumatology at the Cleveland Clinic Foundation, under supervision of doctors at the FDA and consultants from the National Academy of Sciences. Dr. Scherbel carried out these studies and saw changes in a treated hand, as compared to an untreated hand. In three months there was a marked improvement that was statistically significant. When Dr. Scherbel came to the FDA for acceptance of his study, it was refused. The NDA was denied.

By 1983, the NDAs tossed aside by the FDA included 1,500 medical studies performed on approximately 120,000 patients with a variety of health problems. Moreover, four more international symposia were held by health scientists to accumulate more information on DMSO. The second symposium conducted was under the auspices of the New York Academy of Sciences, in March 1966 in New York City. The third was sponsored by the University of Vienna, Austria, in November 1966. The fourth and fifth were again in New York, under the sponsorship of the New York Academy of Sciences, in January 1974 and September 1982. All of these symposia reported favorably on the drug.

Because of the ongoing differences among DMSO pioneers and the medical bureaucrats, Charles C. Edwards, M.D., then Commissioner of Food and Drugs, asked the National Academy of Sciences in 1972 to review all available information on the effectiveness and toxicity of DMSO. He wanted the National Academy members to provide the FDA with an independent judgment on these matters.

The Academy appointed a committee of experts, with six subcommittees, to conduct the review. The committee ran an active review until 1974. The Academy was actually a semi-governmental body, not really independent at all. As it received its financing under an FDA contract, it tended to agree with the FDA position on DMSO. Specifically, the report finally presented by the National Academy of Sciences stated that there was inadequate scientific evidence of effectiveness of the drug for the treatment of any disease, that the toxicity potential was sufficiently great that the drug should remain an investigational drug, and that controlled clinical investigations were necessary to demonstrate the effectiveness of DMSO.

In light of continued lack of evidence of eye damage in humans from the time it laid down regulations against DMSO, the FDA has concluded that the regulation is no longer necessary. Thus, finally, on September 21, 1979, the agency published a *Federal Register* proposal to revoke the regulation. Yet, Jere Goyan, Ph.D., former head of the entire FDA, continued to make public statements about the dangers of eye toxicity. It may have been to justify these statements that he sent investigators to grab files wherever they could, searching for reports on DMSO and its relation to the human eye.

Also by 1983, the FDA had sixteen active investigational new drug applications for DMSO on file. Conditions under study included scleroderma, joint injuries, and spinal cord injuries. There were no active INDs for the study of DMSO in the treatment of rheumatoid arthritis or osteoarthritis, which seems unusual as DMSO use for these conditions is the most popular.

THE PUBLIC REBELS AGAINST THE FDA REGULATIONS

Despite the FDA restrictions on the use of DMSO, tens of thousands of

Americans still manage to obtain it. Some use a form of the medicine that has been approved for veterinary use. Some resort to the industrial solvent. Others travel to DMSO arthritis clinics in Mexico. The drug is passed from person to person, especially among victims of arthritis.

Even though there is no existing IND arthritis application pending before the FDA, osteoarthritis and rheumatoid arthritis are the two main health problems being treated by layperson exponents of DMSO. The public is rebelling against the imposition of what it considers nonsensical regulations for limited use of DMSO. People ask, if it is safe enough for internal treatment of interstitial cystitis, why isn't it safe to paint it on the skin for arthritic joints?

An underground market for supplying the substance has developed. Pharmacies sell the pure medical grade on a doctor's prescription at a cost of anywhere from fifteen to twenty dollars for four ounces. Technically, once a drug gets FDA approval for certain uses—such as for interstitial cystitis—it is not illegal in any state for a doctor to prescribe it for other purposes.

The thriving nationwide black market in DMSO is also operating, unfortunately, across the counters of hardware stores, in gasoline stations, at mail-order houses, on the backs of trucks operating near shopping centers or parking lots, and even out of ice cream parlors. For example, according to a published article in the *Chicago Tribune*,[3] the industrial grade dimethyl sulfoxide solvent has appeared in such unlikely spots as an ice cream parlor and a locksmith's shop in Chicago. A solvent retailer based in Seattle, Washington, offers a toll free mail-order number and has opened stores in Milwaukee, Chicago, and Evanston, Illinois.

The sales pitch for the substance is careful not to make medical claims about DMSO. "We're selling this to you as a solvent; what you do with it is up to you. It's against the law any other way," one salesperson says.

Billy Williams, president of the solvent retail firm, says that the DMSO he sells is pharmaceutical grade. It's safe, he assures people, though he technically sells it as a solvent.

"We're marketing this stuff because it sells," Williams said. "And we assume people use it. We get orders from doctors, chiropractors, and dentists." He opened a packaging and distribution plant, and buys a pharmaceutical grade DMSO in bulk from an undisclosed medical laboratory, then packages it into smaller bottles in his Seattle plant. "We buy it third-hand from the medical lab," Williams said. "They 'back door' it to us.

"As to the medical usage, we can't help but be aware that people actually are using it to reduce the pain of arthritis. I have read many letters that people are using it, because they imply that they have arthritis or muscle strain or a number of medical disorders.

"I know what we're selling it for: we're selling it for a profit. That sounds crass, but that's what people are in business for. The stuff works! We're not profiteering in the sense that we're going to profit from somebody's misery."

Another typical source of public sale is a hairstyling salon in Chicago. The manager said he stopped selling the solvent because of the controversy over its legality. "I only sold it for a few days," he said. He had purchased a case of industrial DMSO from a Chicago police officer who had also supplied the ice cream parlor.

Research Laboratories, Inc. of Salt Lake City, Utah is often referred to by the United States Food and Drug Administration when inquiries are made by physicians and other health professionals for a source of dimethyl sulfoxide for human therapeutic purposes. Research Laboratories sells a 50 milliliter (ml) ampoule of DMSO to health professionals for injection purposes for $28.00.

Specifically for the consumer, the finest source of acquiring DMSO products is Dr. James Critchlow, proprietor of American Pharmaceutical Enterprises, Inc., P.O. Box 12543, Scottsdale, Arizona 85267; telephone (602) 998-4142 or call toll free (800) 345-3391. American Pharmaceutical Enterprises (APE) provides a deodorized, pharmaceutical grade of DMSO quite suitable for human therapeutic application. A purified pint by mail order costs $60.00 and Dr. Critchlow's slightly lemon-scented DMSO Solvent Creme in a four-ounce jar is $29.95.

He also furnishes DMSO products for medical doctors, osteopaths, podiatrists, chiropractors, naturopaths, homeopaths, dentists, nurses, physical therapists, and other types of health professionals who utilize DMSO as part of their therapeutic reserves. Under the Critchlow company name, Phyne Pharmaceuticals, Inc., P.O. Box 12543, Scottsdale, Arizona 85261 or 14325 North 79th Street, Scottsdale, Arizona 85260; telephone (602) 998-4142 and toll free (800) 345-3391, health professionals are offered medical grade products for topical or internal application. For instance, the Phyne Pharmaceutical pint quantity of liquid DMSO is so pure that many doctors use it for intravenous infusions of patients. Product prices are considerably less for health professionals when they purchase in quantity.

Federal studies, according to former FDA Commissioner, Jere E. Goyan, indicate that industrial grade DMSO is not suitable for treating humans. It does not have to pass the same quality control as the medical grade. When the solvent is transferred to smaller containers, it increases the chances of impurity. The FDA official warning states that the "risk that may accompany use of the industrial grade . . . is its potential as a carrier chemical capable of delivering harmful substances into the bloodstream if they are present in impure DMSO or on the skin."

"People are taking a risk whenever they use a substance of unknown quality and effect," Commissioner Goyan said. "It's risky business to drink, inject, or apply to the skin any substance not intended for that purpose."

The black market in DMSO, pure grade and industrial grade, continues simply because the FDA keeps the drug off the market for any use except the treatment of interstitial cystitis. Arthur Scherbel, former senior physician at the Cleveland Clinic's Department of Rheumatic Disease and Immunology, declared that the FDA is holding back approval of the drug "for no good reason. People are using it without proper guidance, and that is a mistake. The sooner it is released the better."[4]

LEGISLATORS ACT ON BEHALF OF THE PEOPLE

No fewer than six resolutions to legalize the public use of DMSO and to override the ruling of the FDA have been introduced into the United States Congress. United States Senator Mark O. Hatfield (R-Ore.) said: "Since I have no scientific expertise, I cannot make an absolute statement that DMSO is indeed the wonder drug of our century, but every bit of evidence I encounter reinforces the premise that it is.

"After over 1,200 scientific publications on the merits of DMSO, after international symposia in Germany, the United States, and Austria—all concluding that DMSO is safe and effective—after three separate pharmaceutical firms have submitted four new drug applications to the FDA, DMSO is still not available to Americans, though it is available in many other countries. I have urged the Senate to support my legislation on behalf of all Americans who are suffering today from diseases untreatable by any other known substance and those who may have need of this drug in the future."

The Honorable Wendell Wyatt (D-Ore.) reintroduced legislation in the United States House of Representatives aimed at getting a fair hearing for DMSO. "Since the FDA action against DMSO has been taken on the flimsiest of evidence," said Wyatt, "we have been unable to get even a hearing for DMSO. The whole issue has been submerged under a bureaucratic cloud."

The Congressman's efforts, and the efforts of other members of the United States legislature, have paid off. Senator Edward M. Kennedy (D-Mass.) held a Senate subcommittee hearing on the drug's status at the FDA on July 31, 1980. Congressman Claude Pepper (D-Fla.) chaired a hearing (under the title "DMSO: New Hope for Arthritis?") before the House Select Committee on Aging on March 24, 1980.

Since those hearings, the Inspector General of the Department of Health and Human Services has been conducting an investigation into the regulatory procedure DMSO has undergone at the FDA.

Furthermore, some state legislatures have overridden the FDA ruling against dispensing DMSO and altered state laws to allow its use by authorized health professionals. Currently Texas, Washington, Montana, Oklahoma, Florida, Oregon, Louisiana, and Nevada are the eight states in the nation that have authorized prescribing the medication. Legalization of DMSO in Florida is another example of the people rebelling against FDA regulations. The difference here was that the legalization of DMSO in Florida was pushed by a legislator whose wife was forced to travel to Mexico for DMSO treatments.

In 1977, the Florida legislature legalized the drug for intravenous, intramuscular, oral, and topical human therapy. The Florida law reads:

> Section 1. No hospital or health facility shall interfere with the physician-patient relationship by restricting or forbidding the use of dimethyl sulfoxide (DMSO) when prescribed or administered by a physician licensed under chapter 458 or 459, Florida Statutes, and requested by a patient unless the substance as prescribed or administered by the physician is found to be harmful by the State Boards of Medical Examiners and Osteopathic Medical Examiners in a hearing conducted under the provisions of the Administrative Procedure Act, Chapter 120, Florida Statutes. Furthermore, no hospital or health facility shall remove the staff privileges of a physician solely because said physician prescribed or administered dimethyl sulfoxide (DMSO) to a patient under the conditions set forth in this act.

Section 2. No physician licensed under chapter 458 or 459, Florida Statutes, shall be subject to disciplinary action by the State Boards of Medical Examiners and Osteopathic Medical Examiners for prescribing or administering dimethyl sulfoxide (DMSO) to a patient under his care who has requested the substance unless the State Boards of Medical Examiners and Osteopathic Medical Examiners, in a hearing conducted under the provisions of the Administrative Procedure Act, Chapter 120, Florida Statutes, has made a formal finding that the substance is harmful.

Section 3. The patient, after being fully informed as to alternative methods of treatment and their potential for cure and upon request for the administration of dimethyl sulfoxide (DMSO) by his physician, shall sign a written release, releasing the physician and, when applicable, the hospital or health facility from any liability therefor.

Section 4. The physician shall inform the patient in writing if dimethyl sulfoxide (DMSO) has not been approved as a treatment or cure by the Food and Drug Administration of the United States Department of Health and Human Services for the disorder for which it is being prescribed.

Section 5. This act shall not apply to conditions for which dimethyl sulfoxide (DMSO) has been approved as a treatment by the Food and Drug Administration of the United States Department of Health and Human Services.

Following passage of this new law, the potential for abusing it, spurred on by paid advertisements of DMSO clinics as well as broad media coverage, prompted the Florida Medical Association (FMA) to issue a statement in the form of a "letter to the editor," in October 1980, to all newspapers throughout Florida. A *60 Minutes* television broadcast had stimulated an almost daily stream of inquiries, both by letter and telephone, to the FMA headquarters in Jacksonville, Florida. Most of the in-state queries were from the press, while the majority from out of the state were from individuals with a variety of symptoms seeking a physician to provide them with the "miracle cure" called DMSO. The FMA official position is this:

Without an approved new drug application, the drug cannot be marketed or distributed in Florida for indications other than the treatment of interstitial cystitis. However, legally, a doctor may prescribe an approved drug for other indications.

The Florida Legislature passed a law in 1978 which permits a physician to use DMSO after advising the patient of alternative treatment and any potential for cure. The law requires that upon request to the physician for DMSO treatment, the patient shall sign a written release of liability to the physician and, when applicable, the hospital or facility. The physician shall inform the patient if DMSO has been approved by the FDA for the disorder for which it is being prescribed in writing.

The Florida Medical Association does not condone going outside of the approved and responsible mechanism for the introduction of a new drug. As a matter of fact, physicians covered by professional liability insurance under the FMA-sponsored plan have been warned regarding the drug. They will not be covered by the plan if they use DMSO for any symptom other than the relief of interstitial cystitis for which, as previously stated, it is approved by the FDA.

At the same time, FMA does encourage its physician members who are interested to take part in the FDA investigational program in this and other areas. Assistance is available for obtaining from the FDA an Investigational New Drug Application (IND) plus sterile nonpyogenic DMSO solution. In order to participate in this research, the physician must agree to keep the necessary records. The DMSO solution will be supplied free of charge and assistance given to the physician in developing the necessary protocol.

As to the law passed during this year's legislative session allowing for the manufacture, distribution, and sale of a DMSO ointment in Florida, FMA has no direct knowledge and no participation in any way in this matter. We are informed by officials in The Department of Health and Rehabilitative Services (DHRS) that they are in the process of developing rules and regulations to govern the manufacture of such a product and that at this time one formal application to do so has been submitted.

We are also informed by personnel in the DHRS that there

is a serious question in their minds as to what constitutes a "safe" product for human consumption. This question could lead to an Attorney General's opinion being sought prior to anyone being allowed to manufacture a DMSO product in Florida.

Consumer inquiries concerning DMSO or any other new experimental drug should be directed to the FDA Bureau of Drugs, Advisory Opinion Board HFD 35, 5600 Fishers Lane, Rockville, Maryland 20852. Physicians interested in working in the experimental drug program should contact the FDA Bureau of Drugs, Division of Oncology HFD 150, Radiopharmaceuticals Branch, 5600 Fishers Lane, Rockville, Maryland 20852.

On January 28, 1981, the Public Health Committee of the General Assembly of the State of Connecticut held a committee meeting to consider whether the state should encourage physicians to use DMSO to treat painful and sometimes fatal diseases. A bill submitted by Wolcott, Connecticut Representative Eugene Migliaro would relieve medical doctors of their professional liability if they prescribed DMSO. Migliaro explained that the public may receive DMSO through the mail.

"We know that DMSO is not a cure," Migliaro said. "And I understand the things that can happen to you if you use it wrong. I'd like to protect it. This will say to doctors, 'protect your people without fear of being sued.'"

State Senator Regina Smith, Public Health Committee co-chairperson, noted that doctors are liable for all other drugs they prescribe. She indicated that it would be a dangerous precedent to exempt this experimental drug.[5] The Connecticut bill was defeated, but DMSO supporters said that they planned to submit a revised version in the future. They did not.

I agree in principle with Senator Smith, but the FMA has gone to the opposite extreme. Florida medical liability policies won't cover the use of DMSO for anything other than interstitial cystitis.

Between the time the FMA issued its official statement about DMSO and the State Legislature of Connecticut introduced a bill to get physicians off the hook in the event something went wrong with any patients for whom they had prescribed DMSO, the State of Florida spoke up. James T. Howell, M.D., State Health Officer in the Department of Health and Rehabilitative Services of Florida, felt it necessary to respond on DMSO. Through the press Dr. Howell expressed a grave concern that an industrial solvent-type of DMSO was made available for human consumption. He was also worried about the veterinary product. He said that neither of these had been refined for human consumption and could be extremely harmful.

Two programs with a tremendous viewing audience broadcast over CBS-TV, one in March 1980 and a repeat in July 1980, seem to have caused people to throw caution aside. The public insisted upon getting hold of this painkilling drug whether it's surrounded with controversy or not. All that people want is relief of pain whatever the cause. Interestingly, some prominent figures in sports, politics, acting, and other occupations are submitting to DMSO treatment, too, without regard to whether its use is legally admissible by the judgments and standards of the FDA.

The various applications of DMSO in clinical practice and for home use as a self-care remedy for such problems as arthritis, shingles, headaches, cataracts, herpes simplex, burns, Down's syndrome, spinal cord injuries, bursitis, sprains, and many other conditions, make it an ideal product. The various modes of treatment such as skin applications, intravenous therapy, and oral and intramuscular therapy are desperately wanted by the famous and unfamous alike.

THE NEW PAINKILLER BECOMES A MEDIA CELEBRITY

When Governor George Wallace traveled across the country to find pain relief from DMSO administered by Dr. Stanley Jacob, this new painkilling drug got a big boost. He began treatment July 1, 1980, to relieve discomfort associated with paralysis.

Wallace had been confined to a wheelchair since he was wounded in a 1972 assassination attempt while campaigning for the Democratic nomination for President at Laurel, Maryland. Doctors described Wallace's discomfort as occurring in the "flank," a medical term referring to the area between the lowest rib and the waist. While his pain was not excruciating, it was persistent and limited Wallace's everyday activities.[6]

The governor's flank discomfort reportedly disappeared, especially by faithfully dabbing DMSO on the painful area from time to time during the course of a month. As Wallace was a well-known public figure, his success in relief from pain has had an impact on the promotion of the drug as a painkiller and anti-inflammatory agent that works.

An even greater booster was the television news show that Wallace watched that featured DMSO as the definitive but controversial product for eliminating pain when all else failed. Wallace was controversial himself at one time and he knew the incongruity of such a label. The TV show stimulated the governor to seek treatment with DMSO.

On March 23, 1980, and again on July 6, 1980, the popular television program *60 Minutes* reported on DMSO. In a broadcast segment titled "The Riddle of DMSO," CBS news correspondent Mike Wallace gave broad national attention to this chemical. On the program, Dr. J. Richard Crout, the chief FDA opponent of DMSO, said that double-blind studies were mandatory before approval would be forthcoming from his agency. Yet, researchers can't conduct double-blinds because of the distinctive odor of the product. Within a few minutes of putting it on your skin, you can taste it on your tongue; it penetrates the skin and runs through the blood stream so effectively.

There is a lot more to the issue of DMSO, however, and on *60 Minutes* Mike Wallace brought in the human factor in which the relief from pain is of primary importance. He showed Emily Rudich playing the piano in spite of her severely deformed fingers and years of searing, unrelenting pain from arthritis.

Referring to DMSO's effect on her condition, Mrs. Rudich said, "I have some very badly gnarled fingers from arthritis, and the DMSO eases the arthritis right away. It's not a miracle drug, doesn't really cure it, but it eases it . . . I had a fever blister on my lip. I used DMSO three times, and the fever blister went away immediately. I've cut myself in the kitchen, and sometimes quite badly, and have used DMSO on it and the cuts begin to heal right away."

Most dramatic was the case of Sandy Sherrick of Riverside, California, who had suffered severe whiplash and nerve damage in an automobile accident two years before. In November 1979, Mrs. Sherrick writhed in an agony of back, neck, and shoulder pain. "No painkiller, no therapy, no doctor, it seemed, could help," said Mike Wallace.

"Oh, the pain was extremely bad," Sandy Sherrick confirmed. "I was to the point where I cried continuously. I did not cook meals. I did not clean. I barely got myself dressed. . . . They finally got to the point where they just told me, 'You're going to have to live with it. The weather's going to affect you, and you're just simply going to have to live with it.'"

Upon learning about DMSO, Mrs. Sherrick grasped at it as a last resort. Feeling awful pain throughout the trip, she flew to Portland,

Oregon, for treatment by Dr. Jacob. By the third day of intravenous and topical application of DMSO, the patient began to feel somewhat better, reported Mike Wallace. *60 Minutes* followed her progress on videotape. Before she left for home, Dr. Jacob showed her where and how to apply DMSO topically to her neck and back.

The television camera then switched to Mrs. Sherrick in her Riverside, California, home. She was feeling comfortable, smiling, and taking no medicine for pain relief. She said, "Oh, the pain's gone. The pain is totally, completely gone from my neck. . . . I'm telling the truth, the honest-to-God truth." She ,could do her housework, drive a car, lift packages. "I have not found anything I can't do."

Mike Wallace pointed out that a story like Sandy Sherrick's does not take the place of a scientific test, which the FDA requires.

"Well, that's fine. I can understand their feeling," said Mrs. Sherrick. "But they've got to be able to look at the test results and take me as an individual. I have no reason to say it does work or it doesn't. All I can say is what it's done for me personally. It worked for me."

This powerful presentation reached 70,000,000 TV viewers. Dr. Jacob's office was immediately swamped, with up to 10,000 people figuratively crying, "Save me, save me from pain!"

Pain victims also came to other physicians around the United States, Canada, and Mexico who were known to utilize DMSO. They arrived in droves. Telephones in the offices of doctors and pharmacies in Florida, Oregon, Louisiana, and Nevada rang busily for several days following the Sunday evening broadcast of *60 Minutes.*

A subsequent wire service report about the FDA's refusal to approve the drug appeared around the country in Tuesday's newspapers.

In his program footnote, Mike Wallace stated: "Tomorrow morning in Washington, the House Committee on Aging begins an inquiry into why DMSO is not available to all Americans for any appropriate ailment, including plain and simple pain." The numbers of letters and telephone calls that came into congressional offices inquiring about the cause of DMSO unavailability were massive. A sampling of the letters sent to just one congressman, Claude Pepper of Florida, are found in Chapter 4.

The disclosures that came out of this and other Congressional investigations were shocking to an already embarrassed scientific medical community. The apparatus by which the Food and Drug Administration studies the efficacy of a new drug was turned upside down. As fully discussed in Chapter 13, revelations about ignorance of the scientific method or fraudulent tests in relation to the drug's effectiveness caused not only DMSO opponents to discontinue clinical trials but even made its proponents back off. And this disconnection to the product's therapeutic effects also included its chief proponent, Dr. Stanley Jacob.

As you will read in more detail later on, FDA investigator Dr. K.C. Pani allegedly took money from Dr. Jacob to pay off his wife's exceedingly high medical bills for cancer treatment. Dr. Pani lost his standing and his job with the FDA. Dr. Jacob was indicted by the Federal Grand Jury on three counts of improper payments to an FDA official and one count of criminal conspiracy. In May 1982, mistrial was the result of these courtroom trials.

Then the government went after Dr. Pani and Dr. Jacob again. This time, Dr. Pani plea-bargained and accepted conviction of a misdemeanor as his crime. Dr. Jacob not only was let off, but the FDA, on October 29, 1982, offered him an apology for their incorrectly bringing the charges against the pioneering surgeon.

More than that, it was learned by Congress that poor or fraudulent investigative techniques employed during the trials of DMSO for interstitial cystitis, the only condition for which it is approved in the United States, almost had the FDA recall such approval. Not this or any other internal or external condition would have been allowed as acceptable in the United States for DMSO application. Research Industries Corporation (RIC), the manufacturer of Rimso-50, a major retail-selling brand of DMSO, apparently played a big role in causing the FDA to have its breach of confidence in the drug. In a semi-confession to U.S. Senator Edward Kennedy, the president of RIC admitted his company's complicity in the mismanaged interstitial cystitis clinical trials.

And there were more adverse findings, which will be revealed near to my book's ending. However, almost all of the fallout during these Congressional investigations occurred from human foibles, greed, and/or inappropriate behavior and not from physical, chemical, or biological faults of dimethyl sulfoxide. The drug remains as efficacious as ever—a true medicinal from nature that continues to astound both holistic and conventional medical scientists as a new and powerful healing principle.

Still, the result from exposure of these scandals of ten years ago is that very few clinical studies on DMSO have been carried out and published since that 1982–83 period. Compared to prior decades, the relatively few journal papers—perhaps 100 of them, which are cited throughout these pages—are all that remain of the tremendous effort originating at the University of Oregon Medical School. If DMSO experiences a resurgence of interest among researchers, it will happen more from prompting of doctors by medical consumers who are reading magazine articles and books such as this one. Because of its dramatic remedial properties, dimethyl sulfoxide deserves more respectful attention than mere public interest. Scientists must be the ones to take up the challenges presented. The public should have access to the remarkable therapeutic principle of DMSO about which I report in the next amazing chapter.

CHAPTER 3

The Therapeutic Principle of DMSO

A married couple arrived in Sarasota, Florida, directly after the *60 Minutes* television broadcast. They had driven all night from Hamilton, Ohio, to keep a 9:00 A.M. emergency appointment to receive the new wonder drug for pain at The Douglass Center for Nutrition and Preventive Medicine (no longer open). They considered their quest for DMSO to be a last-ditch try after a full year and $10,000 worth of unsuccessful treatments with other remedies.

Mrs. Fred Dabbelt explained that her husband's left hand had become stiff and claw-like after surgeons operated to remove a blood clot in his arm. The hand was unusable. Nothing helped the muscles regain their normal capacity, and, after a series of unsuccessful procedures, the doctors began to suggest that the problem was psychological.

After three intravenous injections of DMSO, Fred Dabbelt was able to open and close his hand—something he had found impossible to do before.

Altogether, the patient had five days of treatment. When contacted nine months later he said, "The pain has completely disappeared. My hand is still numb but usable. Before DMSO, the hand looked like a claw; it now looks normal."

"We'd tried everything. This was the last resort," said Mrs. Dabbelt. "It's just amazing. Before this, nothing worked."

How *does* dimethyl sulfoxide work? It may best be summed up in the words of Dr. Stanley W. Jacob, co-discoverer of the therapeutic properties of the drug: "We've barely scratched the surface, for this is a new principle in medicine. We've had only three new principles in our century—the antibiotic principle, the cortisone principle, and now the DMSO principle—and the DMSO principle is the only new one of our generation. Despite all the controversy, my guess is that history will record it this way!"

This chapter explores the *modus operandi* of DMSO and discusses its penetration power and the rationale for its use. We will be taking a highly technical biochemical science and simplifying it as much as possible without changing the hypotheses upon which DMSO actions are based.

Students of biophysics and biochemistry will find the following information useful for their purposes. Others may wish to skip to page 37 for a summary.

STRUCTURE AND PHYSICAL PROPERTIES
OF THE MOLECULE

The dimethyl sulfoxide molecule is ten-sided with a center occupied by a sulfur atom. Two methyl groups, an oxygen atom, and a nonbinding electron pair are located at the points of the tetrahedron. See Figure 3.1 for a depiction of the molecular formula.

DMSO's molecular weight is 78.15. The drug is capable of entering into a chemical reaction characterized by the development of heat, and it releases 60 calories (cal) per gram (g) of DMSO when mixed with water. The boiling point at 760 millimeters (mm) mercury (Hg), degrees Celsius (°C) is 189.0; vapor pressure at 20°C, mm Hg is 0.37; specific gravity at 25°C, grams per milliliter (g/ml) is 1.0958; melting point, °C is 18.55; heat of combustion, cal/g is 6,050; flash point in an open vessel, °C is 95; viscosity at 20°C, centipoise (cP) is 2.473; surface tension at 20°C, dyne/centimeter (cm) is 46.2.[1,2,3,4]

Because DMSO has a freezing point of 68°F, one is able to tell its approximate concentration, if a bottle of the liquid solvent is acquired from an unknown source. Put the unopened bottle into the refrigerator (not the freezer). Within two hours the liquid will turn solid, like ice. You now have 99.5 percent DMSO, the purest and highest concentration made. Leaving the bottle cap on will prevent hydrolyzation (decomposition) so that the liquid will freeze at 68°F or less.

If, when the frozen bottle is turned upside down, little rivulets of

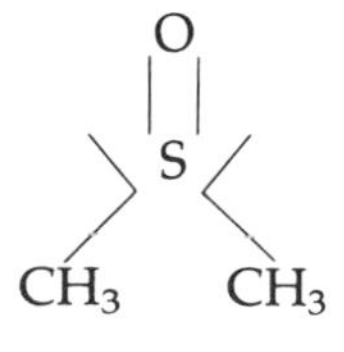

$$\begin{array}{c} O \\ \| \\ S \\ CH_3 \quad CH_3 \end{array}$$

Figure 3.1 Molecular formula of dimethyl sulfoxide.

water flow through the ice, you probably possess the veterinary grade DMSO. This is a 90 percent concentration. Ten percent is distilled water.

If the DMSO doesn't freeze while standing in the refrigerator, put it into the freezer compartment. If it does *not* turn solid even after standing at below 32°F, it probably indicates a 50 percent mix of DMSO and water. If it *does* turn solid in the freezer, this liquid is not DMSO, or is almost all water with just a small bit of the solvent mixed in. Fifty percent DMSO is an antifreeze; it will work well in automobiles for winter driving.

To reliquify DMSO that has turned to a block of ice in the bottle, merely put it into a pan of warm water. In pure form, the life of the solvent is indefinite. DMSO may be used for years.

Many other physical properties of DMSO could be discussed, but those given here provide enough of a representative sampling, since this is not a text exclusively on the chemical and physical characteristics of the solvent. Almost all the known chemical and physical properties of DMSO are found in Crown Zellerbach's *Dimethyl Sulfoxide Technical Bulletin*.

The crystalline structure of this solvent indicates the presence of a weak hydrogen bond that contributes to the molecular forces in DMSO.[5] In liquid state DMSO seems to assume a chainlike structure held together by the alignment of the two sulfur-oxygen poles.[6,7] This structure is believed to suffer a partial breakdown between 40°C and 60°C since certain properties of the liquid, such as the refractive index, density, and viscosity, exhibit distinct changes in their temperature coefficients in this temperature range.[8]

Chemists find that DMSO's ability to associate with molecules that have a thick layer of hydrogen ions and with neutral molecules as well as ionic species is a fascinating property. It makes DMSO an excellent solvent and penetrant through organic and some inorganic material.

Interactions between DMSO and other substances increase in proportion to the polarizability of the substance. Solubility of the substance into DMSO is promoted not only by this type of molecular interaction but is also favored by the degree to which the energy of a system or substance is available for work. The greater the packing of spherical molecules in the "free volume" of liquid DMSO, the better solubility of cyclic unsaturated hydrocarbons as compared to that of noncyclic saturated hydrocarbons. The solubility of a substance increases with the decrease in the electronegativity of the atoms that constitute the substance with which the solvent is mixing.[9]

DMSO has a strong hydrogen bonding with hydroxyl groups. The significance of DMSO as a scavenger of hydroxyl radicals is that *this chemical ion is dominant in arthritis.* Hydroxyl radicals are responsible for breaking down the synovial fluid and the cartilage of the joints. One of the few known substances responsible for detoxifying this radical, DMSO forms a dimethyl sulfone plus water with the hydroxyl ion. These are readily excreted out of the body. Neutralizing this highly toxic free radical causes the reduction of inflammation and the diminishing of pain in arthritis. *It is probably the primary mechanism that allows DMSO to work effectively against arthritis.*

Incidentally, DMSO acts in a similar therapeutic way against the pathological biochemical changes in cancer, atherosclerosis, and any other set of circumstances where there would be a preponderance of free-radical generation.

If superoxide anions are present in quantity as a result of ecological alteration such as radiation toxicity, water pollution, chemotherapy, or other stressors, the body's ability to detoxify is affected. Instead, superoxide and superoxide dismutase form hydrogen peroxide. Lipid peroxidation takes place. More hydroxyl radicals develop and bring on cellular damage with degenerative disease. DMSO offsets these effects and brings the body back to a more normal state.

Free-radical pathology is an intricate part of virtually every metabolic dysfunction you can think of. To illustrate, cancer manufactures prodigious quantities of hydrogen peroxide, which then generate the hydroxyl radical. This is probably part of the reason why DMSO has proved to be valuable in the treatment of cancer. Holistic physicians are using it clandestinely all over the country for that purpose. It is no "magic bullet," but in the total metabolic program against cancer, DMSO is quite useful as an adjunct.

DMSO also has an effect on proteins and nucleic acids. It has excellent solvent properties for dyes, starch, cellulose and its derivatives, lignin, vinyl polymers and copolymers, polyvinyl alcohol, acetate, halides, and other things too numerous to mention in this cursory description of its pharmacological effects.[10,11,12,13,14,15,16]

Superior to water in associations based on the solvent's induction of two poles in aromatic rings, DMSO is able to exchange sites with "bound" water molecules in relatively immobile protein structures. It has the unique property of transferring through the skin barrier without attendant tissue damage. There seems to be a loosened protein structure that results from the replacement of water in the skin.[17,18,19,20,21]

In a conference call lecture delivered to the semi-annual meeting of the American College of Advancement in Medicine in May 1980, Dr.

Jacob said, "DMSO is literally water's alter ego. It moves through membranes and substitutes for water so that it pulls substances through cells that ordinarily would not move through them. This is its basic mechanism of action. The DMSO-water bond is 1.3 times stronger than the water-water bond." This attribute of bonding with water better than water molecules themselves is highly significant. *It probably is what makes DMSO an entirely different healing power than anything medical science has known before.*

THE HEALING POWER OF DMSO

The New York Academy of Sciences sponsored a 1967 conference on the forms of water in biological systems and the changes induced in its structure by the presence of different solutions such as DMSO. The participants in the conference were greatly concerned about the biological implications of the different states of water.

DMSO stabilizes ice-like water clusters. It is probably capable of displacing the equilibrium between the less and more highly structured water, in favor of the latter. The chemist Dr. H. Harry Szmant says, "Since the hydration of cell constituents and the activity of water in general are not necessarily the same in the different states of water, it follows that DMSO may exert an indirect effect on biological systems by virtue of the changes that it causes in the liquid structure of water. Among the more important biological consequences of this indirect effect of DMSO, one can mention changes in the conformations and associations of proteins and other molecules. More direct biological effects caused by DMSO, without a profound change in its chemical identity, may include changes in ion-pairing equilibria and in the specific solvation of hydrogen-bond donors."[22]

In brief, Dr. Szmant is saying that the basic therapeutic principle of DMSO is that cellular damage can be altered—the cell healed and restored to near normal—by changing the water structure within the cell. Cell membrane permeability by DMSO also alters what normally goes into and comes out of the cell.

As a unique nutrient substance, DMSO tends to cause a build-up of white blood cells and more immune production of the migration inhibitory factor (MIF) of macrophages. White blood cells surround any foreign particles in the blood thus helping the body to fight infections. Macrophages are large wandering white blood cells that eat and destroy foreign proteins including microorganisms and other cells in the blood and tissues. Thus, the immune system is made more effective by DMSO, which allows macrophages to move around and through the tissues faster. The MIF, or the factor that holds back macrophages from wandering away from where they are needed, immobilizes and activates bystander macrophages. Such activated macrophages have specific and nonspecific death-dealing properties against germs and are poisonous to tumor cells. MIF is a kind of natural chemotherapy for cancer present in the body all the time.[23,24]

By its ability to modulate the lymphocyte form of white blood cell, DMSO potentiates its immune production of MIF. In conjunction with immune stimulation, DMSO can enter the cell to prime or activate the subcellular mechanisms involved in the production and release of MIF. Also, it produces a cofactor that enhances MIF or has MIF-like activity.

DMSO diminishes allergic reactions by unfolding the cell membrane and making more cell receptor sites available to attachment by specific antigens, the substances that stimulate the body's production of antibodies. When antigens appear in the blood or tissue, antibodies that are produced or are already present move into action against them and neutralize them. This process helps to produce immunity to infectious diseases and prohibit the growth of malignancies.

The modulating effect of DMSO on lymphocytes also tends to increase the production of other lymphokines (stimulators of the circulation of lymph through the vessels) such as interferon and lymphotoxin, as well as enhance the direct toxin diluent effect of sensitive lymphocytes. Such a diluent reduces the potency of a toxin. This activity has application in the control of microbiological infections and tumors. It could be effective in breaking the body's tolerance that may be associated with cancer, and could also affect the tolerance associated with the acceptance of organ transplants. DMSO may eventually be used as a cancer preventative or as an agent helping to prevent transplant rejection.

DMSO tends to potentiate cell-mediated immunity in diseases reported to be associated with the decrease of cell-mediated responses, such as multiple sclerosis, systemic lupus erythematosus, rheumatoid arthritis, sarcoidosis, lymphoid thyroiditis, ulcerative colitis, lepromatous leprosy, cancer, and congenital diseases associated with T-cell deficiency or dysfunction. For all these problems, DMSO could be quite effective in healing or useful in their metabolic treatment.

Furthermore, DMSO could also potentiate the cell-mediated immunity that accounts for autoimmune diseases.[25]

All of this potential activity of DMSO may be due to its property of affecting cell membranes. It is a true therapeutic principle that has yet to be investigated to its full potential. Medical science and biochemical study have hardly begun to penetrate the metabolic mystery of this new healing power.

In a paper published on DMSO's usefulness in treatment of headache, Dr. Jacob wrote: "DMSO readily crosses all the membranes of the body thus far studied without apparently destroying the integrity of these membranes and permits the passage of a number of compounds across the membrane barriers. The mechanism is not understood. . . . Dimethyl sulfoxide in the laboratory blocks conduction in an isolated nerve when a 25 percent concentration is employed. Conduction returns when the fiber is washed free of DMSO. This blockade may be an osmotic effect."[26] Nerve blockage is the way a local anesthetic works and accounts for why DMSO takes away pain.

DMSO, representing a new therapeutic principle, is not a drug in the usual sense. Dr. Jacob told the House Select Committee on Aging: "The difference between a therapeutic principle and a drug is that a drug is useful in treating a disease or a dozen diseases or even one hundred diseases. But a therapeutic principle is an entire new means of treating illness."

By the end of 1991, the medical literature throughout the world had been enriched by more than 3,000 scientific studies involving approximately 500,000 clinical patients on this new therapeutic principle, carried out in the most important university centers and published in renowned medical journals in the United States, Russia, Germany, Japan, England, Scandinavia, Switzerland, Chile, Argentina, and many other countries in Asia, Europe, South America, and North America.

NONTECHNICAL SUMMARY
OF MOLECULAR CHARACTERISTICS

Setting aside the physical and chemical properties of the DMSO molecule and translating what we know into easily understood language, here is a non-technical summary:

- DMSO is a simple, small molecule with truly amazing chemical, biological, and physical characteristics.
- One interesting property that all users should be familiar with is the "exothermic reaction." When DMSO is diluted with water, heat is

released. The bottle containing the medication will be warm to the touch. This is a temporary, harmless reaction.

- Hydroxyl radicals (OH) are ubiquitous and highly injurious to health. DMSO combines with, and thus neutralizes, these dangerous little time bombs that can literally explode your individual cells. The DMSO combines with the hydroxyl radical, adds water, and then the kidneys excrete this chemical complex into the urine.

- The generation of "free radicals" such as hydroxyl, chloride, and others is one of the major factors in the disease process no matter what the state of the disease. This is a major reason that DMSO, a "free radical scavanger," is useful in the treatment of many conditions such as cancer, arthritis, and arteriosclerosis.

- DMSO substitutes for water in the living cell and, because of this remarkable property, can heal the sick cell by destroying free radicals within the cell.

- DMSO also increases the permeability of cell membranes, allowing a flushing of toxins from the cell.

- Allergic reactions are diminished by DMSO, which increases the body's resistance to infection by a number of complicated mechanisms.

DRUG TRANSPORT PROPERTIES OF DMSO

Numerous drugs dissolved in DMSO retain their therapeutic activity and their specific properties over a long period. DMSO not only maintains but strengthens and multiplies the action of the drugs dissolved in it, thus permitting the administration of lower doses than normally required to obtain a satisfactory response. Certain drugs dissolved in DMSO, such as insulin, corticoids, antibiotics, pyrazolic derivatives, and cystostatics, may be used in lower dosage than usual without reducing their therapeutic efficacy. Furthermore, their undesirable side effects are greatly diminished when they go into DMSO solution.

In organ banks around the world, organs and tissues are stored and preserved in DMSO so that they are available for transplanting and grafting. Tissues such as red blood corpuscles for transfusions and semen for artificial insemination are preserved in this manner.

As a penetrating carrier of drugs, DMSO is unsurpassed. It easily carries necessary pharmaceuticals to any part of the body for a therapeutic effect. It passes through cellular membranes and tissues. It is invariably able to penetrate endothelial coatings of the arterial walls, meninges of the brain, healthy skin, mucous membranes, and other tissues.

Intravenous or intramuscular injection of DMSO passes into the fluid of the head and spine. When injected within a sheath such as that surrounding a muscle or nerve, it appears rapidly in the blood stream. The central nervous system has a response to DMSO different from that to other drugs because DMSO passes the blood-brain barrier, easily penetrating it and flowing out again. Other drugs will pass through this usually impenetrable blood-brain barrier along with the solvent when they are molecularly mixed with it.

Basic chemical processes at the nerve cell level are stimulated in the central nervous system by use of DMSO. It permits the transport of amino acids to the brain where they take part in the synthesis of glutamic acid and other elements that, incorporated in the metabolic cycle in the brain, energize the functional activity of the neurons and the brain. This functional stimulation permits the correction of many neurological syndromes characterized by mental deficiency, slower brain activity, loss of memory, and depression and anguish.

On an experimental basis, DMSO has been administered topically, subcutaneously, intramuscularly, intraperitoneally, intravenously, orally, intrathecally, and by inhalation. It has been instilled into the eye, on the mucous membranes, and into the urinary bladder. It has been given to laboratory animals including rabbits, hamsters, rhesus monkeys, chickens, dogs, pigs, guinea pigs, rats, mice, and goldfish, as well as humans.

In the United States DMSO is currently an experimental drug for human use and has been released as a veterinary prescription drug for the treatment of acute musculoskeletal injuries and inflammations of horses. At the time of this writing, DMSO remains approved by the FDA only for use in interstitial cystitis, a relatively rare bladder disease. It has been prescribed for humans by clinics in parts of Europe and South America for three decades.

DMSO'S PRIMARY PHARMACOLOGICAL ACTIONS

DMSO has a wide range of pharmacological actions including membrane penetration and anti-inflammatory and local analgesic effect. It inhibits the growth of bacteria, promotes the excretion of urine, holds back the secretion of cholinesterase, changes the action of a concomitantly administered drug, acts as a solvent for collagen, provides a specific or nonspecific increase of immunity, and produces local vasodilatation. Moreover, DMSO will effectively carry local anesthetics into the deeper layers of skin and into the eardrum, permitting incision without pain.

In controlled studies veterinarians report a wide range of efficacy for their animal patients in multiple problems involving musculoskeletal injuries and acute inflammations, including skin problems.

When integrated with other drugs, DMSO is more efficacious than when it is used as the sole medication. For instance, Dr. Jacob told the assembly of the American College of Advancement in Medicine: "We have treated a number of patients with cellulitis [the inflammation of cellular or connective tissue] but DMSO alone has limited effect on the condition. Rather, I would combine DMSO with an antibiotic, although the solvent by itself has anti-bacterial properties. It will convert bacteria which are resistant to a given antibiotic to being sensitive to that same antibiotic." This DMSO characteristic of resensitizing bacteria could possibly restore an entire group of obsolete antibiotics to the armamentarium of medical practitioners.

In 1968, based on two years of animal experiments, the first clinical investigations were begun on people in hospitals and health centers of Santiago, Chile. DMSO, combined with many different drugs, was administered for various diseases such as mental retardation, senility, rheumatic and cardiovascular disorders, chronic respiratory insufficiency, skin infections, and other problems. These clinical studies integrating individual drugs with DMSO gave excellent results that widely surpassed those obtained in the United States and in Europe up to that time. DMSO previously had been administered alone, not in the form of an integrated DMSO therapy.

Further observations of the primary pharmacological actions of DMSO indicate that administered parenterally (by some other means than through the intestinal canal, particularly by injection into veins and subcutaneous tissues), it has a more rapid and efficacious therapeutic effect than oral or topical (on the skin) applications. For example, after both one-time and repeated topical application of DMSO on the skin of rats, rabbits, and dogs for as long as several weeks, there was no accumulation of the labeled DMSO found in the organs. (DMSO was labeled with a dye.)

Autoradiograms (photographs detecting radioactivity) taken of rats twenty hours after skin application showed no accumulation in the brain, spinal cord, vertebral disks, fatty tissue, or adrenal glands. In dogs, skin application for three weeks resulted in no accumulation of radioactivity except in those regions of the skin that were directly treated with DMSO and in the muscle underneath the treated areas.

In contrast, intravenous injection of DMSO into laboratory animals resulted in its permeation of almost all organs of the animals' bodies. Yet, DMSO administered intravenously, intramuscularly, or intraperitoneally has an extremely low index of toxicity. Hence the therapeutic dosage is far below the toxic dose (see Chapter 5).

Topical and oral absorption in humans is different from that in animals. DMSO is readily absorbed when administered on human skin, with peak levels occurring after 4 to 8 hours. The orally administered drug was rapidly absorbed, reaching a blood serum peak in 4 hours, and serum levels of DMSO were undetectable after 120 hours. Both unchanged DMSO and its metabolite dimethyl sulfoxone ($DMSO_2$) were isolated from the urine. $DMSO_2$ appeared in the blood after 48 hours and stayed in the blood for as long as 400 hours.[27]

Scientists have concluded that the pharmacological action of DMSO lasts in the body even when it is applied to the skin or swallowed. It is excreted partly as the unchanged drug and partly as $DMSO_2$. DMSO is rapidly absorbed in humans when applied on the skin or given by mouth. Since blood levels are lower after skin administration than after oral administration, skin absorption is probably less complete than absorption from the gastrointestinal tract.

While the solvent readily crosses most membranes of the body without destroying the integrity of these membranes, it will not rapidly penetrate the nails, the hair, or the enamel of the teeth.

Steroids dissolved in DMSO, including hydrocortisone and the hormone testosterone, will increase threefold in skin penetrability.[28]

DMSO will carry hydrocortisone or hexachlorophene into the deepest layers of the skin, producing a reservoir that remains for sixteen days and resists depletion by washing the skin with soap, water, and alcohol.[29,30,31]

DMSO significantly lessens inflammation and swelling by reducing inflammatory exudate and enhancing the development of granulation tissue. Within tissues such as the membranes of cells or their organelles, it renders steroids in the body more available to their targets.[32,33,34]

Keloids show softening and increasing return to normality when exposed to DMSO therapy. A concentration of 50 to 80 percent put on two or three times a day will flatten the raised scar after several months. Microscopic changes seen in the skin will show loosening of collagen bundles.[35]

A medical journal review article published in January–June 1985 discussed the drug interactions, therapeutic use, metabolism, and toxicity of dimethyl sulfoxide. The author, Dr. B.N. Swanson, gave a rather complete summary picture of the substance. He described DMSO as a clear odorless liquid, inexpensively produced as a byproduct of the paper industry that is widely available in the United States as a solvent, but whose medical use is currently restricted by the FDA to the palliative treatment of interstitial cystitis and to certain experimental applications. Cutaneous (skin) manifestations of scleroderma appear to resolve following topical applications of high concentrations of DMSO. A limited number of clinical trials indicate that intravenous DMSO may be of benefit in the treatment of amyloidosis, possibly by mobilizing amyloid deposits out of tissues into urine. (Amyloidosis is the accumulation of amyloid in the tissues, in amounts sufficient to impair normal function. Amyloid is a glycoprotein, resembling starch, that is deposited in the internal organs.) Topical application of DMSO provides rapid temporary relief of pain in patients with arthritis and connective tissue injuries.

Dr. Swanson, in his balanced evaluation, said that claims for anti-inflammatory effects or acceleration of healing by DMSO seem to be currently unwarranted. There is no evidence that DMSO can alter progression of degenerative joint disease, and, for this reason, DMSO may be considered for palliative treatment only and not to the exclusion of standard anti-inflammatory agents. The safety of DMSO in combination with other drugs has not been established; neurotoxic interactions with sulindac have been reported.

In experimental animals, intravenous DMSO is as effective as mannitol and dexamethasone in reversing cerebral edema and intracranial hypertension. An initial clinical trial in eleven patients tends to support this latter application. DMSO enhances diffusion of other chemicals through the skin, and, for this reason, mixtures of idoxuridine and DMSO are used for topical treatment of herpes zoster in the United Kingdom. Adverse reactions to DMSO are common, but are usually minor and related to the concentration of DMSO in the medication solution. Consequently, the most frequent side effects, such as skin rash and pruritis (itching) after dermal application, intravascular hemolysis (breaking up of the blood elements) after intravenous infusion, and gastrointestinal discomfort after oral administration, can be avoided in large part by employing more dilute solutions. Most clinical trials of DMSO have not incorporated the components of experimental design necessary for objective, statistical evaluation of efficacy. Randomized comparisons between DMSO, placebo, and known active treatments were rarely completed. Final approval of topical DMSO for treatment of rheumatic diseases in particular will require a multicenter, randomized comparison between high and low concentrations of DMSO and an orally-active, nonsteroidal anti-inflammatory agent.[36]

HOW DMSO IS ADMINISTERED TOPICALLY

The substance is usually administered in liquid or gel form on the surface of the skin; the liquid may be more effective though people seem to prefer the gel. It is not rubbed in but merely painted or patted on in a thin coating. When Dr. Jacob showed Sandy Sherrick how to apply the solvent to her neck and back, as shown on *60 Minutes,* he said, "Now, when you put it on, don't rub it too hard. You just have to apply it to the skin and it goes in. Let it dry over twenty minutes to a half an hour. It won't be totally dry, but anything left you can just wipe off."

Treatment must be individualized. The optimal concentration varies from 50 to 80 or even 90 percent. In general the face and neck are more sensitive to DMSO than other parts of the body and no higher concentration than 50 percent should be applied there. Topical concentrations of DMSO should be kept below 70 percent in areas where there is a reduction in circulation. Not all clinicians agree that this lesser concentration is necessary. It is preferable to begin treatment with lower concentrations until the skin tolerance builds up. Look for skin irritation before advancing to the higher concentration.

For some rare conditions such as scleroderma or Peyronie's disease (where plaques or strands of dense fibrous tissue encircle the penis, causing deformity and painful erection) the treatment periods are more than a year. How often you administer the DMSO solution depends on the judgment of your doctor and the particular clinical problem.

If the solvent is applied for long periods where there is a lessened blood supply, antibiotics should become part of the therapy, despite their bacteriostatic qualities.

The most common set of health problems for which people will apply topical DMSO at home probably involves acute musculoskeletal injuries and inflammations. The earlier the drug is put onto the injured site, the more dramatic the result. For example, a fourteen-year-old boy was punched in the face. A one-inch laceration with swelling broke open over the bridge of his nose and extended to his eye. Six milliliters (ml) of DMSO were applied to the area. Fifteen minutes later the pain, swelling, and skin irritation started to diminish and disappeared completely within four hours.

The skin must be clean, dry, and unbroken, not only for musculoskeletal problems, but for any topical use of the medication. Remove any excess skin oil or perspiration. Make sure heavy metal or insecticide material has not been allowed to dry on or coat the skin. The medical conditions that respond best are acute post-traumatic soft tissue injuries to the neck, shoulders, and back, sprains and strains of the larger joints of the upper and lower limbs, acute post-traumatic soft tissue injuries associated with subcutaneous and intramuscular bleeding involving the trunks or the limbs, and acute bursitis involving the large joints of the body.

A 70 percent concentration of DMSO mixed with water in volumes ranging from 8 to 12 ml, applied on and around the injury in a wide area at least three times daily, will provide effective healing response for four out of five people. Some benefit will be experienced within twenty-four hours.

Measure out the amount of DMSO you judge is required to cover the affected area. Paint on the solution with a cotton-tipped applicator. As an example, to treat gout of the big toe, apply about 6 ml of the material to the toe and the entire forefoot. Usually it requires several minutes of painting and repainting before an adequate dosage is achieved. Allow the treated area to remain uncovered for thirty or forty minutes; any remaining solution should then be wiped off with an absorbent material to prevent injury to your clothing. Relief from gouty swelling and pain occurs in thirty minutes and lasts for one to four hours. Repeated applications up to four times daily will adequately control the pain of acute gout.

When 60 to 90 percent DMSO is applied to the skin, warmth, redness, itching, and sometimes local hives may occur. In most cases this local irritation disappears within two to three hours. The skin surfaces behind the knee and elbow joints and the skin of the face, neck, and armpit are sensitive to strong concentrations of the solvent. When 60 to 90 percent concentration is applied to the palm of the hand, the skin may wrinkle and stay that way for several days.

Some liniments give pain relief, decreased muscle spasm, and increased mobility of affected arthritic joints through a counterirritant effect. Ordinary liniments take pain away only as long as counterirritation lasts. This is not how DMSO works. In contrast, with DMSO the skin reaction of hives and irritation disappears while the beneficial effects last for several hours.

An interesting observation is that the application of DMSO to one affected joint or area often leads to pain relief in some other location. DMSO has systemic effects. It is a depressant to the central nervous system and, of course, it reaches all areas of the body when absorbed through the skin and into the blood stream.

HOW DMSO IS SUPPLIED

The only DMSO solution of sufficiently pure grade for medical purposes, available commercially, has been Rimso-50 manufactured by Terra Pharmaceuticals, Inc. of Buena Park, California and distributed by Research Industries Corporation, Salt Lake City, Utah. Recently other distributors have been marketing DMSO in gel and solution in strengths other than the 50 percent concentration of Rimso-50.

The brand Domoso is a 90 percent, pharmaceutical grade DMSO suitable for injection and for mixing with water to lower its strength for topical application and oral ingestion. Thirteen distributors across the United States make Domoso available. Until the FDA stopped its production, Demso, another brand-name product, which had a 75 percent concentration, the ideal strength for use on the skin (other than the face and neck), was produced by Commercial Laboratories of Florida, an ethical drug company producing DMSO for prescription by doctors. It was licensed by individual states under the stringent rules and regulations that cover all pharmaceutical manufacturers. DMSO is available legally to veterinarians and for research purposes with humans in states where such investigational use is allowed by law.

Rimso-50 comes in 50 cubic centimeter (cc) vials. Domoso is supplied in pint bottles and in gallon bottles for veterinary use. These products are sold mainly to doctors and pharmacists, but many businesses have acquired supplies for resale to the public. Veterinary DMSO gel comes in a 120 gram tube of 80 percent concentration. There has to be some water mixed in to dilute pure DMSO, otherwise it tends to freeze at around 68°F. Adding one part water to 10 parts solvent will drastically lower the freezing temperature. The material is exceedingly hard to handle without water in the solution.

Many of the industrial grade DMSO solutions have an acid or acetone contamination of several percent. Although this solvent grade is being used for pharmaceutical purposes from one end of the country to the other, there is some hazard involved. Human skin reacts to the contaminants and to too high a DMSO concentration. Acetone contamination can lead to serious medical consequences. Because of its small molecular weight, acetone is readily carried into the blood by acetone-contaminated DMSO. Prolonged exposure to acetone can lead to liver damage and death. So *caveat emptor*—let the buyer beware—when he buys crude DMSO from his friendly local dealer.

While DMSO side effects and toxicity will be discussed in Chapter 5, we advise here that the most efficacious remedy for acid burning or skin rash resulting from DMSO usage is to coat the topically treated skin with aloe vera cream. Aloe vera is a transparent mucilaginous gel derived from the leaf of the aloe, a cactus-like plant. It is useful as a follow-up to any topical DMSO application—its use is recommended after each DMSO treatment, with or without skin irritation occurring. Aloe vera is a good preventative for such external irritation.

The usual oral dosage of DMSO is one to two teaspoons per day. The drug is mixed with tomato juice or grape juice, since it is quite foul tasting by itself. Arthritics benefit from taking 50 percent DMSO orally as well as applying it topically.

Some physicians give patients as many as three injections of DMSO intravenously per day. This is not the intravenous infusion or drip technique, but is a slow push into the blood stream all at once. This method is reported to be useful for treating the more serious degenerative diseases such as cancer, atherosclerosis, crippling arthritis, multiple sclerosis, parkinsonism, and others. As much as 20 cc DMSO in injections have been given as a push. The drug is diluted to approximately 25 percent concentration with sterile water.

The slow intravenous drip procedure is carried out over a two- to three-hour period. Then 50 cc to 100 cc of DMSO are placed into a 500 cc glucose or saline solution and dripped into a vein in the patient's arm.

EDTA (ethylene diamine tetraacetic acid) chelation therapy, the intravenous injection of a synthetic amino acid that removes ionic calcium from the blood stream, may be administered at the same time with the chelating agent being a portion of the same DMSO intravenous solution for infusion. EDTA itself will often relieve the symptoms of arthritis.

Please note that these injection procedures must be performed by a physician trained in the use of DMSO and EDTA. There are some possible side effects, which are completely reversible and harmless but can be frightening to someone unacquainted with how to counter them. As with any other medicine, the doctor should be properly trained and experienced in the use of these compounds.[37,38]

CHAPTER 4

General Medical Uses for DMSO

Ruth P. Lewis of Sarasota, Florida, age sixty-four, was in so much pain from rheumatoid arthritis she couldn't walk without the aid of a four-legged walking device. Suffering from her joint complaints for over twenty years, she had also recently sustained a back injury and was told by her physicians that she must have complete bed rest for at least six months. It was the only thing to do, they emphasized.

Mrs. Lewis realized that remaining in bed for so long could cause her never to walk again, even with the aid of her walking device. So, rather than give her life over to remaining flat on her back, the woman had her son and her husband physically carry her into the Douglass preventive medicine clinic, then located in Marietta, Georgia (the clinic has since been moved to Clayton, Georgia), to undergo a course of treatment with DMSO.

"I had previously experienced many months of severe pain in my hips and legs, visiting specialists, diagnostic clinics, hospitalization in traction, and other procedures," said Mrs. Lewis. "When I entered the doctor's office for DMSO treatment, I was unable to put both feet on the ground. After two-and-a-half weeks of intravenous DMSO treatment, I walked out of that office without any help whatsoever—no cane—no support at all.

"I had not been able to close my right hand completely for over a year. It even kept me awake at night with severe pain. But after the IV, topical, and oral DMSO treatment, I can now close my hand tightly. The arthritis has not returned," said Ruth Lewis.

"I cannot put into words what this drug has done for me. I highly recommend it. I saw many people come and go during my clinic stay; all walked out well," she said.

* * *

"In January 1980, I injured my knee and was in terrific pain, at times immobile," wrote a retired schoolteacher, sixty-two-year-old Gertie D. Brown of Port Charlotte, Florida. "My orthopedist stated that I had a torn ligament, and that this would require surgery. But I refused to have the knee operation. Six months later I heard of Dr. William Campbell Douglass through the media (television) and of the wonderful results his patients were getting from the use of DMSO. I immediately contacted Dr. Douglass's clinic and started receiving treatments. I received at least eight intravenous DMSO treatments and got wonderful results, too."

Mrs. Brown's IV doses of DMSO were quite small. Most of her direct comfort came from topical application of DMSO to her injured knee and to other joints that had given her aching pain over the years.

"The knee is not fully strong, so when I do quite a bit of walking it feels weak," said Gertie Brown. "Before retiring, I apply a small amount of the topical DMSO and the next morning I am ready to return to my daily activities. For those who seem to have great problems with joint pain, I strongly recommend [that they] try DMSO."

*   *   *

A handsome man, six-foot-tall Marvin Combs of Bradenton, Florida, doesn't look his sixty-six years. He still works hard in construction as a building contractor.

Mr. Combs said, "Being in an auto accident with a terrific whiplash that also aggravated other existing health problems, DMSO gave me decided improvement over the back pain and for my other troubles. Medicine prescribed by other doctors had given me no results at all. But lawyers fighting my accident case thought I should continue with my original doctors. So I stopped the DMSO treatment. Again I got no results from the numerous pain pills prescribed and just built up high prescription costs.

"The way I know how I now feel, I surely will return for additional DMSO treatment [after this accident claim is concluded] as it is the only thing I can honestly say gave me relief even to the aggravated problems I already had. To me it is wonderful there is something to help folks besides stuffing a lot of pills into one's system."

Unfortunately, payment for medicine like DMSO is not reimbursed by health or liability insurance policies because it is not considered a legal form of therapy. This, despite Combs's medical record that says: "Arrived with severe pain in his neck, left arm, lower right arm, some tenderness in both legs, and general arthritis. After five days, he 'sleeps like a baby because I have absolutely no pain.' Relief was obtained after the third IV. He was able to return to his normal routine directly after the conclusion of DMSO treatment."

One of the ways to determine progress from using DMSO for weak, arthritic joints is to measure grip strength in the hands before and after receiving DMSO treatment. The technique involves inflating a rolled-up sphygmomanometer cuff, the same instrument used to measure blood pressure, to 20 millimeters of mercury (mm/Hg). The patient then grabs hold of the cuff and squeezes it as hard as possible to raise the mercury reading on the attached pressure gauge as high as he or she is able. A normally strong man's hand should be able to put out between 200 mm/Hg and 300 mm/Hg of pressure; a normally strong woman might squeeze the blood pressure cuff in a range from 100 mm/Hg to 200 mm/Hg.

Before DMSO treatment, Combs could raise the mercury reading only to the 40 mm/Hg level with either hand. In three days of taking intravenous DMSO he doubled his grip strength reading to 80 mm/Hg with either hand. He will probably grow stronger when he returns to using DMSO.

* * *

Another building contractor, sixty-one-year-old Russell Whitney of Arcadia, Florida, is a severe arthritic who consumes an exceedingly high daily amount of sugar—fifty-one teaspoonsful in his refined foods. This high sugar intake is quite significant, for it may contribute to the patient's arthritic disability. Sugar's deleterious effect on the body will be discussed at length in Chapter 7.

Mr. Whitney had excellent results with DMSO usage. His consumption of overly refined foods and sweets did not prevent the solvent from exerting a beneficial effect. The man's ability to sleep without pain improved greatly; the swelling of his finger joints went away; he tapered off all pain medication within five days of the start of DMSO treatment.

The patient is a sportsman and hunter. Immediately following his DMSO intravenous infusions, he left on an African hunting safari that lasted for three months. The DMSO treatment allowed him to lift, cock, aim, and shoot a heavy hunting rifle and enabled him to tramp jungle trails without pain.

GENERAL MEDICAL USES OF DMSO

First listed in the *Physician's Desk Reference* of 1980, the editors' statement for DMSO says: "There are no known contraindications."[1]

Of all the areas in which dimethyl sulfoxide might be used, the public seems to be most interested in using it for various forms of arthritis; however, informed physicians know that the solvent has a vast array of applications. In fact, in the medical and pharmaceutical literature *this drug is declared to have the widest range and greatest number of therapeutic actions ever shown for any other single chemical.* DMSO shows approximately 40 pharmacologic properties that may be advantageous in the prevention, symptomatic relief, or pathology reversal of human organic disease.

Following are sixteen of its major therapeutic properties:

1. It blocks pain by interrupting conduction in the small c-fibers, the nonmyelinated nerve fibers.
2. It is anti-inflammatory.
3. It is bacteriostatic, fungistatic, and virostatic.
4. It transports numerous pharmaceuticals across membranes.
5. It reduces the incidence of platelet thrombi in blood vessels.
6. It has a specific effect on cardiac contractility by inhibiting calcium to reduce the workload of the heart.
7. It acts as a tranquilizer even when simply rubbed into the skin.
8. It enhances antifungal and antibacterial agents when combined with them.
9. It is a vasodilator, probably related to histamine release in the cells and to prostaglandin inhibition.
10. It inhibits the release of cholinesterase.
11. It tends to soften collagen by its peculiar cross-linking effect.
12. It scavenges the hydroxyl free radical.
13. It stimulates various types of immunity.
14. It is a potent diuretic, especially when administered intravenously.
15. It brings about interferon formation in the organism.
16. It stimulates healing of wounds.

The medicine is prescribed in many parts of the world. For example, in the United States it became prescriptive in veterinary medicine in 1970 and in human medicine in 1978. It is prescribed in Canada for scleroderma; in Great Britain and Ireland for shingles; in Germany and Austria for a whole host of disorders including bursitis, tendinitis, and arthritis; in Switzerland for a variety of disabilities; and in Russia for the widest range of medical uses.

Certain fair-skinned people such as those with red or blond hair and blue eyes are more sensitive to DMSO. For them, the topical, oral, or intravenous concentration should be 50 percent or less, particularly around the face and neck.

DMSO seems to grow cumulative in its effect. Experts have observed and reported that less DMSO is needed to achieve results as time passes. This is a "different" quality in a drug, since most pharmaceuticals require increasingly heavy doses. DMSO attacks the disease itself rather than just the symptoms.

DMSO encompasses an entirely new method of treating disease and therein lies its difficulty with the traditional medical community and the watchdog bureaucrats. It has been classified as a drug that is useful for a single disease or class of diseases, but DMSO really is something more than a drug.

On the *60 Minutes* television broadcast in which Mike Wallace questioned Stanley Jacob, M.D., Wallace asked: "Dr. Jacob, isn't a drug that has so many alleged uses from arthritis to tennis elbow, from burns to spinal cord injuries, from mental retardation to baldness—isn't a drug like that automatically suspect?"

Dr. Jacob replied: "No question. And I think that that's one of the reasons it's having problems. And if I had it to do all over again, maybe the major mistake that I made, Mike, in the beginning was to tell it the way it was. I think if I would have said it was good for a sprained ankle, but only if the ankle sprain were on the left side, DMSO maybe, might be approved today."

Indeed, DMSO has been too dramatically therapeutic to be believed. For instance, a January 11, 1981, news report in the *Ocala Star Banner*, Ocala, Florida, carried the headline: "DOCTOR CLAIMS DMSO SAVED 11." The story read:

> SAN DIEGO (AP)—A doctor at the University of San Diego credits the controversial drug DMSO with saving the lives of 11 people who suffered severe head injuries.
>
> Dr. Perry E. Camp, a UCSD Medical School neurosurgeon, said Friday that dimethyl sulfoxide was effective for 11 of 30 people judged near death and for which other life-saving methods have proved useless.
>
> "To take patients like that and have even one out of 10

survive is phenomenal," Camp said. "The fact that we have any survivorship at all . . . doesn't sound like much, but it is extremely encouraging," Camp said.[2]

"A few researchers claim this painkiller may be the aspirin of the 21st century," said the New York *Daily News.*[3]

Such drama reported in the press doesn't make DMSO more popular among the orthodox medical community. It puts too much pressure on doctors to use a pharmaceutical they're not well acquainted with.

Without question, any legitimate scientific resistance to the general medical uses of DMSO is at a minimum. Possible therapeutic doubt exists merely in the minds of those physicians who have not informed themselves of the published medical studies in scientific literature. If you hear a doctor downgrade the drug, usually you'll discover that he has not actually used it or has done little literature research on it.

Resistance is purely political. DMSO got a bad press in 1965, and the FDA disapproved of it then. Once the bureaucracy does that, it has trouble backtracking on its original objections. Today, there are still pockets of resistance within the FDA. The political opposition is not based on anything solid but on emotion and the greater ease in saying something negative.

Also, economic opposition may be generated by the large pharmaceutical firms, because DMSO is not patentable in the general sense. Its broad medical usage would dilute the value of the vast quantities of pharmaceutical agents on which the pharmaceutical companies hold patents. It is natural, therefore, to find little enthusiasm for such a nonpatentable therapeutic substance that is able to be produced and marketed so cheaply.

Consider, for instance, the four "wonder drugs" now being pushed for arthritis by the drug companies and the doctors: Motrin, Tolectin, Nalfon, and Naprosyn. All of them have proved to be ". . . about as effective . . . as aspirin . . . clearly any differences are small," according to the February 1977 issue of *The Resident and Staff Physician,* page 109.

What about the cost and safety of these pretenders? At the time of this writing, Nalfon cost the patient a minimum of $175 a month. This is about *twenty times* the cost of equally effective aspirin and *ten times* the cost of topical DMSO—a tough pill to swallow.

Tough to swallow indeed. Consider the following possible side effects of Nalfon as compared to non-toxic DMSO:

- Gastrointestinal bleeding and possible hemorrhagic death
- Ulcers
- Gastritis
- Clotting abnormalities causing hemorrhage–possible stroke
- Hemolytic anemia (destruction of blood cells)
- Meningitis (brain inflammation–possible death)
- Kidney failure
- Vasculitis (inflammation of the blood vessels)
- Heart failure
- Fatal aplastic anemia

Side effects of Nalfon were reported in the April 4, 1980 and February 6, 1981 issues of *The Medical Letter*. They include personality changes, paranoia, and rage. The latter two side effects are serious psychiatric signs that may lead to murder, suicide, or both.

DMSO has proved to have interesting and valuable biological properties. Some of them are discussed briefly in this chapter and others are explored in greater detail in the chapters that follow. These later chapters will be devoted exclusively to particular disease conditions or body systems where DMSO is found to be useful.

PROTECTION AGAINST RADIATION, FREEZING, AND THAWING

When DMSO is painted on the leg of a rat, the leg is shielded from the effects of X-rays.

The radioprotective properties of DMSO were originally reported in 1961.[4] DMSO safeguards a number of cells, cellular systems, and whole animals against the lethal and mutagenic effects of X-rays.[5]

Whole-body protection against radiation occurs at the cellular level rather than as an indirect pharmacological mechanism. At the cellular level, amounts of glycerol and DMSO that defend against freezing damage also protect against X-irradiation damage. This was demonstrated for bacteria,[6,7,8,9] human kidney cells,[10] and mouse tail bones[11] irradiated into the living organism. Topical application of DMSO to the skin of sixteen-day-old nestling rats protects them against X-ray-induced damage.[12]

A method for the prevention of radiation injuries of the urinary bladder and rectum for cervical cancer patients was worked out by medical researchers in Russia. Reported in March 1985 in the Russian radiological journal, *Meditsinskaia Radiologiia*, the method was based on the local application of dimethyl sulfoxide as a radioprotective agent before a session of interstitial irradiation with the AGAT-B X-ray apparatus was carried out. Accompanying radiation therapy with DMSO as the protectant was provided to twenty-two cervical cancer patients. The control group included fifty-nine patients who received similar treatment without DMSO. The expression of early reactions and late injuries of the rectum and urinary bladder were significantly lower in the DMSO group. The DMSO-protected patients did not get radiation burns, while the unfortunate control group of patients did.[13]

There is evidence that DMSO sustains red blood cells during freezing and thawing. Evidence of preservation against cellular freezing by DMSO was published in a 1959 report.[14] Little doubt exists that the solvent, at concentrations between 5 percent and 10 percent, offers excellent protection to a number of very different cellular systems from the damaging effects associated with freezing and thawing.

INJURIES OF THE BRAIN AND SPINAL CORD

An important possible advance in the prevention of paralysis after injuries to the brain and spinal cord, DMSO is being studied for this purpose at four centers of learning. One of them is the University of Miami School of Medicine, where Jack C. de la Torre, M.D., is Associate Professor of Neurosurgery and Psychiatry and Chief of the Department of Neurological Research. By 1992, he had been working with the compound for about twelve years. Dr. de la Torre first illustrated his findings at a November 1980 scientific conference of the DMSO Society of Florida, Inc. held in Sarasota, Florida.

Studying monkeys that were given an occlusion of the middle cerebral artery, the blood vessel in the brain that controls motor function, Dr. de la Torre prevented their paralysis by dosing them with DMSO. The DMSO-treated monkeys didn't suffer from the severe neurological damage from cerebral stroke that would occur if they were left untreated or were treated with corticosteroids, the current conventional treatment. Stroke, which causes half a million deaths or more each year among Americans, is the second most common cause of death from cardiovascular disease. There are many facets to the pathologic process—pressure, lack of oxygen, inadequate blood flow, release of enzymes—and DMSO is well equipped to arrest them.[15] The DMSO must be administered within four hours to be effective, and within ninety minutes is best, reports Dr. de la Torre.[16] I provide a full discussion of his DMSO research with head and spinal cord injuries in Chapter 9.

At the University of Oregon Medical School where Dr. Jacob works, intravenous DMSO was given to patients following severe head injury. For a group of patients receiving barbiturates and mannitol, brain pressure remained elevated. When 40 percent DMSO was administered (one gram of DMSO per kilogram of body weight) the pressure came down to normal within three to five minutes. Barbiturates and mannitol are at present considered the best available treatment in traditional medicine for such brain injuries, but DMSO proved better, said Dr. Jacob in an interview.

In separate animal studies with cats, rats, and dogs done at three universities, DMSO given intravenously to the spinal cords of the animals within an hour of injury brought about reversal of the injuries, which ordinarily would have been irreversible.

"We have had experience at our medical school in Oregon with two patients in which DMSO was given as early as an hour after what was considered an irreversible injury—an immediate, complete quad-raplegia—and in both people there was total recovery with them walking out of the hospital," said Dr. Jacob. For optimal therapeutic effect it is considered critical to give DMSO intravenously within ninety minutes of a head injury.

"Since the grey matter of the brain seems to deteriorate after any injury, at least in experimental subjects, DMSO has to be given very quickly. Every emergency room and every ambulance should carry it. For paralysis, the drug should be administered in the dosage of one gram per kilogram of body weight. Forty percent concentration for paralysis is recommended even though it extends the bleeding time," Dr. Jacob said. "We have had three patients come into our medical center paralyzed after injury: one five hours, a second six hours, and the last nine hours. Historically, we thought their chances of recovery were just about zero. Two of those three are now walking as a result of our administering IV DMSO despite the time being beyond an hour-and-a-half of the injury." The Douglass Center recommended, and Dr. de la Torre concurred, that 2 grams per kilogram patient body weight should be given for the first dose in these trauma cases.

HEMORRHAGIC STROKE AND HEAD WOUNDS

Even though 40 percent DMSO does cause a prolongation of bleeding time, it is still indicated for use in treating embolic or hemorrhagic stroke. Hemorrhagic stroke is the rupture of a weakened blood vessel in the brain often causing headache, nausea, and ringing in the ears just before the onset of this type of cerebral vascular accident. Embolic stroke is the plugging of a vessel by a clot.

DMSO is superior to any other treatment for high velocity missile wounds of the brain where a great deal of hemorrhage is present. The key to success with DMSO for hemorrhagic stroke or any other problem, as has been shown, is to use it as soon as possible after the stroke or head wound occurs. The healing qualities of DMSO work to bring the injured tissues back to normal. See Chapter 9 and Appendix I for more extensive information on DMSO's use in embolic and hemorrhagic stroke.

BRAIN-DAMAGED CHILDREN

DMSO has been useful in cases of mental retardation and Down's syndrome. As a penetrant it carries drugs across the blood-brain barrier, always a major problem in treating the brain. It has also been used to combat certain forms of psychosis.

Brain-damaged children are given oral DMSO in 50 percent strength. It's especially advantageous for impaired babies, who are provided with a quantity of one half of a gram per kilogram by mouth. Efficacy will be noticed by the child's parents, although measurable changes may not reach the level of statistical significance for the person administering therapy. A cholinesterase inhibitor, the drug may stimulate central nervous system transmission, which is certainly worth a try even over several years to restore a brain-damaged child.[17,18]

See Chapter 10 for greater detail on the response to DMSO therapy of children with mental retardation, Down's syndrome, and learning difficulties.

SCIATICA AND LUMBAR DISC PROBLEMS

In aching backs, particularly disc diseases that cause excruciating spinal pain and often end with surgery, European reports show treatment time and techniques can be reduced by 50 percent with DMSO use.

From 20 to 50 ml of 20 percent DMSO combined with the local anesthetic Xylocaine injected intramuscularly into the painful area daily is a valid adjunct to other treatment. The injections should be given for three to five days in a row.

The following is part of a letter written by Patrick J. Potter of Beavercreek, Oregon, and sent to Chairman Claude Pepper of the House Select Committee on Aging March 25, 1980:

> I, myself, have realized almost complete freedom from pain since being injected with DMSO by Dr. Stanley Jacob. My pain was due to scar tissue formed around the sciatic nerve as a result of two lumbar disc surgeries and would drop me by surprise to the ground—thus causing a constant need for pain medication and the use of a cane, for walking. After two (2) shots of DMSO I was able to quit using the cane, and after about six (6) shots of DMSO by Dr. Jacob I was able to stop using the pain medication. I now feel better than I have since before I got hurt, and owe it all to Dr. Jacob and DMSO. . . .

Unfortunately, not everyone treated for these difficult back problems gets such an excellent result.

KELOIDS, SCARS, AND BURNS

Applied topically and repeatedly, DMSO will flatten the raised, nodular, lobulated linear mass of scar tissue in keloids and take away some of the discoloration. It won't cause the parallel bands of densely collagenous material to disappear, but it does have a positive effect. It could also be an aid in reducing scarring from chronic acne where the fibrous papules have developed at the site of hair follicles, usually on the back of the neck at the hairline.

In one study of ten people with keloids, applying up to 80 percent DMSO a couple of times a day induced scar flattening with loosening of the collagen surrounding the fibrous bundles.[19]

DMSO may be useful in preventing adhesions secondary to previous surgery. This would be accomplished by instilling a dilute solution of DMSO in the abdominal cavity at the time of surgery. More research needs to be done on this.

Thus, DMSO reduces, dissolves, or prevents the formation of scar tissue, a feature important in burns as well. It prevents the contracture of the scar tissue left after burns.

DMSO was used for the local treatment of surface burns by Russian burn specialists in March 1985. Dr. Fil'iula administered the skin penetrant to burned adolescents under bandages and did a comparative study with it against other therapeutic burn agents: nitrofurazone, trimecaine, and monomycin. He found that DMSO was superior in its therapeutic effect.[20]

Dorothy S. Ludwig of Lake Grove, Oregon, wrote to the Honorable Claude Pepper March 25, 1980, and said in part: "I have used it for severe burns and had the pain stopped at once, and somehow, the DMSO prevents the heat of the burn from penetrating further into the body and damaging more tissue. No blisters, scars, or infection."

When Dr. William Campbell Douglass practiced medicine in Sarasota, Florida, his experience involved a little six-year-old girl, Penelope Pappas of Sarasota, who slipped her finger into a live light socket for a prolonged period of time. Her index finger was cooked through and burned ash white at the tip. Within thirty minutes, Dr. Douglass was able to have the finger soaking in full-strength DMSO solution as the child screamed with the pain of the electrical burn. By the end of twenty minutes' immersion in the liquid, the girl had stopped crying because she felt no more discomfort. She slept undisturbed all night, and the next day showed a pink and healing index finger—a truly amazing sight considering the severity of her injury. At the time of the accident, it was felt that she would probably lose the tip of her finger from gangrene. Today, you would never know she had sustained an injury.

ANTIFUNGAL, ANTIBACTERIAL, ANTIVIRAL EFFECT

DMSO stops the spread of fungus. It has been found effective when combined with the oral antibiotic agent, griseofulvin, to kill ringworm, especially mycotic toenails. The solvent can be mixed with other usual antifungal ingredients, too, such as iodine or one of the commercial preparations, to form a 90 percent solution. I do not recommend treating in this fashion except under the supervision of health professionals' advice, which, of course, applies to all treatments described in this book. Applied to fungus toenails or tinea pedis, a paste of griseofulvin and DMSO works well to clear the condition. When I practiced as a doctor of podiatric medicine, this was a treatment I developed and used successfully. The solvent carries various fungicides deep into the skin badly infected with fungi.

In a lower concentration ranging from 30 percent to 40 percent, DMSO is bacteriostatic against *Pseudomonas, Staphylococcus aureus,* and *Escherichia coli.*[21,22] The substance in 12.5 to 25 percent concentrations causes complete inhibition of growth of highly pleomorphic bacteria regularly isolated from human tumors and leukemic serum. In the body of the tumors, twenty-seven such isolated organisms were inhibited from growing without affecting the intact red blood cells.[23]

Many doctors are excited because the drug shows itself able to make antibiotic-resistant bacteria sensitive to antibiotics again. By adding penicillin or streptomycin to DMSO for an inhalant, tuberculosis resistance to these antibiotics is partially avoided. It also carries antibiotics to reduce middle-ear infections in children.

DMSO acts synergistically with other drugs to provide a combination therapy against bacterial infections of the lungs, reported four Russian physicians in 1986. It proved useful for the treatment of lung abscess and pneumonia when combined with other antibiotics.[24]

The solvent alone combats viruses and carries antiviral drugs into the tissues for such infections as fever blisters or painful shingles.

It is thought that DMSO dissolves a virus organism's coating of protein and leaves it unprotected with only its core of nucleic acid exposed to the immune mechanism of the host animal. It did just that to a murine virus-induced leukemia.[25]

MUSCULOSKELETAL INJURIES

It is in the field of musculoskeletal disorders that DMSO showed some of its first and most exciting uses. Originally, Dr. Jacob painted it on the ankle of a colleague who had sustained an accident, and relieved both pain and swelling—only to find out later that the bone was broken. The orthopedic surgeon on the case said he'd never seen so severe a fracture with so little swelling. For another laboratory worker who had sprained his ankle, DMSO wiped out both swelling and pain, and he walked away in comfort.

Sports has proved the medicine's most adaptable area—removing bruises and relieving sprains and strains. DMSO has been employed successfully for thirty professional baseball players on one team, their time loss from injuries only a third that of those treated by conventional methods. DMSO is the treatment of choice in soft tissue injuries.

The drug facilitates the healing of almost any type of traumatic occurrence to the musculoskeletal system. When applied to the back immediately after an injury, it starts complete healing. Without DMSO, paralysis could result. This has been shown repeatedly in tests on dogs.

A clinical journal review article published in August 1988 confirmed that DMSO is an inorganic compound with many interesting *in vitro* properties (occurring in laboratory apparatus), including the ability to scavenge oxygen-free radicals. The four authors had used this substance to treat a variety of clinical conditions, especially musculoskeletal trauma, but they stated that valid data regarding its effectiveness were lacking. Their paper, published in *Clinical Orthopaedics & Related Research*, reviewed the pharmacology of dimethyl sulfoxide and reported on its effectiveness in reducing post-traumatic limb swelling and ankle joint stiffness in a rabbit hind limb model. The left and right hind limbs of the test and control animals were fractured identically in the laboratory. Then, DMSO was applied daily to the skin of only one limb in the test animals. The investigators advised that DMSO reduced postinjury ankle stiffness in both ankles of the test rabbits by 41 percent but had no effect on limb swelling compared to control rabbits. Their postulated mechanisms of decreased joint stiffness included oxygen-free radical scavenging and reduction or stoppage of fibroblastic growth and spread. (A fibroblast is the cellular element that creates connective tissue.)[26]

One criticism of the compound, leveled by Sarasota rheumatologist Ronald Weitzner, M.D., in a newspaper article, is that DMSO, when used in injuries such as ankle sprains, can be dangerous because the relief from pain encourages the patient to use that ankle when he should be staying off it. In actual practice this has not been a problem at all.

Surprisingly, in musculoskeletal disorders and in other conditions where DMSO is applied topically, it is better tolerated in higher concentrations below the waist than above the waist. Yet, DMSO is apparently more effective above the waist, with the quickest response for problems involving the face, neck, shoulders, upper limbs, and upper back and trunk. It should be used cautiously, with a concern for side effects. Concentration should be lowered if any occur.

Distilled water is usually the preferred liquid to mix with DMSO to make up a solution. And no contraindications for any generally acceptable solution or pharmaceutical to be mixed with DMSO are known. It seems compatible with any drug. Furthermore, the substance is not derived exclusively from trees; it can be made from nearly any organic base and probably is naturally present in human beings, although it has not been identified as such.

CANCER

DMSO is an excellent adjunct in metabolic cancer therapy, for it potentiates chemotherapy. There are now twelve tumor-cell types in the test tube in which DMSO tends to stimulate the tumor cell toward changing into a more normal cell, Dr. Jacob told me.

In Chile, Jorge Cornejo Garrido, M.D., Head of the Oncological Department of the Military Hospital and Oncologist of the "Lopez Perez" Foundation, Santiago, and Raul Escobar Lagos, M.D., Head of the Department for Radiotherapy of the "Caupolican Pardo Correa" Institute, University of Chile, used chemotherapeutic agents and DMSO in sixty-five patients with different cancerous localizations. All the people were diagnosed as incurable and previously subjected to conventional treatments. This DMSO combination of drugs had a strengthened antiblastic activity (destroying cancer cells) due to the potentiating and penetrating property of the DMSO. It reduced considerably the toxic side effects of Cyclophosphamide, the chemotherapy agent employed, especially in prolonged treatments.

The doctors divided their patients into three different cancer classifications: lymphomas, breast cancer, and miscellaneous cancers. They reported the following:

- The best results in regard to clinical improvement were obtained by the lymphoma group.
- The beneficial effect on the patients' anemia was significant, as they appeared more lucid and more disposed to resume their habitual activities shortly after the treatment had been initiated. Moreover, there was a definite mitigation of pain and, in many cases, it was not necessary to use morphine.
- There exists a clear synergism of DMSO-Cyclophosphamide when the latter is dissolved in DMSO with amino acids, which permits the application of lower daily doses and lower total doses of Cyclophosphamide than those generally used, without impairing the therapeutic activity.
- Patients who do not otherwise tolerate Cyclophosphamide in saline solutions have good tolerance of the DMSO medication.[27] A cancer researcher has found a way to make cancer cells behave more normally by bringing about a mitotic "turnabout." Charlotte Friend, M.D., of New York's Mt. Sinai Hospital, injected DMSO into leukemic mice and was astonished to discover that the cancer cells started to perform normal cell functions because of the injected solvent. She saw that 90 percent of the cancer cells started making hemoglobin, which leukemic cells do not. The DMSO had somehow caused the cells to "grow up."[28]

In a paper presented at a New York Academy of Sciences meeting, Dr. Joel Warren and his associates at Nova University in Fort Lauderdale, Florida, said: "Treatment of human cancer with combinations of oral DMSO and antitumor compounds is both feasible and attractive. Because of potential toxicity problems, it must be approached, however, not only with caution but also under circumstances in which the maximum amount of information can be obtained on the mode of action of DMSO."

Building on the Mt. Sinai Hospital research and the Nova University research, William Campbell Douglass, M.D., has developed a certain therapeutic approach for malignancy. It is based on the premise that neoplasms (cancer) are signs of a chronic metabolic dysfunction. Therefore, after testing for blood chemistries and trace minerals, analyzing the diet, and determining immune status and other aspects of physiology, orthomolecular-DMSO cancer therapy is instituted. Possible toxicity is stringently monitored. The treatment for cancer consists of intravenous injections of vitamin C, amygdalin, and DMSO. The patient's relief from cancer pain and the patient's return of appetite has been impressive. He or she has a chance for self-healing through resurgence of the body's immunological defenses.

Orthomolecular cancer therapy is a non-toxic approach that combines intravenous DMSO injections with optimal nutrition and lifestyle changes, when indicated. Dr. Douglass observed that he possibly had prolonged life in many of these patients; how much, of course, is difficult to measure.

It has been known for half a century that certain murine (pertaining to mice) and human cancers can spontaneously mature to benign tissue. These observations have stimulated investigators to attempt to induce a state of more normal or benign differentiation in cancer cells using biologic substances or chemicals. Polar solvents including dimethylsulfoxide, dimethylformamide, and monomethylformamide have proven to be good inducers of maturational events in murine and human cancer cells. Moreover, several laboratories have demonstrated that polar solvents inhibit the growth of human tumor xenografts (human tissue grafted into the tissues of animals) in nude mice. These findings have resulted in the entry of monomethylformamide into phase I clinical trials in the United States and Europe.

In 1984, two researchers published a significant paper in the *Journal of Clinical Oncology* about their preclinical work on polar solvents such as DMSO as useful agents in combination with conventional treatment modalities for human cancers. The use of drugs like DMSO can convert neoplastic cells (with abnormal formations of growth or tissue) to benign cells rather than kill the tumor cells. (See the research of Eli J. Tucker, M.D., reported in Chapter 11, on the potent combination of hematoxylon and DMSO against cancer.) Such conversion represents an important conceptual departure from standard cytotoxic chemo-therapy (treatment using poisonous chemicals). The use of matura-tional-agent therapy should be considered as a vital new tool in the design of cancer treatment protocols.[29]

To determine whether dimethylsulfoxide can induce antitumor activity of cyclophosphamide (CYC) in patients with squamous cell carcinoma of the lung, five investigators working cooperatively in 1981 treated fourteen patients who had that disease. The patients were administered a 5-percent solution of DMSO over three days and 1,500 mg CYC/m^2 intravenously as a 60-minute infusion on the third day of treatment. Serial blood, cerebrospinal fluid, and urine samples were collected from the patients to assess the pharmacokinetics (the actions of drugs on human tissues) of CYC. Courses of treatment and testing were repeated every four weeks. No antitumor responses were observed, but the twenty-four-hour urinary excretion of CYC, which is a highly toxic anticancer agent, was much lower than previously reported by the same investigators.[30]

In the journal *Clinical Pharmacology and Therapeutics* in July 1982, medical researchers in oncology reported that ten patients with brain tumors and indwelling ventricular reservoirs were pretreated with up to 10 percent dimethylsulfoxide (intravenously, orally, or both) and were then treated with 1.25 gm/m^2 of CYC. All patients were also receiving anticonvulsant drugs and dexamethasone. CYC and alkylat-ing activity in plasma and accompanying ventricular cerebrospinal fluid were measured by gas chromatography and p-nitrobenzyl pyri-dine assay. CYC entered the cerebrospinal fluid without difficulty and was lost from it more slowly than from plasma.[31]

In Japan, in January 1987, a middle-aged man with multiple myeloma—a cancer of the kidney—was successfully treated with DMSO during the course of an exchange of his blood plasma.[32]

Also, the July 1983 issue of the *British Journal of Dermatology* published a report on the successful treatment of skin cancer in hairless mice using DMSO and an enzyme called methylcholanthrene.[33]

DIABETES

For diabetics, the importance of DMSO comes when it lessens the incidence of diabetic neuropathy, the classical sensory nerve function loss seen frequently in older people with the disease.

In one out of four juvenile diabetics using the topical DMSO, there will be a reduction in the need for insulin, Dr. Jacob told the American College of Advancement in Medicine. It tends to improve blood supply by dilating the smaller blood vessels, especially of the lower limbs. The drug probably should be made a part of presurgical preparations when the surgeon wants to increase the blood supply to a part of the diabetic's body.

NASAL SINUSITIS, TIC DOULOUREAUX, HEADACHE

Placed directly into the nostrils, DMSO can open blocked sinuses in a few minutes. It accomplishes this through its ability to cross all the membranes of the body without destroying the integrity of these membranes, as we've noted before. It also permits the passage of a number of compounds across the membrane barriers.

Sixty patients treated with DMSO for various types of head pain received marked relief. Thirty-five of these people were diagnosed as having tic douloureaux, an involuntary repeated contraction of the trigeminal muscles in the face causing excruciating pain. Seventeen of the patients had headache with cervical osteoarthritis (arthritis of wear and tear in the neck). In five people the headache was associated with sinusitis. Two patients had temporal arteritis, with superficial pain in an artery of the temple.

For the last two patients, simple analgesics were not effective; both required codeine for the pain in the temporal artery. When a dose of 20 ml of 50 percent DMSO was applied twice a day to the entire forehead area and back of the neck, within half an hour the pain in both these patients disappeared and did not recur for at least four hours. Both continued DMSO treatment for one month, at the end of which time pressure on the temporal artery no longer served as a trigger mechanism for setting off pain. These two people have not had recurrence of their headache pain for eighteen years. It should be emphasized, however, the DMSO alone is not the complete treatment for temporal arteritis. Cortisone must be employed along with DMSO.

Initial results for thirty patients suffering from tic douloureaux were similar. Pain relief lasted indefinitely and took place in three or four days.[34] Topically applied DMSO works well for tic douloureaux, but there is an even better result when the drug is injected directly into the spasmed muscles' trigger points. DMSO is not, unfortunately, effective in all cases of tic douloureaux.

A letter mailed to the House Select Committee on Aging, dated April 11, 1980, written by Joyce Louise Ratliff of Selah, Washington, said in part:

> I have read a great deal about DMSO and have also used it and seen it used. The relief my mother-in-law received by the use of DMSO was fantastic. After years of surgery and drugs (approved), she applied DMSO and within a short time obtained relief from (all) pain. She has tic douloureaux in which there is no cure, just pain and suffering. Even the prescribed approved drugs are of little value, especially with the side effects and possible overdose and addiction. I personally administered the DMSO and saw the relief she had. Thereafter she applied DMSO as needed for her pain and always got relief with no side effects. Now, out of DMSO and no place to get more, she is back to being drugged and suffering.

SKIN DISEASES, ULCERATIONS, AND HERPES

In the form of a spray, DMSO was coated on the skin lesions of 152 patients by Lazaro Sehtman, M.D., dermatologist of the Alvear and the Jewish Hospital and of the Railroads' Central Polyclinic, Buenos Aires, Argentina. The skin complaints had been treated with other remedies and had failed to respond, even after treatment for quite a long time.

Except for a pain with a sensation of burning and a strong odor, none of the patients experienced any undesirable side effects of an objective or subjective nature. The best and most spectacular results were achieved in people suffering with herpes zoster (shingles). Shingles is a painful inflammation of the sections of the nerve emerging from the spinal cord. The illness comes from the same virus that causes chicken pox. Here, seventeen patients had regression of symptoms in forty-eight hours with just two spray applications per day. The only side effect, redness, developed and persisted for ninety-six hours.

The November 25, 1981 issue of the *New Zealand Medical Journal* told of forty-six patients with herpes zoster who were randomized into two groups. One group was treated with DMSO alone and the other was administered 5 percent idoxuridine (IDU) in DMSO. Both had their treatments rendered within forty-eight hours of the appearance of the shingles rash. In the IDU/DMSO group, the interval before pain improved in a significantly shorter time than in the control DMSO group. And compared with the control group, significantly fewer new vesicles (tiny blisters) developed at the three-day follow-up interval in the active group. These findings are in agreement with previously published work and confirm the usefulness of 5 percent IDU in DMSO (known as Zostrum) in the treatment of herpes zoster.[35]

In four cases of genital herpes, a form of herpes simplex, the patients were able to have sexual intercourse after only two days of treatment. As in most conditions, DMSO is more effective in genital herpes if used early.

A 100-percent success was obtained for tinea versicolor, a form of fungus infection, among forty-two cases treated by Dr. Sehtman. Tinea versicolor, usually a recurrent problem, is difficult to cure most of the time, but not in these patients treated with DMSO. Using the Wood's lamp as a test, complete recovery was noted in one week.

In cases of inflamed and infected toenails, the analgesic and anti-inflammatory effect of the DMSO spray began within twenty-four hours. These nine patients had previously been treated with antibiotics and anti-inflammatory preparations without any result.

Two people in Sehtman's group with Gilbert's pink pityriasis of unknown cause, ordinarily requiring at least two months for it to heal itself spontaneously, had their lesions disappear within one week, also by spraying on the DMSO solvent.

For another sixty-seven people victimized by severe varicose veins, the DMSO spray proved highly effective. Many of these patients had undergone vein ligations, resections, skin grafts, and removal of their saphenous veins. Some were relapses, but these had the most rapid healing of the skin dermatitis connected with the condition. The patients also had reduction of swelling and pain, and could resume normal functioning. People who had difficulty walking found themselves able to return to work only seven days after DMSO treatment began. A remarkable and surprisingly fast scabbing of varicose ulcers took place in a shorter time than with any other dermatological method, including surgical intervention, which is often used for this type of disorder, reported Sehtman.[36]

Furthermore, Rene Miranda Tirado, M.D., Assistant Professor of Nutrition and Dietetics, Faculty of Medicine, University of Chile, reported quick healing in skin ulcerations of the legs, feet, and upper limbs, infected wounds, other skin lesions, and in second and third degree burns for 1,371 patients. They all received exclusive therapy of topical applications of a medicinal DMSO spray similar to that used in Sehtman's cases. Three times weekly the medicine was sprayed directly onto the lesions after they were cleaned with only sterile water. At the Douglass Center, these conditions were treated on a daily basis, at least at first, and then three times weekly.

Of the 1,371 patients treated in the Tirado study, 95.04 percent were discharged as completely cured and able to resume their usual activities. For instance, those with chronic diabetic ulcers of the feet and legs were completely healed after daily DMSO spray applications for twenty days. Some of these ulcers had been on the patients' limbs for fifteen years. Rapid healing occurred in chronic varicose ulcers, which had not responded to the traditional treatments employed by dermatologists over several years.

Pain and discomfort from these burns, ulcerous lesions, and skin wounds abated almost immediately after the first few applications. Some people who had been suffering intense pain from lesions located in areas at a distance from the affected part where the DMSO was sprayed expressed happy surprise that these pains also disappeared.

Second degree burns on both arms healed completely without leaving any ugly scars. Chronic ulcers that had plagued patients for years, including those from varicose veins or mycotic infections that had not healed in spite of hospital treatment for prolonged periods on several occasions, healed completely. "The DMSO spray did the job," said Dr. Tirado.

"No collateral effects nor undesirable symptoms were observed during the applications of DMSO spray," the doctor reported to the New York Academy of Sciences, "with the exception of a few cases of deep wounds where, during the first few applications, a more or less intense pain occurred which was localized and of short duration, and was no impediment to continue subsequently with this very efficacious therapy."[37]

In the Tirado study, diabetic perforating ulcers were treated with local applications of DMSO, both painted and sprayed with the substance. Perforating foot ulcers constitute a major problem in diabetics with peripheral neuropathy (loss of nerve sense at the extremities) for which no specific therapy is available. In January 1985, as described in the *Journal of the American Geriatrics Society*, twenty patients with chronic, resistant, badly perforating ulcers were treated by such DMSO applications. The solution brought about complete healing of the ulcers for fourteen patients following four to fifteen weeks of daily treatment. Partial resolution was observed in another four patients, and in the remaining two there was no effect. A control group, equal in number, was treated conventionally. Complete healing of the ulcers took place in only two of these control patients. The therapeutic effect of DMSO most probably results from an increase in tissue oxygen saturation via a combined mechanism of local vasodilatation (expansion of the blood vessels), decreased thrombocyte aggregation (clumping of blood platelets), and increased oxygen (absorption of extra oxygen from the blood).[38]

Accidental subcutaneous extravasation (leakage out of a vessel into the tissues) of several antineoplastic agents (agents against tumor creation) are so toxic that they may provoke skin ulcerations for which there has been no simple and effective treatment. Writing in the March 1987 *European Journal of Cancer and Clinical Oncology,* a group of four oncologists advise, "Since January 1983 we have treated all patients in our institution sustaining extravasation by a cytotoxic drug with a combination of DMSO and alpha tocopherol [vitamin E]. During the first 48 hours after extravasation, a mixture of 10 percent alpha tocopherol acetate and 90 percent DMSO was topically applied. The bandage was changed every twelve hours. Eight patients with extravasation of an anthracycline or Mitomycin [two toxic anticancer drugs] were treated on this protocol. No skin ulceration, functional or neurovascular impairment, occurred in any of these patients. The only toxic effect observed by this treatment was a minor skin irritation. The combination of DMSO and alpha tocopherol seems to prevent skin ulceration induced by anthracyclines and Mitomycin."[39]

CATARACTS AND OTHER EYE PROBLEMS

In ophthalmology, DMSO was put into the intraocular area of the eye and was beneficial in the treatment of corneal swelling.[40]

An ophthalmologist reported to the American College of Advancement in Medicine (ACAM) in May 1980 that he had great success using DMSO in treating cataracts and other eye problems. "I've treated two hundred patients in the last year for macular degeneration [deterioration of the macula lutea, an area of the retina], macular edema [swelling of the macula lutea], and traumatic uveitis [an inflammation of the pigmented area of the eye]," the eye specialist said. "I instill 5 mg of DMSO in 1 cc of normal saline placed retrobulbar under Tenon's capsule behind the equator or to wherever the area of activity is. Strictly for cataracts, all we need to do is put one drop of DMSO directly onto the eyeball."

Other ACAM physicians told of instilling one drop of a solution consisting of 25 mg of DMSO with 2 cc of superoxide dismutase (SOD) once or twice a day for clearing cataracts and glaucoma.

The ophthalmologist said, "In using DMSO, glaucoma drugs are potentiated, including those required for treating wide-angle glaucoma. But DMSO alone is better for macular degeneration. In dropping it, we may combine 5 mg of 2 cc DMSO with 5 mg of 2 cc SOD for a 4 cc solution."

The first clue to the possible efficacy of DMSO in retinal disease, variously called deterioration, degeneration, dystrophy, and abiotrophy, all non-inflammatory types of disturbances of the retina, was discovered inadvertently. The retina is the part of the eye that is sensitive to light, a delicate film covering about two-thirds of the inner surface of the eyeball. It is closely attached to an underlying layer, the choroid. Some patients with retinitis pigmentosa, a retinal disease, who were taking DMSO treatment for certain musculoskeletal disorders, sensed that their vision had improved while they were taking the drug. The patients told this to Robert V. Hill, M.D., of the University of Oregon Medical School, and he undertook a preliminary investigation into the effectiveness of DMSO in the treatment of retinal diseases.

"Such an investigation was begun after one patient suffering from retinitis pigmentosa had a rather spectacular recovery of vision after treatment with DMSO," Dr. Hill explained to the Science Writers–Research to Prevent Blindness seminar in Los Angeles in February 1973. "At the time his DMSO treatment was started this patient could see hand motion only with his right eye and had a visual acuity of 20/200 (Snellen) in his left eye. Five days later (February 15, 1972), his vision was measured as 20/70+1 in the left eye, and he could count fingers at five feet with his right eye. Three months later, his visual acuity was 20/50 in the left eye.

"An additional fifty patients with retinal deteriorations (macular degenerations as well as retinitis pigmentosa) were then treated similarly with DMSO, and the subjective evidence gathered was still encouraging," continued Dr. Hill. "This subjective evidence consisted of improved or stabilized visual acuity, improved or stabilized visual fields, and improved night vision. (It is considered 'subjective' because it requires subjective responses from the patient.) Of the fifty patients treated with DMSO, twenty-two improved in visual acuity; nine improved in visual fields; and five improved in dark adaptation. Two patients have continued to regress, and the rest have had no measurable or personally-noted changes in vision."[41]

THE ASTHMATIC SYNDROME

In a paper presented at the Latin American Congress of Asthma and

Allergies, in Santiago, Chile, in 1969, three medical experts, allergist Zoltan Bernath, M.D., internist Norman Bennett, M.D., and pulmonary disease specialist Ernesto Chacon, M.D., gave the results of their research in the treatment of the asthmatic syndrome. The medium used was DMSO as the solvent for an anti-inflammatory steroid, an antihistaminic preparation of recognized efficacy, and a strong bronchodilator, all administered by intramuscular injections.

The treatment was applied in 153 adults, 84 male and 69 female, who were divided into two groups. The 43 people in the first group suffered from frequent asthmatic crises but with more or less prolonged asymptomatic periods. The second group of 110 patients had more intense and more frequent crises, but without asymptomatic intervals, despite the treatments previously received.

The results of the treatment were evaluated by frequent examinations of the patients, including their chest sounds, chest movement, ability to exhale, vital capacity, and other tests. See Table 4.1 for how the DMSO solution aided the patients.

PREGNANCY AFTER TUBAL OBSTRUCTION

Thousands of animals have been impregnated with spermatozoa preserved in the DMSO substance—and had normal offspring.

Like other drugs to be avoided during pregnancy, it probably should not be used. However, women who want to conceive are finding success with DMSO hydrotubation treatment. Hugo Venegas, M.D., head of the Gynecological Department of the Valparaiso Naval Hospital, Valparaiso, Chile, reported that a solution containing one gram of Chloramphenicol plus the contents of one 5 cc ampoule of DMSO with Dexamethasone and Chlorpheniramine, the total diluted with 20 ml of distilled water, was injected by means of ascendent hydrotubation through a canula into

Table 4.1 *How DMSO Solution Aided Asthma Patients*

Results	Number of Patients	Percentage of People
Excellent	37	24.5
Good	92	60.0
No change	24	15.5

women sterile because of inflammatory tubal obstruction. A series of six hydrotubations, one every third day, was carried out.

When a good tubal function was obtained, the woman was asked to lead a normal sex life. If after three months pregnancy did not occur, treatment was repeated in the same form. An analysis based on the results obtained in forty-seven patients was reported.

Dr. Venegas said, "The results we have obtained with this new procedure largely surpassed those obtained with traditional methods of tubal infertility treatment. Possible limitations of this new treatment are minimal, as no significant undesirable side effects were observed, except for the characteristic smell, which is exhaled by the patients during treatment with DMSO therapy."

Of the forty-seven women who were sterile, twenty-seven became pregnant—a success rate of 57.4 percent. Twelve had their babies full term, healthy children, representing 25.5 percent of the total. Three women had spontaneous abortions; four others had voluntary abortions for their own reasons; the remaining seven were normally pregnant at the time of Dr. Venegas' presentation to the New York Academy of Sciences in January 1974.

Note that these pregnancies occurred in the wives of members of the Chilean Navy, who had only short periods ashore. The gynecologist said, "We are convinced that the gratifying results obtained do not represent only a transitory improvement."[42]

MISCELLANEOUS USES OF DMSO

I could continue giving descriptions of conditions cleared or greatly improved by employment of DMSO. In fact, every body system, most physical disorders, and many mental disorders are affected in some way helpful to the patient. Instead, I will devote entire chapters to those health problems where more investigation has been recorded, and I will sum up in the present section some additional findings.

In dental practice in Poland, DMSO has cleared up gum conditions, and has been effective in cases where decay has reached the dental nerve. In the case of decay, DMSO attacks both the infection and the inflammation, wiping out both of these and the pain as well.[43]

Russian physicians, in the November–December 1988 issue of *Stomatologiia*, told how adolescent patients as well as the aged were successfully treated with DMSO and procaine to get rid of chronic parenchymatous parotitis (an inflammation of the parotid salivary glands).[44]

In additional Russian research, DMSO was combined in a 1981 study with two drugs for their evaluation in the treatment of dry socket. The dry socket is an unhealed wound at the site of a tooth extraction, characterized by intense pain, discharge of pus, and sequestra. It is most often associated with a difficult extraction. DMSO acted as a synergistic penetrant for the two drugs, resulting in increased speed of healing.[45]

A German study has shown that women who applied DMSO topically for a month were relieved of a painful breast condition, chronic cystic mastitis.

Conditions of the urinary tract, unaffected by any other known medication, have responded to this medicine. In some cases, it has made it possible for men to resume sexual intercourse where previously pain or urethral blockage made it impossible.

DMSO speeds blood flow by causing vessels to dilate. South American studies indicate it is effective in heart attacks or angina pectoris. It has been credited with preventing damage to heart muscle. There is a crying need for research on the use of massive doses of DMSO (2 gm. per kilogram body weight) in the treatment of heart attacks.

Simply by soaking his patient's hands and forearms in the drug, Cleveland Clinic's former rheumatologist, Arthur L. Scherbel, M.D., had been having great success against scleroderma, also known as "hidebound disease," in which the skin becomes thickened, hard, and rigid.[46] More about the use of DMSO for scleroderma is found in Chapter 13.

DMSO has a history similar to ether. Ether was known for 600 years before it was recognized as an anesthetic. Dimethyl sulfoxide waited on the laboratory shelf for nearly 100 years before it was learned that it had medicinal properties.

Exhaustive tests to determine more therapeutic uses and possible toxicity or unknown side effects are continuing daily in both clinical trials and laboratory experiments. Reports on DMSO are continually funnelled into the University of Oregon central clearinghouse. New information and more journal references are being sought. What is recognized as toxicity or side effects needs recording and broadcasting to the scientific community, including the FDA. The following section sets down all the information about side effects and toxicity as they relate to DMSO. As you'll see, there aren't many, but research is continuing under the watchful eye of the FDA.

CHAPTER 5

The Toxicity and Side Effects of DMSO

The ABC-TV program *Good Morning America* interviewed Robert Herschler, the co-discoverer of the pharmaceutical effects of DMSO, at 8:17 A.M., February 5, 1981. Viewers watched this chemist, a former employee of the Crown Zellerbach Corporation, now Director of the DMSO Research Center, say on the broadcast, ". . . the toxicity of DMSO is very low. It's not true that it is dangerous. Compared to aspirin, DMSO is a much safer drug. People are killed taking aspirin; no one has ever been killed taking DMSO."

The program host, David Hartman, asked, "If this is the case and you are so sold on it, why has the FDA not approved its use?"

"In 1964, the FDA complained bitterly about DMSO because it was both a commercial solvent and a drug," replied Herschler. "They could not control it. Beyond that, we had a meeting with Francis Kelsey of the FDA where she raised her hands and said, 'We simply cannot cope with a product like DMSO. We envision hundreds of applications [NDA's] coming in, and we simply don't have a budget or staff.' From then on they took a hard line against DMSO . . . There are many controlled studies that prove it is both effective and safe. And the FDA knows it! The FDA has at least 100,000 clinicals [patient reports], and if they statistically evaluate them, and they have, and if they try to prove it is not safe and effective, they simply cannot do it. They have been using this gambit of 'double-blind'—being able to use the 'double-blind' as the reason for rejecting it."

Herschler added that it is a situation of "bureaucratic Mickey Mouse" that is keeping DMSO out of the hands of the people.

Hartman's other television guest, J. Richard Crout, M.D., Director of the FDA's Bureau of Drugs, took exception to being aligned with Mickey Mouse. "It's true that there's been quite a bit of initial inquiry—scientific dabbling—certainly a lot of patients have used DMSO," Dr. Crout said.

"There's no question about that! But it hasn't gone through the rigorous, disciplined, controlled kind of evaluation that all the drugs do."

"Why not?" asked David Hartman.

"I think there are probably two main reasons. One is that it has really not attracted the attention of a number of experts. It's not dramatically effective, and a number of people have recognized that. Secondly, I think the manner of its promotion has tended through the years to scare off the establishment in science. Regrettably! A lot of people who ordinarily would be engaged in drug research and study new drugs simply have neglected DMSO."

"What evidence do you have that it is harmful? Do you say that DMSO is harmful? Mr. Herschler says it is safer than aspirin," said Hartman.

Dr. Crout admitted, "It's really quite safe when put on the skin. I don't believe I would raise scare tactics about when people put it on and use it for a few days. Anybody who uses it for a month or more in doses of an ounce or more is getting into the unknown. There simply is not much experience with its toxicity there."

The drug has been in public use underground since 1964, employed by tens of thousands of Americans, and up to now no toxicity has been reported in consumer reports, at medical meetings, in the scientific literature, during the four international DMSO symposia, or anywhere else. The approximately 2,000 people for whom physicians in medical practice have personally prescribed DMSO have not advised of any serious deleterious reactions. Yes, there are minor side effects, which I will discuss, that are outweighed by the many DMSO benefits. But toxicity or ill health arising from its use? None at all!

THE LABORATORY INVESTIGATIONS OF DMSO TOXICITY

Scientists have studied DMSO with eight species of mammals, including humans, as well as some fish and birds, with almost universal agreement as to its low toxicity.[1] Short- and long-term administrations of the drug to many animals have shown they tolerate it well. When fed to, injected into, or applied to the skin of animal laboratory subjects and human clinical subjects over periods of weeks, months, or years, there have been none or very few signs of any noxious response. People want the painkilling properties that DMSO offers. Even if mild side effects are present, people say they are worth the improvement this substance brings.

One of the statements J. Richard Crout, M.D., made on *Good Morning America* is that DMSO "is not dramatically effective, and a number of people have recognized that." What he said is directly at variance with the official declarations of Dr. Crout's own Bureau of Drugs of the Food and Drug Administration. Indeed, a rating that the FDA posted on drugs and published in *Consumer Reports* shows that the agency frequently contradicts itself.

The FDA is secretive about the kinds of studies it requires in order to approve a drug for market use. The agency declares publicly that if a drug is safe and effective it will be approved, but this does not always carry. For example, a number of drugs have been classified by Dr. Crout's bureau as to effectiveness. The classification places drugs into the following categories: 1A—this drug is a breakthrough discovery; 2A—this drug has potential uses; 3A—this drug is probably useless. Out of thirty-seven drugs that the FDA classified within these categories, only four were rated 1A. DMSO was one of these four. Yet, the FDA does not approve DMSO for general medical use, and Dr. Crout says "it's not dramatically effective."

Since DMSO dissolves many materials and can be absorbed through the skin, combinations of the solvent and many other substances have been investigated. Some materials dissolved in DMSO have shown a change in toxicity or rate of absorption. Many were unchanged. DMSO merely heightens their therapeutic effectiveness.

Toxicity of a substance is indicated in science by the LD_{50}, meaning the number of milligrams (mg) of DMSO per kilogram (kg) of body weight of the test animal that results in the death of half of the animals being tested. The period of observation is commonly from one week to four weeks. Thus, 100 guinea pigs may be administered DMSO for one or more weeks in a dosage of 2 mg per kg (1 pound equals 0.45 kg), so that a 3-pound guinea pig receives about 3 mg of DMSO. Raising the dose to a point during this period where half the animals die determines the toxic dose, or LD_{50}.

The toxic dose divided by the therapeutic dose is the therapeutic index. This therapeutic index tells researchers and physicians how dangerous a drug or other substance is to living organisms, especially people. The higher the number representing the therapeutic index, the safer the compound or drug. If it is a small number, the substance is toxic. Swallowed, the LD_{50} of aspirin for monkeys is 558 mg/kg. The LD_{50} of DMSO for monkeys is 4,000 mg/kg.[2] Thus, DMSO is more than seven times safer than aspirin.

In the case of laboratory mice being tested, the LD_{50} of DMSO when applied to their skin is reported to be 50,000 mg/kg. Mice survive complete dipping in up to 60 percent DMSO. Rats survive dipping in 80 percent DMSO, and they survive repeated dippings in 60 percent DMSO three times per week for twenty-six weeks.[3] See Table 5.1 for the single-dose toxicity of DMSO as LD_{50}.[4]

In humans, DMSO's concentration on the skin usually produces some reddening,[5,6] but the effect is often no longer noticeable after repeated applications.[7] In 35 percent of people using the compound, a burning sensation at the area of contact is noted.[8] Smaller numbers of patients report skin roughness, mild itching, blistering, dermatitis, thickening, and scaling. None of these are toxic reactions but only side effects. Some of these effects are probably due to dehydration and removal of fats from the skin.[9] In most cases an odor is apparent on the breath and skin. (See more detailed descriptions of side effects from DMSO intravenous use later in this chapter.)

There may be toxicity if the drug is inhaled. DMSO evaporates very slowly since its vapor pressure is 0.6 mm/Hg at 77°F. Therefore, when it is applied to the skin, the concentration of DMSO in the air is very low under most conditions. When heated or sprayed, however, normal precautions should be taken by the user against inhalation as with any organic solvents.[10,11]

The addition of DMSO to blood gives varying reactions determined by the concentration and the method of administration. The effects of skin applications of DMSO to the membranes of small blood vessels of New Zealand White Rabbits are shown in Table 5.2.

Table 5.1 *Single-Dose Toxicity of DMSO as LD_{50}*

Species	Applied to Skin	Taken by Mouth	Into Blood Stream	Beneath Skin	Into Body Cavity
Mouse	50,000	16,500–24,600	3,800–8,900	13,900–20,500	14,700–17,700
Rat	40,000	17,400–28,300	5,200–8,100	12,000–20,500	13,000
Guinea Pig	–	>11,000	–	–	>5,500
Chicken	–	14,000	–	–	–
Cat	–	–	4,000	–	–
Dog	>11,000	>10,000	2,500	–	–
Monkey	>11,000	>4,000	4,000	–	–

Further live animal studies showed that the blood stream soon became normal after direct administration of DMSO into a vein. Dogs showed rapid recovery after intravenous injection of DMSO at a level up to 10,000 mg/kg.[12,13,14]

In the scientific literature no cases of any toxicity to the offspring of humans or animals from the skin applications of DMSO have been reported. Tests have been performed on hamsters[15] and chickens[16,17] where direct DMSO injections were made into the embryo or the area of the fetus and malformations resulted. But 50 percent DMSO given orally at a level of 5 grams per kg per day to male and female rats for four days prior to mating produced no abnormality or infertility. The pregnant females were then given DMSO throughout the gestation period, and the litters were born normal.[18]

DMSO shows no cancer-causing activity.[19,20] Furthermore, the drug does not promote allergic tendencies.[21,22] Common allergies that already exist in people, such as those from house dust, animal hair, dander, mixed grasses, and weeds, are not increased by DMSO.[23] Still, be warned that the skin irritation produced in some people by the solvent may enhance the activity of some allergens, the substances that bring on an allergic reaction.

Administered in any manner, DMSO is absorbed and enters the blood stream by way of the skin capillaries. These tiny blood vessels distribute it into the circulatory system so that it enters tissues throughout the body. Most DMSO is excreted unchanged in the urine, and laboratory studies on rats and rabbits indicate that 85 percent of the compound is disposed of this way.[24,25] Some is oxidized to dimethyl sulfone;[26,27] while a study on cats produced evidence that 3 percent of the DMSO is excreted in the breath as dimethyl sulfide.[28,29] This dimethyl sulfide product of the body's metabolism is what gives a DMSO patient the malodorous smell on the breath. Such metabolized products are not toxic in the measurable quantities found in the body. It is

Table 5.2 DMSO Skin Application Effects on New Zealand White Rabbits

Percentage of DMSO Concentration	Observed Effect
20	White cell sticking.
30	Granular pasty consistency.
50 or greater	Instant solubilization of the red corpuscles; white cell sticking; fibrinogen precipitation.

noteworthy that the source of halitosis, dimethyl sulfide, is also found naturally in milk, cooked corn, tomatoes, tea, coffee, asparagus, and clams.

EYE CHANGES THAT BROUGHT THE FDA BAN

Research on DMSO in the United States came to an abrupt halt on November 11, 1965, because lens changes had been observed in a number of mammalian species. A conference was called between the FDA and the pharmaceutical companies that were involved in the research and they agreed to discontinue the clinical studies. This, despite no changes being observed in humans or any primates. A possible flaw in the pretreatment examinations of the large number of patients under DMSO therapy at that time was that their eyes had not been checked routinely beforehand.

The consequence of withdrawing DMSO from clinical investigation is that it acquired a reputation of extreme toxicity, comparable to that of thalidomide and some other drugs that had previously run into major toxicology problems. It was an FDA medical bureaucrat, Dr. Francis Kelsey, who became famous by allegedly keeping thalidomide from invading the United States with birth defects in 1962. (At least that is the popular version. The real truth is that thalidomide was used in the United States for *six years* and was available to 1,200 physicians in the United States. There were American thalidomide babies, many of them the children of doctors![30]) She is the same FDA official who threw up her hands with alarm and frustration against DMSO in the years following the ban on its testing in 1965, as reported by chemist Robert Herschler on *Good Morning America.*

A statement of Congressman Steven D. Symms (R-Idaho), made during the Hearing before the Select Committee on Aging of the House of Representatives, March 24, 1980, points out part of the bureaucratic problem faced here. Congressman Symms said, "I think what we really need is a broad attitude which would not only cover DMSO but would cover other products. We have had the problem with valferrate. We have had the problem with erythrocin for tuberculosis which took so long to get them on the market in the United States where other places in the world people were using these products very well.

"Part of this is because of our overrestrictive amendments which passed in 1962. They have most certainly delineated a cause for a slowdown in the ability of the FDA to make those judgments and make them expeditiously . . .

"The overall question of what has happened to the FDA since 1962, if one will study it, and I have spent a great deal of time looking into it," continued Mr. Symms, "we have a general drug lag, a slowdown because of the efficacy requirements of being able to prove that something is effective."

As mentioned, in November 1965 there had been no cases of confirmed human eye damage or significant complaints among any of the patients using DMSO. None of the studies by any of the pharmaceutical firms showed eye problems. Instead, there were refractive index changes in the lenses (not an opacity) of dogs, rabbits, and pigs. After being dosed with approximately 5 g/kg of DMSO for three months, the animals became slightly nearsighted. No microscopic or chemical differences could be found between the lenses of the treated animals and the control animals.

In the affected animals, there appeared two distinct zones of different refraction. This could easily be observed with an ophthalmoscope and with the slit lamp. It appeared to be related to the dose, and the problem diminished as the dose was reduced. These animals were exposed to 50 to 100 times the usual human therapeutic dose.

Yet, pretreatment examinations of the eyes of human patients had not been performed. The researchers felt that to reexamine at this late stage all the people who had been under treatment would be fruitless. Many of the patients were elderly and had begun their DMSO treatment with preexisting eye trouble. All the researchers were able to do, therefore, was to check long-term DMSO patients on high doses.

In Portland, Oregon, Dr. Jacob and Edward E. Rosenbaum, M.D., Clinical Professor of Medicine and Head of the Department of Rheumatology at the University of Oregon Medical School, had thirty-two patients examined by ophthalmologists connected with the medical school. These patients had been treated for from three to nineteen months, at an average dose of 30 grams of DMSO per day. None of them showed any of the characteristic lens changes that had been seen in the animals.

One of the thirty-two patients was a nineteen-year-old man from Seattle, who had by chance received a complete pretreatment examination by an ophthalmologist a few months prior to his neck injury. The neck was treated with 60 grams of DMSO per day for twenty months. His follow-up eye examination showed no changes of the lens even with careful tonometry, visual field, refraction, and slit lamp examinations.

At the Cleveland Clinic, Dr. Scherbel had forty-four people under treatment for scleroderma. Some patients received as much as 3 g/kg per day and were treated for as long as twenty-three months. None of them showed the characteristic lens changes that were observed in the DMSO-treated animals.

When 11 g/kg of DMSO was applied to the skin of monkeys and 5 g/kg was given to them to drink each day for a full year, no lens changes occurred. The laboratory workers suspected that the eye changes were specific only for dogs, rabbits, and pigs.

Meanwhile, the pharmaceutical companies continued to collect case reports in which no real toxicity of any kind was being observed. Merck and Company gradually collected 17,000 patient reports. Syntex collected approximately 7,000 and E.R. Squibb and Sons around 3,000. The FDA seemed to turn a blind eye to these human case studies, although DMSO was officially banned from human experimental use.

Then, Richard D. Brobyn, M.D., of the Bainbridge Medical Center, Bainbridge Island, Washington, was retained as a consultant to the Squibb laboratories to develop a program to reestablish clinical research on DMSO. With the FDA's permission, in the latter part of 1967 to February 1968, Dr. Brobyn conducted human toxicological studies of dimethyl sulfoxide, especially as it relates to the lens of the eye.

DO LENS CHANGES OCCUR IN HUMANS?

Sixty-five healthy prisoners in the state institution at Vacaville, California, volunteered to have DMSO in an 80 percent gel applied to their skin at one gram per kilogram for fourteen days. There were no toxic effects.

Next, for three more months, a second group of forty healthy prisoners allowed themselves to be coated with DMSO and had no toxicological result. Their eyes were examined with slit lamps, ophthalmoscope, and tenometry; they were examined for lens refraction and visual fields, and underwent many blood, urine, liver, and other analyses. There were pulmonary function studies, neurological and other physical exams, and electrocardiogram studies. They were the most exhaustive series of toxicological studies that had been carried on for some time. See Table 5.3 for studies showing no harm to human eyes from DMSO.

The conclusion by Dr. Brobyn was: "A very extensive toxicology study of DMSO was conducted at three to thirty times the usual treatment dose in humans for three months. DMSO appears to be a very safe drug for human administration, and in particular the lens changes

Table 5.3 *Observations Showing No Harm to Human Eyes From DMSO*

No. of Human Patients	Period of DMSO Treatment	Note
Extensive	Up to 2 years	31
160	–	32
52	9 months	33
9,521	–	34
38	12 weeks	35
108	Up to 15 months	36
Further studies[37,38,39,40,41]		

that occur in certain mammalian species do not occur in man under this very high prolonged treatment regimen. I am very glad to be able to present these data at this time so that we can permanently dispel the myth that DMSO is in any way a toxic or dangerous drug."[42]

As an aside, the investigator added that DMSO appears to be so effective that it could justifiably be used for hangnail.

When you consider the enormous amount of DMSO that the first group of prisoners received over two weeks and the second group for three months, the lack of toxicity is proved. If the typical subject weighed 90 kg (with 1 kg being equal to 2.2 pounds) and he used up 1 g/kg, then at least 8.1 kg (8,100 g) were taken during ninety days of testing. Any other compound such as sugar, salt, coffee, or tea taken in such huge quantities would kill the subject during this three-month period. Or, he would suffer from some severe metabolic problems. Not so with the prisoners taking DMSO through the skin.

DMSO has been instilled directly into eyes[43] and has been used for preservation of eyes during freezing.[44,45]

Jack C. de la Torre, M.D., of the Department of Neurosurgery, University of Miami School of Medicine, and his colleagues gave 3 g of 40 percent DMSO per kilogram of body weight by intravenous infusion into monkeys for nine days. They were monitored before and after DMSO treatment for 120 days for any kind of physiological changes from normal. He found no such changes whatsoever in the urine and serum chemistry tests, cardiovascular and neurological examinations, or any other of the exhaustive health studies in these animals. Following up at the end of four months, the animals were sacrificed and pathologists performed post mortem examinations on the monkeys' organs. They found absolutely no pathology existing in these primates from taking such high concentrations of DMSO. Also recorded during the time they were alive, as in humans, no pathological eye symptoms showed up in the monkeys.

All the ophthalmologic and pathological examinations were done on a double-blind basis. All other tests and evaluations performed by the examiner were single-blind. Routine tests such as weighing, cardiac examination, respiratory rate, temperature, funduscopic, and other examinations were performed daily before and after each drug administration, then periodically throughout the study.

Dr. de la Torre concluded: "No changes in refraction or translucence of the lens or any other abnormalities were noted in any animal before, during, or eighteen weeks after any drug administration." This toxicological study, which was published in the *Journal of Toxicology and Environmental Health*, volume seven, March 1981, is available as a reprint from Dr. J.C. de la Torre, Department of Neurosurgery (R-35), University of Miami School of Medicine, P.O. Box 076960, Miami, Florida 33101.

In other animal studies of the effect of large doses of DMSO on the eyes, the variation depends on the particular species. Oral administration of 5 to 10 g of DMSO per kilogram per day to dogs caused alteration of the eye lenses after treatment periods of nine to sixty-three days. For a 30 lb dog, 5 g/kg/day would be equivalent to approximately one-third cup per day. Skin application at 4.4 g/kg/day to rabbits and 9.0 g/kg/day to swine produced effects after ninety days of treatment. Lines of discontinuity are produced and sometimes opacity of the lens. When DMSO administration is discontinued, some but not all of the changes disappear.[46,47]

It is true that reports of different investigators show a certain variation in animal eye effects but this seems to be due to the differing means of their evaluation. What is not variable is that lens changes in animals are specific to certain species and that humans are not among these species.

The dosage and number of days before any change is noticeable in animals' eyes are indicated in Table 5.4. One investigator did say that a change in the eyes of monkeys occurred after he dosed the experimental animals with 9.9 g/kg/day DMSO for nine weeks and 3.3 g/kg/day for fourteen weeks.[48] However, the scientist who reviewed this study later suggested the study was invalid. It appears that the significance of the lens changes was difficult to assess since the monkeys in this

Table 5.4 DMSO Effect on Eyes of Animals

Level	Animal	Time to Affect Eye	Note
5 g/kg/day oral	dog	9–20 days	49
10 g/kg/day oral	dog	28 days	50
5.5 g/kg/day oral	dog	9 days	51
5 g/kg/day oral	dog	63 days	52
4.4 g/kg/day skin	rabbit	90 days	53
9.0 g/kg/day skin	swine	90 days	54
10 g/kg/day oral	rabbit	7–10 days	55
1 g/kg/day skin	rabbit	11 weeks (slight)	56
6 g/kg/day oral	monkey	100 days, *no effect*	57
11 g/kg/day skin	monkey	6 months, *no effect*	58
0.9, 2.7, 8 g/kg/day skin or oral	monkey	3 months, *no effect*	59
1, 3, 11 g/kg/day, skin	monkey	185–200 days, *no effect*	60

study had been previously utilized in other research involving a study with the drug phenolphthalein.[61]

In summary, human and animal studies to determine the toxicity of DMSO showed no adverse changes in the chemical and physiological parameters carefully investigated by clinical and laboratory methods. No gross pathology or eye changes were found in the humans and no gross or microscopic pathology was found in any monkey.

There are a few unpleasant side effects from the use of DMSO, but none are dangerous. The obnoxious side effects seem to be far outweighed by the marvelous benefits, as shown by the case history of Patricia McClenathan who experienced nearly every known side effect and still uses DMSO.

THE UNPLEASANT SIDE EFFECTS

Patricia McClenathan of Cheektowaga, New York, a homemaker then thirty-nine years old, had been receiving treatment from rheumatologists for spondylitis for more than six years. Spondylitis is an inflammation, from injury or disease, such as arthritis or tuberculosis of one or more of the vertebrae of the spine. For Mrs. McClenathan, it was a chronic, crippling condition leading to some degree of stiffening of the spinal joints and slight deformation. Since 1964, she had suffered with deep aching pain and loss of mobility.

She went through the full gamut of antiarthritis drugs, which caused her exceedingly uncomfortable gastrointestinal problems. She also took muscle relaxants, painkillers, and nerve blocks into the spinal area by ethyl chloride spray and injection. The nerve blocks helped half the time, and the painkillers knocked her out all the time so that she coped with pain but couldn't perform her household chores.

Ruptured disc problems later arose as well, which gave her additional back pain and kept her confined to bed for long periods. In April 1980, she was referred to a neurosurgeon who hospitalized her for a laminec-tomy operation to remove the involved vertebra. She underwent the computerized axial tomogram (CAT scan) and the myelogram diagnostic procedures. But the myelogram didn't coincide with what the surgeon expected, and he couldn't find the exact spot where he thought there was a ruptured disc blockage in the spinal cord. Therefore, the neurosurgeon did not perform the operation, and Mrs. McClenathan was sent home still suffering in agony. Extended bed rest and painkilling drugs were the only regimen available for the balance of her life.

The patient fell into the depths of depression. Her hopes were completely dashed. She thought that the laminectomy was going to solve all her pain problems, but now she was confined to bed, felt extreme discomfort constantly, couldn't perform as a wife and mother, and recognized that the last door of relief was finally closed. She was absolutely immobilized with depression.

When her sister-in-law, who lived in Port Charlotte, Florida, con-tacted Pat McClenathan in June 1980 to explain that DMSO had become legal for use in Florida, the patient jumped at the chance—any chance—to find some kind of relief from her back pain. She decided that there was nothing to lose by giving DMSO a try. She was afraid to hold out hope for herself, but Mrs. McClenathan is a fighter and refused to give in to lifelong pain. She flew to Florida from upstate New York and was driven each day from Port Charlotte to Sarasota for DMSO treatment.

The treatment that started on a Monday provided no immediate relief. Tuesday, she even felt increased pain, which is a common but unexplained side effect. She became depressed all over again and believed she was wasting her time, money, and the tremendous effort that went into her daily automobile commutation.

Her pain relief first came on the third day of treatment. "Wednesday night I felt a lifting of pain," Mrs. McClenathan said. "I was lying on a recliner when an easing of the sensation came over me. That night I tested my relief by standing up and sitting down repeatedly, because I could do it for the first time in six years without pushing off using my hands. The next day it was even better. I was elated! I was free of the pain I had lived with for years. The fifth day, the last of my treatment, there was just no pain at all from any movement." Even sitting during the automobile ride didn't trouble her as it had at the beginning. Sitting in a car while somebody else drove had always been most difficult for her, but no more.

Undergoing the DMSO intravenous injection procedure didn't feel uncomfortable unless the solution dripped into her vein a little too quickly, Mrs. McClenathan explained. Then she would ask the nurse to slow the rate of drip, or she would merely reach up and reduce the speed of flow herself. The drip could go into the arm vein faster than into a vein on the top of the hand. Most of the time she took it in the hand alongside the thumb. Occasionally, the patient asked for a board on which to rest her hand when the IV was given there. Soreness remained in her arm for about a month after the IV treatment had concluded. The intravenous sensation was one of tingling and burning that subsided as soon as the flow was lessened. She felt nauseated but she learned that eating a good breakfast before going for the IV prevented the nausea. Each treatment lasted between three and four hours during the five days. The drip solution contained in the pint IV bottle consisted of 50 percent DMSO in 500 cc of dextrose, a sugar water.

Admittedly overweight, Mrs. McClenathan said, "I had a total loss of appetite while I took the treatment. I had to force myself to eat a supper. The distinctive sweet taste of DMSO came on my tongue almost simultaneously with the nurse opening the IV. It was really fast—a sensation more than a taste, like tiny little burps and a dryness to my mouth. Even now, just putting DMSO on my skin causes me difficulty with quenching my thirst. Also, it brings on the urge to urinate.

"I was very self-conscious about the odor that I carried," continued the patient. "The odor emanated from my skin pores over my whole body. I think I could almost see the substance in my bath water. The DMSO seemed to have a yellowish tint to it. I don't know if I'm exaggerating about this, because my brother-in-law made me paranoid about my odor. I'm uncertain as to the validity of my feelings on the smell, but if I ever have to return to Florida for treatment I won't stay at his house. In five days he used up almost four cans of Lysol deodorant spray. If I walked through a room it was sprayed. Remembering it now, I don't think it was all that bad, but at the time I was completely obsessed with my body and breath odor and consequently did not leave the Port Charlotte house. Flying home, I was really worried about how I smelled."

Mrs. McClenathan described the DMSO taste as not salty or garlicky as some do. She said it's a mild indigestion or gastric repeating taste that you can compare to clams, oysters, and other raw seafood tastes.

As a general reaction since having the intravenous infusions, she now experiences a mild diarrhea anytime she uses DMSO either on the skin or by mouth. "When I return to applying DMSO at home, the diarrhea gets bad. My bowels and stomach kick up in protest worse than they did when I was on the antiarthritic drugs. This causes me great discomfort such as gas, heartburn, and stomach cramps. This is just from putting it on the skin," she said. But, she uses the veterinary grade in a 99 percent strength that she brings down to a 70 percent concentration by adding three parts water to seven parts solvent. This DMSO veterinarian grade full strength produces no hives on the skin for her as it has for others, though Mrs. McClenathan does encounter redness, an irritation, and an occasional rash. Applying veterinarian grade DMSO to her back causes more burning, a warmer sensation, but less odor in the bottle. When mixed with water, the heat reaction between the two substances seems to bring out the odor.

The DMSO odor has definitely interfered with Pat McClenathan's sexual relationship with her husband, she said in our interview. And he is the person who assists his wife with applying the solvent. He is a patient and tolerant man, she said, but he found it exceedingly difficult to remain close to her body no matter how much they desired each other. "I felt rejected," she confessed, until they discovered how to overcome the problem of body odor. Leaving off DMSO usage for a few days allows the McClenathans to express their married love sexually. It's a bit of knowledge they are willing to share with other couples in the same predicament.

DMSO emanates from the skin pores for from twenty-four to forty-eight hours, although it isn't clear from the body completely for about seven days. When Pat McClenathan is feeling especially well and doesn't have her occasional bouts of discomfort she goes off the skin application. "I use the topical for a three- or four-day period and can then discontinue applications for approximately two weeks. During the fall of 1980, I functioned with relative ease through the constant air pressure changes. Previously, this was the worst time of year for me," she said.

Patricia McClenathan has consented to reveal this full case history including its more intimate details to assist other people who suffer with pain and wonder about the DMSO side effects.

She wrote: "Since taking DMSO, I am now a functioning person where previously I had not been, spending much of the time in bed accomplishing nothing. I can do most normal things now by relying on DMSO. At this time, I take no painkillers or muscle relaxants [both used quite heavily before] and find for this reason I can cope with everything very well. I am finally physically, mentally, and emotionally much better and attribute this to DMSO. I feel that the problems DMSO has caused are by far outweighed by the new life it has given me—a life other than just surviving in constant pain. Again, I thank you."

OVERCOMING THE MALODOROUS DMSO SIDE EFFECT

Mrs. McClenathan has experienced practically all of the unpleasant side effects of using DMSO routinely. The pharmaceutical and the veterinarian grades have their individual ways of bringing about the body's counteraction, and each person responds in his or her own unique manner.

"In all the time I have incorporated DMSO as part of my treatment program, I have seen no serious side effects except for possible redness, burning, and itching of the skin with the topical application," said Robert L. Harmon, M.D., who was medical director of the Mattie Evans Alderman Foundation for Preventive Medicine, part of the Desert Holistic Health Center of Palm Desert, California. Dr. Harmon had used DMSO as an arthritic therapy for a number of years. "The skin reaction is much more noticeable in certain persons than it is in others. There is no other relationship you can make. It's strictly an idiosyncrasy of the individual.

"We have not encountered any toxic reactions intravenously even though we have given people over 50 cc of pure DMSO in 500 cc of Ringers lactate solution within a period of two hours. There have been no toxic effects either immediately or delayed," Dr. Harmon added. "We've applied it wherever there have been skeletal problems with joints, muscles, and connective tissues involved."

The biggest problem of DMSO—the odor that occurs when the drug is injected intravenously or intramuscularly, taken orally in juice, or subcutaneously by painting it on the skin, has not been completely solved. Chemist Robert Herschler has combined DMSO with a series of complex substances, including urea, salt, and other items, for topical application. He has reduced the DMSO odor with these complexes by around 75 percent. When intravenous DMSO is given to seriously injured or ill people in a hospital such as the medical center affiliated with the University of Oregon Medical School, the endotracheal tube of an unconscious patient is hooked up to the wall suction to cut the odor. Exhaust fans are installed and run in regular hospital or doctor treatment rooms where DMSO is being infused.

In other instances, the oral administration of DMSO may have its odor modified if the patient eats cheese, ice cream, milk, and other dairy products beforehand. Raw milk seems especially able to reduce mouth odor when one is drinking DMSO. Raw milk is the main beverage of children in Chile. When Chilean youngsters are given DMSO in any of the three common ways, their body and breath odors are less objectionable, perhaps because of the raw milk in their diet.

United States Representative Robert Duncan, a member of Congress from the State of Oregon, agreed that odor remains the main problem with using DMSO. Congressman Duncan told the House Select Committee on Aging: "With respect to my own use of it, the most serious side effect is a threatened divorce by my wife because she doesn't like the odor. Dr. Jacob has removed some of the odor and he has masked it in another preparation by a wintergreen flavor.

"I asked my wife if she didn't like the wintergreen flavor, and if that wouldn't remove her objections. She said no. Instead of smelling like the tidal flats at Bayonne, New Jersey, when the tide is out, she said, you now smell like the locker room of the Green Bay Packers. But that odor is infinitesimal compared with the relief."

This characteristic odor that escapes as soon as DMSO comes in contact with the water content of the body is the reason there has been no performance of double-blind or single-blind clinical investigations that are so desired by the FDA. The report of the *ad hoc* Committee on Dimethyl Sulfoxide, a Division of Medical Science, National Academy of Sciences–National Research Council, supported by The Food and Drug Administration, Contract FDA 70-22, Task Order No. 14, issued August 1973, came out on the same side as the FDA. Even so, the report clearly pinpointed the reason for the lack of double-blind tests—the odor. This *ad hoc* committee said: "The apparent inability to find a substance producing both the unique breath odor and the skin irritation of DMSO resulted in the absence of double-blind controlled studies in which the *placebo* could not be identified by the participants." So the DMSO odor has been a stumbling block in more ways than one.

CONDEMNATION OF OTHER SIDE EFFECTS

The *ad hoc* Committee came down heavily on the various other side effects as a rationalization for its position against DMSO. Yet, it hedged on any condemnation and even nearly came close to recommending DMSO because of the cost-benefit ratio. It said: "DMSO produces side effects, particularly in the skin, in most persons treated, and there have been sporadic cases in which DMSO has, with reasonable confidence, been linked to acute generalized urticaria [hives] in man. There is also evidence that in some species of laboratory animals DMSO in doses somewhat higher than those contemplated for man produces a unique alteration of the lens. The nature of these side effects, the import of the animal data, and the incidence of adverse reactions alone would not warrant withholding the drug in clinical circumstances in which it gave promise of saving life or in which it would clearly be more effective than currently available treatment in arresting a disease process, reducing disability, or relieving pain."

The committee members, all scholarly physicians or doctors in the health sciences, reviewed most of the evidence of toxic effects of DMSO in man and concluded that the reports "did not conform to modern criteria for the evaluation of the toxicity and safety of drugs. In spite of this, we believe that there is reasonable evidence that, with the exception of the eye effects, the toxicity of DMSO is relatively low . . . we conclude that the use of DMSO to treat diseases for which there is no satisfactory therapy will not be particularly hazardous and that further clinical investigation of the drug in treating such disease is justified."

The members carried forward their continued suspicions relating to animal eye effects and any potential dangers in human beings. They said ". . . the evidence of eye effects in animals in chronic studies is such that the risk in prolonged administration to man should be carefully weighed against anticipated therapeutic results, but that, if evidence of efficacy warrants it, investigations involving two weeks of treatment could be undertaken with little risk of eye effects.

"Further research on DMSO, using modern toxicologic procedures, is an absolute necessity to develop a firm basis for judgment of the safety of prolonged use of this drug by patients with minimal medical supervision and surveillance. Such research in animals, especially monkeys, should include:

- A well-designed and executed study of the lenticular effects in subhuman primates.

- Evaluation of the potential of DMSO for inducing carcinogenic, teratogenic, and mutagenic effects.
- Studies of the biochemical and metabolic aspects of the actions of DMSO on the animal body.
- Comparison of toxicity by oral and cutaneous administration.

"The subcommittee hopes that additional studies of human exposure and tolerance to DMSO involving daily cutaneous application for long periods can be performed. In such studies, attention should be given not only to the lens but to signs of toxicity to the blood cells and various organs."

On the *Good Morning America* television broadcast, FDA Commissioner Crout said, "Those tests are to be done by the promoters or sponsors of the drug. We are in the position of approving the work once it's done. Carrying the ball on behalf of the drug is what the drug companies ordinarily do. And, indeed, some work is going on for DMSO today that is of high quality. We look forward to having those data in a year or so. I think there won't be much change in the coming year from what you see now, but the current fad [for bringing DMSO to the people] will wane and a year or two from now we'll have the data we need."

Michael A. DeLuca, M.D., an orthopedic surgeon dispensing services as Humble Orthopedic Associates, P.A., of Humble, Texas, wrote to Congressman Claude Pepper, May 30, 1980, saying:

> Thank you very much for the fine support you are giving the medical profession in the House Bill H.R. 7023 to legalize DMSO use nationally. . . . I would like for you to know that I, as a practicing orthopedic surgeon and physician of several years in practice, do appreciate your efforts and I furthermore am of the opinion that DMSO has very definite benefit with regard to patient treatment. It is even more imperative that we are able to write this by prescription inasmuch as the side effects are, for all practical purposes, non-existent.
>
> Again thank you very much for your contribution against this inexorable bureaucracy that is presently interfering with the practice of medicine in this field.

CHAPTER 6

The Potent Potion
for Sports Injuries

During his senior year at college, June Jones, III, eventually to become a quarterback for the Atlanta Falcons professional football team, signed a contract to play big league ball after graduation. But he was hoping the team management would not take him out to the football field just then and ask him to display his skill. The reason? He couldn't lift his right arm to throw a football.

Jones was suffering with a calcification in the right shoulder, his throwing arm. Some days he was unable to practice at all. He couldn't put on his jacket because movement of the arm brought him such agony. He spent sleepless nights writhing in a cold sweat, especially if he happened to roll onto his right side. The calcified bursitis of his shoulder was threatening to end his professional football career before it even got started.

"Fortunately I had used DMSO for ankle sprains and contusions in high school but I never thought of using it for my shoulder," Jones told the Select Committee on Aging of the United States House of Representatives. "So kind of by chance I read in the paper about Dr. Jacob's work and went up to see him." Jones is originally an Oregonian, transplanted to Georgia, and most people from Oregon consider DMSO a homegrown state crop—their particular contribution to medical progress.

"I was treated with DMSO," Jones continued. "I used it in my senior year and it got me through the season relatively pain free. . . . I started using it on Thursday and by Saturday I would go five or six hours pain free. I would go through this for six months from July to December. Finally I said, maybe if I just don't do anything with my shoulder anymore, it is going to be all right. So from December until the first part of April I didn't lift a weight or throw a football. But my shoulder still got worse.

"I went up to see Dr. Jacob and he gave me an injection in my shoulder. He told me if I used DMSO for thirty days straight, that that calcification would disappear. It did!

"To say the least, I went to camp in July, pain free, not using DMSO anymore, and the X-rays showed no calcification in my shoulder. I had previously taken cortisone, butazolidin, and all the things the team physicians told me would help my shoulder. They did not. The only thing that helped me was DMSO. Without this drug I would not be playing today."

DMSO treatment for sports-associated conditions such as dislocations, serious cuts, acute sprains, strains, broken bones, tennis elbow, and a wide range of injuries in gymnastics, track and field events, conventional wrestling, football, basketball, judo, diving, swimming, weight-lifting, Greco-Roman wrestling, skiing, cycling, water polo, and fencing has been well received by the athletes, their trainers, coaches, and team officials. In cases of acute trauma, pain is relieved rapidly, sometimes spectacularly. Swelling subsides and function is recovered. Trainers and doctors have said that healing is so spectacular "as to compel us to urge our patients to observe greatest caution in order to avoid further damage to a joint" that may not have healed completely.

Chronic conditions, some of which have become acute again, also respond rapidly, with relief of pain, reduced swelling, and improved function. DMSO also promotes rapid recovery and return to action following immobilization for fractures.

The Institute of Sports Medicine of Italy says: "The complete absence of undesirable collateral reactions, its ease of application, and the few precautions that should be observed, make DMSO a medication for wide use in medical therapy, and also an urgently needed medication in sports-related traumatology."

HEALING IN SPORTS TRAUMA

Is there a reason for such dramatic reduction of tissue damaged in sports and other causes of trauma to the body? "Yes," says Dr. Stanley Jacob. "In the test tube, if you have cells which are damaged by what we call osmotic stress and you add DMSO to those damaged cells, instead of those cells going on to die, those cells will be revitalized and return to a normal state."

DMSO accomplishes this because, as Dr. Jacob explains, "It actually does more than relieve pain. DMSO is not just a substance that reduces pain and relieves inflammation. It actually relieves swelling and this has been demonstrated in good, basic science studies."

Graham Reedy, M.D., of Enumclaw, Washington, former team physician for the Oakland Raiders professional football team, pointed out that his players had benefited markedly from routine use of DMSO. It did just what Dr. Jacob described. In 70 to 80 percent of those who applied it for football injuries, good to excellent results were achieved. The injured players had an immediate reduction of swelling and pain, and consequently, quicker rehabilitation from the particular injury. These benefits were noticed by the athletes by comparing their present injuries, for which they administered DMSO, with previous injuries of a similar nature that they had received. Also, they compared their own injury experience and the experience of others with the same types of current trauma.

Dr. Reedy said, "DMSO, at 70 percent concentration, is an excellent drug which seems to significantly shorten the rehabilitation time for sports injuries to soft tissue or joint defusions. It would definitely make a significant contribution to assist those of us in the field of sports medicine, private practice, and industrial medicine.

"It seems to me that one of our major objectives is to get people back to their activities quickly," the sports physician added. "So the primary significance in use of DMSO may not be just in the relief of pain but in the ability to rehabilitate that person more quickly. Therefore, it might in essence save us millions of dollars as a nation by rehabilitating the industrial-injured patient and getting him back to work.

"In professional football and sports injuries we are interested in rehabilitation time. If, in fact, we can reduce pain, reduce swelling, and more quickly rehabilitate that player or person back to his activity, we can significantly decrease the loss of playing time, the loss of work time, and increase the quality of life."

A PITCHING ARM THAT BECAME REHABILITATED

There are a hundred human interest stories in major league baseball, but a sure-fire tear-jerker is what happened to Washington Senators pitcher Bill Denehy. Denehy was the player who had a 9-10 win record and a big strikeout game in his final appearance. The following spring he tore a muscle in his shoulder and was traded to the Cleveland Indians. But the deal may have been the best thing that ever happened to Denehy because it put him in touch with DMSO to rehabilitate his shoulder.

Denehy had been traded to the Washington Senators by the New York Mets in a $100,000 deal in October 1967. From the time he arrived at the Pompano Beach, Florida, training grounds in the spring of 1968, a lot was demanded of him. Not only had the Senators insisted on acquiring him in the deal, but they also assigned him uniform number 14—the number Gil Hodges had worn as a player with the Brooklyn Dodgers and New York Mets, and as manager of the Mets. Denehy had a lot to live up to.

"I didn't mind at first," said the handsome, wavy-haired righthander from Middletown, Connecticut. "I knew that the Mets had a lot of good young pitchers coming up and I figured with a club like Washington I'd get a chance to pitch.

"And I did at first. That spring, I guess I worked as many innings as any other pitcher on the staff and I had a pretty good record. But then the season opened and they just forgot about me."

Denehy pitched only three games during the season. Then he was sent to Buffalo to pitch in the International league where he chalked up a 9-10 win record with a second-division club. He stayed there two years, and it finally looked like the Senators were going to call him up to start full-time pitching in the major leagues when Denehy tore a muscle in his shoulder.

While he was having the damaged muscle fibers treated, the Senators traded him to the Cleveland Indians. The trade took him to Portland, Oregon, where he came in touch with Dr. Jacob, who cured his shoulder problems using the solvent the surgeon is so closely associated with.

"This doctor introduced me to something called DMSO and it was applied to my shoulder. It's very powerful stuff and you have to know how to use it. It breaks up the scar tissues in the injury and restores strength to the muscles," said Denehy.

"Elgin Baylor has used it on his knee and so has Jerry Lucas. [These were well-known basketball players.] This spring I gave it to Jim Lonborg in Puerto Rico," added Denehy, "and he pitched a ten-inning game in his last start." Lonborg was pitching for the Boston Red Sox.

It was after he began using DMSO that Denehy had a visit from Len Zankie, the baseball scout who originally signed him for the New York Mets.

"When I told him my arm was coming around again, Len must have reported back to the Mets," Denehy remembered, "because a few days later I got a call from manager Johnny Murphy and he told me the Mets might draft me again."

Sure enough they did, and in 1971 Denehy split the year between playing for Memphis in the Southern league and Tidewater in the International league. He had an enviable 10-8 win record. Seeing this, and with pressure from other major league ball clubs who wanted to acquire Bill Denehy, the Mets promoted him to the major league roster.

"I don't know what my chances are of making this club," he said. "It's obvious they've got a lot of pitching. Right now, all I can ask for is a chance. I know one thing. My shoulder is strong again. Among Memphis, Tidewater, and Puerto Rico, I pitched 261 innings this year and struck out 208 batters. I couldn't do that if I wasn't sound."[1]

Bill Denehy got his chance and made the major leagues as a relief pitcher. DMSO gave him the opportunity to show that his shoulder muscle was in good shape and could do the job. Denehy pitched for the Detroit Tigers for several years. Now he has left the major leagues because of age, not shoulder pain. It does not bother him anymore. If ever it should, Denehy feels assured that he could restore his shoulder to good health by the application of DMSO.

PROFESSIONAL SPORTS TEAM PHYSICIANS USE DMSO

During the early months of 1980, the United States House of Representatives Select Committee on Aging solicited responses in the form of a questionnaire to professional sports team physicians. It included such questions as: (1) Have you ever prescribed, or your team trainer used, DMSO for athletes in your care? (2) For what types of symptoms, maladies, or illnesses have you prescribed or seen the drug used? (3) In your opinion, is the drug effective in reducing inflammation, pain, or other arthritic symptoms? (4) In your opinion, should the United States legalize DMSO for the treatment of arthritis and other diseases in humans? Please comment! (5) Would you be willing to testify before the Select Committee on Aging on these matters? Identification of the responding physician was optional.

Staff physicians from the professional athletic teams provided answers to the questionnaire. Of the thirty-nine who responded, only seven admitted to having regularly used the drug for such conditions as inflammation of joints, sprains, swelling, tendinitis, bursitis, muscle bruises and contusions, and gout. An additional five team physicians said they had seen the drug used for the same conditions. Ten of the twelve physicians who had used or seen the drug used found DMSO effective in reducing inflammation, pain, or other arthritic symptoms. Most physicians who responded to the questionnaire believed further study was warranted and necessary to determine its safety and efficacy before DMSO should be legalized in the United States for treatment of arthritis and other diseases in humans.

Following are comments from doctors attending professional athletic teams:

R.R. of Highland Park, Illinois, said, "I was an early experimenter with DMSO and the only side effect was the distasteful breath."

R.C. of Oregon City, Oregon, wrote, "As I indicated in the responses in your enclosed questionnaire, I feel that at least at this point in time, no ill effects have been substantiated, at least with the topical use of DMSO, and I personally find it as effective as most proprietary counter-irritants such as Ben Gay and this type of readily available remedy. My principal concern about the dissemination of DMSO is that if some of the things should happen nationally that are happening locally, I think it would be cause for grave concern. I would like to specifically call your attention to the fact that DMSO is being injected for treatment of a variety of maladies, and I think that this is certainly premature and somewhat adventuresome at this point in time. At any rate, I think that if DMSO is made generally available to the public, it should be done so in a very regulated manner, and at this point in time, limited to topical use only."

D.A. of Atlanta said, "If appropriate studies could be done to see if there is any objective evidence of the efficacy of the drug, then [I] would favor select use."

E.M. of Baltimore said, "Controlled studies by qualified approved investigators have been and are being done. Would suggest you consult these people. FDA should be able to guide you. If Congress doesn't trust or rely on the FDA, they should improve the FDA."

E.V. of Philadelphia wrote, "There is enough anecdotal information suggesting this is a useful drug that I feel proper scientific studies should be carried out. I would not use a drug until it has been so evaluated."

Y.C. of Houston said, "When used judiciously, this can be a very useful and helpful drug for relieving both short- and long-term joint symptoms and pain."

In a summary of the questionnaires sent to professional sports team physicians, the committee staff advised the members of the Select Committee on Aging:

"The Committee learned of the apparently widespread 'bootleg' use of DMSO in professional athletics. Team physicians, however, were reluctant to discuss this with the Committee. Only twenty of the 110 professional sports team physicians have responded to our January questionnaire. Three admitted usage of DMSO, although eight claimed DMSO is effective in reducing pain or inflammation."

Lowell Scott Weil, D.P.M., of Des Plaines, Illinois, who is Professor of Podiatric Surgery and Orthopedics at the Illinois College of Podiatric Medicine and founder of the college's Sports Medicine Center, and who is the sports podiatrist for the Chicago Bears football team and the United States Olympic gymnastics team, uses DMSO on a regular basis for the athletes who are injured. He has been applying the solvent for about twelve years. One of the classic areas treated is in gymnastics.

"I say classic because I was able to spend three full days with the kids during the 1980 Olympic trials, use DMSO every minute, and see exactly how their symptoms went away," said Dr. Weil. "We had a particular gymnast who suffered a severe ankle sprain. Her coach thought there was no chance she would be able to participate in the trials and was about to scratch her. I used DMSO in combination with some other physical therapy modalities, and she went on not only to perform but to make the Olympic team.

"Most of my experience with DMSO has been with using it for tendinitis, myositis [muscle inflammation type conditions], post-injury situations such as muscle pulls, ankle sprains, strains, and tears of the soft tissue. Those types of problems have responded most successfully to DMSO. In addition, I have used it for my arthritic patients, especially those with rheumatoid arthritis, and they've had dramatic relief effects.

"Of the number of patients to whom I've administered DMSO, I've probably had about a 60 percent success rate. The 40 percent rate of failure is in people that just don't show any good or bad effects from the drug," Dr. Weil said. "The only side effects have been some skin irritation and an occasional inflammational blistering on people with sensitive skin. Skin problems are easily treated with ice applications or cortisone cream and do not seem to provide any great problem. I have not noted any other type of allergic reactions or ill effects."

The forms of DMSO that Dr. Weil applies topically are the veterinarian grade in an 80 percent gel and the Rimso-50 pharmaceutical grade 50 percent solution that ordinarily is administered internally for interstitial cystitis. Inflammatory conditions such as nerve excitations in the foot are where he finds it works best.

A Chicago Bears football player who tore a hamstring muscle in his thigh was scheduled to be out of commission for five weeks. "I used DMSO on him every day," said Dr. Weil, "for about a half hour of rubbing it into the injured area. Then I had him apply it before bedtime and keep it on all night. After six or seven treatments, the player found he had full range of motion, virtually no pain at all, and could extend his leg as he wanted. He returned to playing football immediately thereafter."

ARE PLAYERS USING IT ON THEIR OWN?

"Not only have I had the experience of using this drug with my athletic endeavors," said June Jones, "but also I have become emotionally involved with it. . . . I have seen people get amazing results. Most recently I have seen a person who had not walked in close to six years. He had not moved his toes in close to eight years. For the relief of pain he put DMSO on his spinal cord, not thinking it might do anything else—he is walking now within two weeks after using it."

Jones explained that DMSO is used extensively as a healer and pain reliever among the sports figures on a number of athletic teams, and not just in football. They don't permit this knowledge to be commonly disseminated except among themselves, since drug use of any kind is frowned upon in professional sports. Drugs might give a player an unfair advantage through artificial means.

The Atlanta Falcons running back, Haskel Stanback, sprained his ankle in the first game in which he finally had become a starting player. In 1978, he had worked hard in training camp and was named first string tailback for the season. It was his big chance.

In the third quarter of this first game, between the Falcons and the Houston Oilers, Stanback chipped a bone and tore ligaments in his ankle. The team doctors decided he was going to have to wear a cast for six weeks, and the player was put on the injured reserve list.

Knowing the consequences of putting a plaster cast on an ankle, Stanback realized he was finished for the season. His big opportunity was gone. It would take another four or five weeks after the cast came off for his leg to be well enough again to perform on the field. The season would be over before he could run a single step.

The team managers told him to take his gear home. He was heartbroken. There would be no more football for Stanback. Then, June Jones came to his rescue.

"I said, take this stuff home and put it on all night. I said, wake up every hour and put it on. He did it all night," Jones explained. "He came in Monday with no swelling in his ankle. The doctors could not believe it. They went to X-ray it again. The bone chip was still there. They still contended that there was damage done."

The Falcons had Tuesday off. No game and no practice. The doctors said that they would wait until Wednesday to see what happened to Stanback's ankle before making a judgment as to whether he could play. Stanback put DMSO on his foot and leg the rest of Monday and all of Tuesday. He arrived at practice on Wednesday able to walk, run, tackle, throw a football, and do all the other activities demanded of a professional player. He played that next Sunday against the Los Angeles Rams.

"Availability in our business is the most important thing to an athlete," said Jones. "If you get hurt in training camp, your income, your lifetime, everything that sustains your income can be yanked out from underneath you just by an injury."

He said that DMSO "enhances and decreases the time to getting you back to work after an injury."

When he was physician to the Oakland Raiders, Dr. Graham Reedy applied 70 percent DMSO to his players' injuries on an experimental basis, beginning in October 1971. He provided each patient with a careful explanation about its side effects of clam breath and possible skin irritation for up to seventy-two hours past its application. "Our application technique was to apply it liberally all over the affected joint or muscle," he said, "letting it dry for five minutes. This procedure would be repeated up to four times. These treatments occurred from two to four times per day for three to four days.

"Frequently, players were hospitalized for their severe acute joint or muscle problems. They were immobilized, iced, and elevated for forty-eight-hour periods during which DMSO would be applied in the fashion prescribed. Over a total of five years, DMSO was used approximately twenty to thirty times per year," Dr. Reedy said. "Some of the players who used the drug were Ben Davidson, Tom Keating, Daryle Lamonica, Fred Belitnikoff, Jim Otto, and Bobby Moore. Its greatest value was in its application in the first three to four days of an acute injury of a muscle or joint having severe swelling. Our experience was significant reduction occurring 70 percent to 80 percent of the time with these injuries."

Probably the most dramatic reduction of the effects of a sports injury that Dr. Reedy described was a severe elbow contusion sustained by Bobby Moore after a pileup during a football game. Immediately after the game ended, the doctor painted DMSO onto Moore's contusion and all around the elbow area. Practically as the solvent was going on, the patient and doctor saw the swelling go down to the extent that an actual dimpling took place. Robert Rosenfeld, M.D., the Falcon's orthopedist, had seen and remarked on this same phenomenon. Pain reduction is quick, as well, so that the primary benefit the players experience with using DMSO under a doctor's supervision or on their own is a rapidly diminishing swelling of the muscle or joint, with associated pain relief.

When swelling and pain are gone after a couple of days, the doctors can hasten rehabilitation of the part that's injured by instituting other more heroic measures. The players' usual estimate of benefit varies from 50 percent to 75 percent faster results and return to the ball field than from their previous injury treatments.

DOUBLE-BLIND STUDIES IN SPORTS

Double-blind, placebo-controlled investigations have been carried out in order to learn the true characteristics of DMSO for sports injuries. For example, in 1981, the use of DMSO for tennis elbow and rotator cuff tendonitis was tested in such a double-blind study. Over a one-year period, sports physicians E.C. Percy and J.D. Carson treated 102 patients with a clinical diagnosis of either medial or lateral epicondylitis (tennis elbow) or rotator cuff tendonitis with topical applications of dimethyl sulfoxide or a placebo. Their double-blind controlled study was carried out on these patients in the private practice of an orthopedic surgeon to determine how well DMSO treated these two common clinical conditions. Results of this study showed that DMSO improved pain, tenderness, and swelling, and facilitated increased range of motion. Forty patients were treated for each of the two ailments; patients treated with the 70-percent aqueous solution of DMSO did not receive any more beneficial effect from the drug than patients who received a 5-percent DMSO aqueous placebo solution.[2]

Dr. Reedy attempted to perform double-blind studies among the players but found them to be of absolutely no value, due to the particular characteristics of DMSO. He applied a 10-percent solution as a placebo but the effect was much less clam-type breath, only minimal redness of the area treated, and much faster drying time than usual in the 70-percent solution.

Dr. Reedy said, "We had a player, Fred Belitnikoff, who had a shoulder contusion and an ankle contusion in a pileup. Seventy percent was applied in the ankle and only 10 percent in the shoulder. He very quickly told me, 'Doctor, that is not the real stuff; it is not red and it dries too fast.' So double-blind studies were not able to be completed."

PLAYERS SEE A NEED FOR DMSO

Dr. Reedy saw that fair-haired and fair-complexioned players seemed to experience skin reactions sooner than those of darker coloring. But the degree of skin reaction was not proportional to the benefits of reduced swelling. He applied DMSO regularly for acute swelling due to trauma of any joint or muscle, particularly of the limbs, especially the ankle, elbow, hands, or wrist.

The adverse effects he witnessed are the same that have been discussed: clam-oyster breath that is unresponsive to a number of breath deodorizers, and local skin reactions. Skin irritation seemed to come in two separate waves, usually by the third to fourth day or by the ninth to sixteenth treatment session. In fair-complexioned, light-haired players, it came somewhat sooner. However, these symptoms usually disappeared within seventy-two hours after the last treatment session. "I should also state that these effects were welcomed by many of the players to get them back to play sooner," said Dr. Reedy.

Sixteen years ago, Dr. Reedy discontinued his affiliation with the Oakland Raiders when he moved to his present home in Enumclaw. Actively involved in clinical practice and in community education on preventive health maintenance and drug abuse, Dr. Reedy still employs DMSO as a therapeutic tool. "My experience in utilization in my private practice outside the realm of sports medicine has been essentially nonprimary, because I choose to use it within the confines of the field of sports medicine as I had made that decision with Dr. Jacob about it. I would say, however, that I would like very much to use it in my patients with arthritis and acute ankle injuries because about 50 percent of my practice is sports medicine. So I would be very anxious for it to be released so I could use it more extensively."

Daryle Lamonica, former quarterback for the Oakland Raiders, wrote to Val Hallamendaris, Counsel to the Commission on Aging of the House of Representatives, on April 2, 1980, from Walnut Creek, California. This is what the football player said:

> I am writing to express my feelings regarding my experience with DMSO. As a former professional athlete, I had the opportunity to use it because of injuries. The first time was on a jammed thumb on my throwing hand. The swelling was so severe I could not bend it. DMSO was applied and, much to my surprise, the swelling started to leave within minutes.

Although my skin blistered momentarily, within three days I was throwing the ball hard again and was able to compete successfully the following Sunday afternoon. I feel this would not have been possible without the benefit of this unusual drug.

I have had other injuries in which DMSO was used and the results were very positive. It was applied to my swollen and strained left knee, my lower back, my jammed little finger on my throwing hand, and my tender and inflamed right elbow.

I must point out that we had an excellent team physician, Dr. Graham Reedy. I relied on his medical advice and guidance and feel he was most instrumental in my over-all success in the N.F.L. He did introduce me to DMSO.

I have played with many other players who have used DMSO to great success. The only drawback I have observed would be, as my wife referred to it, "gross body odor." It did not add much to my social life, but I understand that this has been corrected.

I personally feel there is a great need for DMSO, not only for professional and amateur athletes, but for all persons who suffer pain. Val, our society is blessed to have drugs like DMSO to help us through our misfortunes.[3]

CHAPTER 7
Arthritis Therapy With DMSO and Diet

A United States Customs Service employee, Roger O. Varga of Bowie, Maryland, was served with divorce decree papers by his wife. The man's personality was so irritating from his inability to accept the pain of arthritis that "my wife can't put up with me anymore," he confessed.

Mr. Varga has been the long-time victim of full-body rheumatoid arthritis and rheumatoid spondylitis (spinal arthritis). His joint pain had become increasingly worse over the last five years to the point that he could not cope with everyday stress.

After taking intravenous (IV) DMSO anti-arthritis therapy, Varga, now fifty-nine, finally found amazing relief in less than five days. He was able to return to his normal work routine. The patient underwent two separate sessions of DMSO IV treatment during the course of fourteen months and left for home both times feeling quite comfortable. He now maintains himself between IV sessions with topical DMSO in the form of a salve—DMSO mixed with cold cream in a 70-percent concentration.

*   *   *

An expert in growing lovely orchards who resides in Mount Airy, North Carolina, Calvin Clayton Vernon, suffered with a combination of rheumatoid arthritis and osteoarthritis, which had lodged mainly in his back, shoulders, hips, and left ankle.

From receiving the oral, topical, and IV-administered DMSO treatments, Mr. Vernon, who had just turned seventy-two, found his joint pains greatly diminished. He could walk better, had less swelling in the ankle, and increased his mobility in all joints. The patient's condition was rated "marked improvement" by the doctor following his conclusion of the standard five-day treatment program. Vernon stated: "I brought home a supply of DMSO to take orally and topically. I am still using it and feel that I can continue to keep up my work."

* * *

A supervisor of quality control, James S. Smith of Marietta, Ohio, developed rheumatoid arthritis in November 1979. It was a severely acute onset in all his joints, but especially in his ankles, feet, wrists, and fingers. He hardly slept at all from the deep, aching pain, which also kept him from working because of his lack of arm strength and his unstable legs.

Five days of IV DMSO, which he received when he was sixty, combined with the application of DMSO on his skin and the administration by mouth, brought relief right away. The pain disappeared to the extent that Smith said, "I am looking forward to playing golf."

* * *

An auto mechanic, James E. Singletary of Porter, Texas, had rheumatoid arthritis of all of his joints at one time or another for over thirty years. He took vast quantities of many different medications for it.

In June 1990, Mr. Singletary took five days of IV DMSO treatment and returned home with a quantity of the topical and oral form. He said, "A month after the IVs and DMSO taken orally, the pain, swelling, and inflammation seemed to subside, although soreness in my joints continues." The mobility in both his shoulders increased and the pain left his knees and feet.

* * *

A retired housewife, Vilma F. Slingerland of Sarasota, Florida, had acquired a gastric ulcer from taking Indocin for rheumatoid arthritis. Since 1978, her knees, hips, neck, and back gave her awful pain.

She took the IV DMSO therapy when she had unusually severe pain in September 1992 and combined it with oral and topical DMSO and also had DMSO combined with Xylocaine injected into both of her knees. These joint injections gave her an excellent result. Her grip strength improved dramatically and neck discomfort disappeared. Mrs. Slingerland's opinion about DMSO includes the statement: "I consider it very helpful in some locations, especially in the sacroiliac region."

* * *

A clerk in a ladies apparel shop, Beatrice L. Luke, from Saluda, South Carolina, suffered with osteoarthritis in the spine and hands. She couldn't tolerate the different arthritis medications and sought DMSO treatment as an alternative.

Ms. Luke experienced fine results from taking IV, topical, and oral DMSO and could return to work full time in August 1992. "My main problem was pain in my back," she says, "and it is much better." She applied topical DMSO thirty separate times before she felt total back pain relief, but the comfort was gratefully accepted when it arrived.

* * *

A housewife from Port Charlotte, Florida, Mary F. Hayes, had osteoarthritis that caused pain in her arms and shoulders for two years. She was limited in her movements, as illustrated by her inability to fasten her bra. "My left arm was inflamed and swollen and very painful," she wrote recently, "so painful I could hardly get a good night's rest. After using one jar of the DMSO cream, I can even fasten my bra."

Mrs. Hayes needed no treatment other than her own administration of DMSO to her skin.

* * *

A highway toll collector in Florida, Fred Flechsig of Fort Lauderdale, was victimized by severe degenerative arthritis of the hips and knees. From inhaling automobile exhaust fumes on the job, Mr. Flechsig suffered from lead poisoning, too, which may have contributed to his terrible joint pains. Where the range of lead in the body of an average American is 0.1 to 2.0, a hair analysis of this man revealed an occupational hazard of 5.0 lead content.

Flechsig didn't need IV DMSO treatment to find arthritis relief, however. He got it immediately from using the DMSO cream on his joints twice daily and drinking the oral preparation regularly starting May 22, 1990.

* * *

A schoolteacher, Marie G. Miller of Randolph, New Jersey, endured osteoarthritis for twenty years. Pain was present in multiple joints, which she attributed to her very active life and her tendency to do too much in a day. She required aid in walking, holding on to the walls and furniture in her apartment.

Mrs. Miller writes: "I went for the DMSO treatment as a last resort for the relief of the constant pain in all joints, shoulders, spine, fingers, toes, ankles, and knees. Knees and feet gave me much trouble. I could not walk without great pain and found it very hard to get up from a chair without turning every which way to grab hold of something nearby to push or pull myself up to stand.

"I had taken gold shots, Indocin, Butazolidine, etc. for two years. I took two aspirin (650 mg) four times a day with some relief but with a number of very bad days every so often, requiring me to spend a half to a whole day in bed under an electric blanket even in the middle of summer in temperatures 80°F and over.

"Then I started to take Darvon, which gave me more relief, taking two a day every four hours during a bad day of pain. After taking DMSO IV in May 1990, I've only had to take perhaps a dozen Darvon until January 1991.

"I still use DMSO on the joints if they become a bit sore or inflamed. I can stretch my fingers out straight without all that previous pain. The joints are still a little stiff but I am able to use them without pain, when I'm careful not to overwork them.

"I have been very happy with the results obtained with the DMSO treatments. I thank God every day since finding DMSO, for the doctors who discovered this treatment and for the doctors who are using it to try and help arthritics," wrote Mrs. Miller.

THE INCIDENCE OF ARTHRITIS

It was reported in a spring 1991 issue of *Medical World News* that at least seven DMSO clinics have opened in Mexico to treat arthritis patients, primarily Americans. One entrepeneur in Mexico is said to have used DMSO in 1989 to treat 30,000 Americans for their arthritic symptoms, and grossed over $20 million.

Rudy Minoot, owner of a Tijuana, Mexico, DMSO clinic, told an audience at the twenty-sixth annual meeting of the National Health Federation in Long Beach, California, January 18, 1981, exactly how he uses American facilities to pack his Mexican clinic with American patients. "We think of the clinic itself as being in San Diego. The patients sleep, eat, and drink in San Diego. Then we take them over to Tijuana by limousine in the afternoon for two hours for them to have the DMSO IV drip. It's on an outpatient basis," said Minoot. "We have another clinic 400 miles down the west coast of Mexico."

The Mexican connection furnishes intravenous pharmaceutical grade DMSO at an average cost of $800 for three days of treatment. People pay their own lodgings and meals. This is big business for the clinic proprietors, because Americans seem especially prone to this arthritis with its exceedingly painful manifestations.

Rheumatoid arthritis afflicts 6.5 million United States citizens, of whom 75 percent are women. At least 66 percent of those afflicted are elderly.

In Ohio alone, over 300,000 people suffer with this one condition, explained Ohio Congresswoman Mary Rose Oakar, a member of the House Select Committee on Aging. "The annual cost to the State of Ohio from arthritic diseases is approximately 450 million dollars, not including 175 million dollars lost in wages. Furthermore," Ms. Oakar said, "in Northeastern Ohio there is a ratio of one physician certified as a rheumatologist to every 200,000 people." With a total state population of approximately 10,000,000, this gives Ohio a disproportionate 5,000 practicing arthritis specialists. They aren't all just for the rheumatoid arthritis patients either; there are plenty of other arthritic types to keep them busy.

Additional forms of arthritis affecting our national population combine to make up more than 41,600,000 victims in this country who have arthritic symptoms severe enough to require medical attention. This comes to 1 in 6 people; for those over age sixty-five the prevalence rate is 1 in 2. Almost 4,000,000 arthritic Americans suffer degrees of full or partial disability. Arthritis diseases comprise 100 types, and osteoarthritis, which is wear and tear to the joints, makes up most of them.

Indeed, arthritis is everybody's disease. If you live long enough, you will have some form of the condition. If you are lucky, you may not suffer acute pain or crippling as have the people I've described, but you will know you have it.

Arthritis is one of those degenerative diseases commonly listed as "having no known cause and no known cure." It has long-term duration and progressively disables and handicaps the patient. The present orthodox treatment for this problem involves the use of anti-inflammatory drugs such as the cortical steroids, gold injections, and analgesics for the relief of pain. Aspirin is taken extensively by arthritics.

In the history of Western man, irrational behavior in political and military leaders has often been attributed to the pain and suffering caused by arthritis. A form of arthritis drove a Roman general to suicide, forced Henry VI to change his wedding date, and made Charlemagne and Alexander the Great difficult to live with. It is also considered a cause of Goethe's despair.

Joanna Jackson of Savannah, Georgia, felt deep despair, for she had been plagued by generalized destruction of her joints, which resulted in severe deformities and swelling. At twenty-nine, she had already gone through nearly twenty years of periodic flare-ups, which had caused progressive and permanent damage to tissues.

For her rheumatoid arthritis, Miss Jackson had taken every conceivable anti-arthritic treatment employed by modern medicine. For weeks, she swallowed thirteen, seventeen, and even twenty aspirin tablets a day until she developed peptic ulcers, slight deafness, and ringing in the ears. She took Indocin until certain central nervous system side effects such as headache, impaired alertness, and poor motor coordination ruled out any more of this drug. Injections with gold worked only when her disease was in its earliest active stages. Steroids in general proved toxic and began to change her features to a moonface. Even the drug Tolectin, a nonsteroidal anti-inflammatory therapy, brought on abdominal pain and discomfort, even nausea and vomiting, and excited her peptic ulcers.

Miss Jackson admitted she was considering ending her misery by suicide, until she saw that Sunday evening *60 Minutes* documentary television program about DMSO. Friends of Joanna Jackson had been cajoling her to cross the state line from Georgia to Florida and take the DMSO treatment. She had shrugged off their requests, believing that the purported arthritis pain-relieving property of the drug was just another "quack cure" that would produce additional side effects to make her life even more unbearable than it already was.

THE OFFICIAL POSITION OF THE ARTHRITIS FOUNDATION

Finally, Miss Jackson was swayed by the stand against DMSO taken by the Arthritis Foundation. Prior statements indicated that its Committee on Unproven Remedies was opposed to the legalization of the drug in the State of Florida, which put the Arthritis Foundation in the position of opposition to use of DMSO for relieving arthritis.

Charles C. Bennett, vice president of public and professional education for the Arthritis Foundation of Atlanta, Georgia, appeared before the House of Representatives Select Committee on Aging. Mr. Bennett said, "The Arthritis Foundation is not against DMSO. We would be delighted if it were established by appropriate scientific procedures to be effective. I don't think the safety question seems to be a major one. That is pretty clear. But the question of effectiveness for arthritis, particularly for inflammatory arthritis, particularly for chronic arthritis, is not clearly resolved. The question [is one] of finding an agent that will deal with the pain problem in a disease that goes on and/or involves a search for something that works not just for a short-term overnight basis, but in a long-term chronic use."

The Arthritis Foundation thus changed its position, in a way. From disapproving legislation in 1977 to permit use of DMSO by individual states and accepting the *ad hoc* Committee on Dimethyl Sulfoxide of the National Academy of Sciences–National Research Council's negative report, the Arthritis Foundation has now endorsed it for limited use as a pain reliever.

"DMSO is by no means a worthless drug," Bennett said. "It appears to work as a local analgesic and therefore might be useful in a host of conditions causing pain. But there is no scientific proof that it reduces swelling and inflammation (which are of such critical importance in rheumatoid arthritis, for example), or that it changes the underlying course of any connective tissue disease."

In summary, the Arthritis Foundation told people who have rheumatoid or other inflammatory arthritis that DMSO was not the drug for them. They needed more than pain relief; they had to have the inflammation suppressed, something even aspirin in proper dosage can do, but DMSO can't, they said.

The Foundation officials wanted the FDA to get DMSO approved for lesser pain problems—without waiting for time-consuming trials needed to clear up questions about the drug's usefulness for serious systemic conditions, Bennett said. He indicated that his organization was taking a neutral stand. He equivocated.

The Mike Wallace television presentation changed Miss Jackson's thinking about having the treatment, no matter what official position was held by the Arthritis Foundation. About a week after the first broadcast she telephoned for an appointment to see a physician who prescribed DMSO. She arranged transportation and also borrowed the necessary funds to pay for the treatment. Average charges in the United States for the entire course of DMSO arthritis therapy under medical supervision, including medication for three months, vary from one physician to the next depending on what geographical area he practices in, but it averages about $950 for the first week and $700 for the second week, if it's needed.

The first thing the patient noticed upon entering the doctor's office was the smell. It was not the antiseptic aroma of alcohol common to most medical facilities; it was the pungent odor of garlic. "Pardon our odor. It's DMSO at work," read a sign in the reception room.

Miss Jackson was introduced to the standard protocol for arthritis therapy, with DMSO and diet as the initial part of her program.

THE PROTOCOL FOR DMSO ARTHRITIS THERAPY

The DMSO Society of Florida, Inc., recommends that any patient treated with the solvent be educated in the full anti-arthritis program of DMSO and diet as well as receiving direct physician care. The program for Miss Jackson, therefore, was a learning experience as well as therapy. The doctor acted as teacher.

A complete nutritional workup was done, including the prescribing of megadoses of nutrients, especially pantothenic acid, niacinamide, ascorbic acid, and other vitamins and minerals in the form of supplements to the diet. A typical patient with inflamed joints, such as Joanna Jackson, follows the specific protocol for DMSO arthritis therapy.

She consulted with the doctor for an evaluation of her existing health problems. A physical examination was carried out, including a number of clinical tests to determine the extent of her limitation of motion in the hands, arms, feet, legs, hips, back, shoulders, neck, and other articulations. Grip strength was measured.

She had a basic series of laboratory blood tests and urinalysis performed. An overly-detailed number of laboratory testings was not done, because as an arthritic, the patient had already gone through too many examinations, probably every one in the book. This overtesting for arthritics is an all-too-frequent practice in most medical establishments. It is a waste of the medical consumer's money. Miss Jackson did have a sedimentation rate, liver function test, hair analysis, computerized diet evaluation, and some other checkups.

It is important to know what the patient eats, since prior observations of arthritic people have shown that sugar taken in excess brings on joint symptoms. (I will have more to say on this topic a little further along in this chapter.) The computerized diet evaluation gave the doctor clues as to what nutrition education was needed.

With completion of the pretesting, the entire treatment program was explained to the patient. She was handed the informed consent state-ment (see Figure 7.1) to read and sign in accordance with the official position of the Florida Medical Association, described in Chapter 2.

For Miss Jackson, intravenous injection of DMSO using a half dose (0.5 g/kg of body weight) was begun the first treatment day. The infusion procedure takes three or four hours depending on the speed of the fluid flow into the vein. The next day and for those treatments administered thereafter, the full dose (1.0 g/kg mixed into 1,000 cc of fluid) was given.

There are five treatment days in a week, extending from Monday to Friday, and one series of a week's injections usually are sufficient, except for people suffering with arthritis of the spine. It takes spondylitis patients longer to respond, so that two weeks of infusions may be required.

Although no health insurance policy was reimbursing the patient for the DMSO arthritis therapy, Miss Jackson financed a second week of treatment herself because of the improvement she saw developing in her joints. At the start of her second week of care, she was feeling more comfortable than any time in the recent past. A tape-recorded treatment room dialogue between the doctor and the patient went like this:

> *Doctor:* Tell me about your progress, Joanna.
>
> *Jackson:* I think I've improved a lot.
>
> *Doctor:* In what areas, specifically?
>
> *Jackson:* Well, when your nurse tested my hand grip with that blood pressure device a few minutes ago, my strength had improved from only twenty pounds of pressure a week ago to sixty pounds today.
>
> *Doctor:* Three times as well; that's one of the best test results we've had this month. Good progress!
>
> *Jackson:* But all my fingers still won't close in a fist.
>
> *Doctor:* Those fingers are quite deformed; they may never fully close.
>
> *Jackson:* But now these two close all the way [index finger and third finger on the right hand] where they didn't before.
>
> *Doctor:* Any other progress to report?
>
> *Jackson:* Yes, my feet are better.
>
> *Doctor:* How can you tell?
>
> *Jackson:* Because I can walk without canes. I can pick my feet up higher and bend my knees without pain. And my ankles don't hurt anymore. I think there's less arthritis in my leg joints, don't you?

Consent Form
for Arthritis Treatment

I, _____, have had explained to me the DMSO form of arthritis treatment, which includes DMSO intravenously and topically (applied to the skin), large doses of Vitamin C, enzymes, such as bromelain from pineapple, and a rigid dietary program. I understand that certain side effects, such as nausea, depression, or skin rash, may occur.

I am aware of the other modes of treatment and I have been advised by Dr. _____ to obtain at least one second opinion from a physician specializing in traditional arthritis therapy. I also understand that DMSO is not approved by the Federal Food and Drug Administration for the treatment of arthritis.

Lastly, in most cases, DMSO IV therapy is not covered by Medicare or other forms of insurance.

WITNESSES:

_____   _____
        (Signature)   *(Signature)*

_____   _____
          (Date)   *(Date)*

Figure 7.1 *Informed consent statement.*

Doctor: Yes, if you're picking up your feet well off the floor, I would say there's less inflammation present. And you've definitely noticed a difference when you walk?

Jackson: I sure have! I can do deep knee bends, where I hadn't been able to since I was nine years old.

Doctor: Be sure to put plastic wrap over your joints below the waist after you've painted them with the solution and place gauze or another wrapping over that. Leave these coverings on overnight. Sleep with them on. The skin is quite resistant to skin reactions from DMSO down there. But don't use Saran or other plastic wrap above the waist because it's liable to produce a blistering from the DMSO application under plastic.

Jackson: I've been painting my knees with DMSO and covering with Saran Wrap. You mean I should do the same to my ankles? For my hands too?

Doctor: Do it for your ankles but not for the hands. You mustn't occlude the air over DMSO on any joint above the waist, because it will cause blistering. Scientists don't know why the skin is more sensitive above the waist than below. Do paint your finger joints with the liquid—all you wish, just as you've been doing.

I will give a complete description of this plastic impervious wrapping technique in the next section, but let us finish following Joanna Jackson through her first week of treatment.

She had been taught how to apply the topical DMSO on the first treatment day and the arthritis diet with its initial supply of supplements was given to her, too. The second day Miss Jackson received a further explanation of the diet. Gentle passive exercises were given to her and more active ones were demonstrated for her own exercising at home.

The third treatment included a demonstration of how to put on the impervious wrapping. The nurses also gave lectures on the significance of hair and diet analyses. Reports in writing about her hair and diet analyses were received by the patient within ten days of the testings. All the while Miss Jackson was being evaluated by the doctor during her physical examinations.

The fourth treatment day consisted of more IV DMSO and the doctor's formal lecture on nutrition. Family and friends were invited to listen to the lecture so that the patient would receive support at home when she attempted to change her eating lifestyle. Miss Jackson had prescribed for her daily doses of flavored cod liver oil for its vitamin A, D, and E contents. She applied it topically as well as taking it orally. At home, the patient was instructed to swallow one teaspoonful of cod liver oil with lemon juice twice a day to keep her blood level elevated. Cod liver oil aids the action of DMSO. Also, more passive exercises were given to Miss Jackson at that visit.

On her final visit she went through the entire diagnostic testing again in order to compare her readings with the baseline record of when she first arrived. Also, if Miss Jackson had not elected to remain another week, she ordinarily would have received a three-month supply of DMSO consisting of four bottles of the oral and two bottles of the topical, with an explanation of when and how to use them. As it was, at the end of the second week she took home a six-month supply.

Every IV treatment procedure was the same. The patient was instructed to eat a good breakfast each morning before the IV hookup except on the mornings when blood was to be drawn for testing. Hookup was between 8:00 A.M. and 8:30 A.M., no later. She brought a snack to eat during the hours of treatment. There was no restriction of bathroom privileges, because anybody could go to the toilet carrying the IV bottle still attached in the vein. One merely needed to hold the IV bottle high in the opposite hand from the IV needle. The IV needle hand had to be kept low and be prevented from getting bumped. There was a hook in the bathroom next to the commode, from which the patient could hang the bottle.

THE IMPERVIOUS WRAPPING TECHNIQUE

Keypunch operator Irene A. Brooks of Bradenton, Florida, had horrible left knee pain from osteoarthritis. Her comfort came merely from the application of topical DMSO under an impervious wrap, the kind of plastic packaging material commonly employed in the kitchen, for example, Saran Wrap, Glad Wrap, and Handi Wrap. For three months Mrs. Brooks followed the wrapping procedure applying it each time her knee flared with pain. Then she felt relief, at least temporarily.

The impervious wrapping technique consists of first putting on the topical DMSO liquid, gel, cream, or ointment to cover the area of discomfort. Do not rub in the medication but apply it lightly with the aid of a cotton ball, wooden cotton-tipped applicator, soft and narrow paintbrush, or just your fingers.

Wrap a thin layer of gauze bandage over and around the affected area. Next, cover the entire bandage and solvent coating with plastic wrap.

Leave the impervious wrapping in place for two hours the first time. If no skin irritation develops, the next time you may leave the wrapping alone for the entire period you're sleeping. Or, you may keep it in place during the day.

Do not wash the treated area with harsh soaps, other solvents, or household chemicals that could contribute to skin irritations. The DMSO alone may bring on a rash or irritation—in which case discontinue the impervious application.

The plastic wrap technique may be used for parts of the body below the waist such as the hips, knees, ankles, feet, or areas in between. Do not use this procedure for the upper body—the arms, hands, trunk, neck, face, shoulders, or back. Plastic seems to be too strong for covering areas above the waist and excludes the air from the DMSO-treated skin.

THE DMSO ANTI-ARTHRITIS DIET
AND FOOD SUPPLEMENTS

For any arthritic person daily diet becomes extremely important. The end products of red meats such as beef, pork, veal, and lamb are particularly antagonistic to inflamed joints. Consequently, red meat should be eliminated from an arthritic's diet at the beginning of treatment and during acute flare-ups.

The Clinica Manner (Manner Clinic) Metabolic Research Foundation, P.O. Box 434290, San Ysidro, California 92143-4290, (800) 433-4962 or (800) 248-8431, recommends the Manner Metabolic Therapy A for use with DMSO. Developed by the late Harold W. Mannner, Ph.D., former professor of biology and chairman of the Biology Department of Loyola University of Chicago, Metabolic Therapy A consists of an anti-arthritis diet and various food supplements. For an overview of the general diet, see Table 7.1, which presents the foods allowed and the foods to be avoided while following the DMSO protocol.

In addition to recommending that certain foods be avoided, the Foundation also advises that pesticides, food additives (especially monosodium glutamate, or MSG, and other additives ending with -*ate*), and artificial colors, flavors, and preservatives be avoided. Furthermore, sugar should be avoided, both by itself and processed into foods.

Prolonged intake of refined sugar (and other refined products) is a major contributing factor in arthritis. Refined sugar depresses vitamin C stores. The highest concentration of vitamin C in the body is in the adrenal glands, and chronic vitamin C deficiency (hypoascorbemia)

Table 7.1 *The Manner Clinic Anti-Arthritis Diet*

Food Category	Foods Allowed	Foods to Be Avoided
Beverages	Herb teas (chamomile, mint, papaya; no caffein), fresh fruit juice, fresh vegetable juice, purified water	Alcohol, cocoa, caffeinated and decaffeinated coffee, carbonated beverages, canned and pasteurized juices, artificial fruit drinks
Dairy Products	Raw milk, yogurt, butter, buttermilk in limited quantities, non-fat cottage cheese, white (Farmer) cheese	All processed and imitation butter, ice cream, toppings, all pasteurized cheeses
Eggs	Poached or boiled (one per day)	Fried or scrambled
Fish	Fresh white-fleshed, broiled or baked	Non-white-fleshed, fried or breaded
Fruit	All dried (unsulfured), stewed, fresh, frozen (unsweetened)	Canned, sweetened
Grains	Whole grain cereals, bread or muffins made from rye, oats, wheat, bran, buckwheat, millet, and other whole grains; cream of wheat, brown rice, whole seeds of sesame, pumpkin, sunflower, flaxseed	White flour products, hull-less grains and seeds such as pasta, crackers, macaroni, snack foods, white rice, prepared or cold cereals, cooked seeds
Meats	Poultry, but never fried or breaded	All red meat products such as beef, pork, lamb, veal
Nuts	All fresh, raw nuts	Roasted and/or salted, especially peanuts

Food Category	Foods Allowed	Foods to Be Avoided
Oils	Cold-processed such as safflower	Shortening, refined fats and oils (unsaturated as well as saturated), hydrogenated margarine or hydrogenated nut butters
Seasonings	Herbs, garlic, onion, chives, parsley, marjoram	Pepper, salt, hot spices
Soups	All made from scratch, such as vegetable, chicken, barley, millet, brown rice	Canned and creamed (thickened), commercial bouillon, fat stock
Sprouts	All, especially wheat, pea, lentil, alfalfa, and mung	None
Sweets	Raw honey, unsulfured molasses, carob, unflavored gelatin, pure maple syrup (in limited amounts)	Refined sugars (white, brown, turbinado), chocolate, candy, syrups
Vegetables	All raw and not over-cooked, steamed, fresh or frozen, potatoes baked or broiled	All canned vegetables, fried potatoes in any form, corn chips

leads to adrenal exhaustion. With prolonged adrenal deficiency, there is a deficiency of endogenous (body-produced) cortisone. Rheumatoid arthritis is the end result of this prolonged attack of sugar on the adrenal glands.

"Demon Sugar" is also a major contributing factor in osteoarthritis, also known as degenerative arthritis. Sugar depresses the blood phosphorus. The blood calcium and phosphorus are kept in a precise balance by the body when in good health. Any stress on the body, such as illness or refined sugar intake, will upset the delicate and extremely important calcium/phosphorus ratio.

Depression of the blood phosphorus by refined sugar causes a *relative* increase in blood calcium. The parathyroid gland, confused by the "low" phosphorus level, thinks the blood needs more calcium and acts, through the release of parathyroid hormone, to pull calcium out of the bones. So now there is even more calcium in the blood. But the body knows that too much calcium in the blood can cause sudden death so, to protect from hypercalcemia and death, the body acts in two ways to eliminate this excess calcium. It eliminates the calcium in the urine and, more germane to our discussion, *it deposits it in soft tissues, such as arteries, and in the joints.*

The prolonged use of refined sugar leads to a veritable army of aggressors released against your body, resulting in arthritis, arteriosclerosis, diabetes, chronic infections, and osteoporosis.

It's popular to believe that "you are what you eat," but this is not entirely correct. The food must be digested and absorbed into the blood stream before nutrients can do the body any good. Arthritis is one of the degenerative diseases, which indicates that digestion is incomplete for ingested materials. The food is poorly absorbed, so that the body joints are insufficiently nourished.

To overcome poor absorption and decrease the stress placed on the gastric glands and the pancreas, a tablet containing hydrochloric acid, pepsin, and enterically coated pancreatic enzymes should be taken at each meal. The Manner Clinic has made such nutritional supplementation a part of its anti-arthritis regime, and I believe in it also. It ensures the proper digestion of food. *Note:* In some people excessive gas might follow gastric juice supplementation, which means that you already have enough hydrochloric acid. In this case, take only tablets containing the pancreatic enzymes.

The Manner Metabolic Therapy A for arthritis also includes the following supplements:

- 2,000 mg vitamin C with each meal
- 400 IU vitamin E with each meal
- 1,000 mg pantothenic acid with each meal
- 2 multivitamin capsules after each meal
- 25,000 IU vitamin A (or 2 teaspoons cod liver oil) twice daily
- 2,500 IU vitamin D three times daily (including at bedtime)

The amounts to be taken of all of the above supplements can be cut in half after symptomatic improvement is noticed.

Vitamin A should be taken in emulsified form to avoid liver involvement. Up to 500,000 IU (International Units) of liquid vitamin A have been given without side effects by physicians practicing metabolic therapy at such places as the Health and Wellness Center of Minneapolis or the Degenerative Disease Medical Center of Las Vegas. If emulsified vitamin A is not available, I recommend instead that you consider using for a few days 50,000 to 100,000 IU of regular vitamin A. *Note:* Observe your skin. If drying or scaling occurs, discontinue vitamin A for one week. If any other signs of vitamin A toxicity, such as headaches, hair changes, or dryness of the mouth, occur, discontinue the vitamin A for a week and resume with a reduced dosage the following week. Continue with a half-dose daily with a two-week-on one-week-off routine. Symptoms of vitamin A toxicity disappear as soon as you reduce your daily dosage.

Vitamin C is quite necessary for an arthritic, and megadoses ranging up to 15 g should be taken daily, according to the Manner Clinic. I suggest a somewhat lesser amount, at least to start. Make sure the vitamin C is in the form of ascorbates, which have a neutral pH (acid–base balance) and, therefore, prevent problems with acidity. Also, ascorbates contain the bioflavonoids that are necessary for the proper metabolism of this vitamin. *Note:* Megadoses of ascorbic acid may cause gastric disturbances such as diarrhea. Acute diarrhea will indicate the body's tolerance level has been reached, and you should reduce your dose until diarrhea no longer is a problem.

A therapeutic vitamin-mineral supplement should be taken morning and evening as well. The tablets or capsules can be swallowed with a Protein Milk Shake, which the Foundation also recommends (see page 120).

In addition to the supplements already mentioned, also recommended on a daily basis are 3 g of calcium, one-quarter pound fresh liver or 15 liver tablets, fresh wheat germ, and 6 tablespoons bran (on morning cereal). A superoxide dismutase (SOD) supplement is also encouraged. Recent laboratory work has indicated that people suffering from arthritic or rheumatic diseases have a decreased amount of SOD in their circulating blood. SOD is a metalloprotein, a natural enzyme. To overcome an SOD deficiency, a tablet or two containing the enzyme could be taken with each meal. Such a supplement will have an anti-arthritic effect.

The anti-arthritic diet and supplement regime may be begun with a two-day juice fast, which is recommended by the Manner Clinic. To

Protein Milk Shake

2 eggs
¼ cup yogurt
4 teaspoons calcium gluconate
1 tablespoon lecithin
1 tablespoon safflower oil
1 teaspoon granular kelp
½ teaspoon magnesium oxide
4 cups skim milk
½ cup powdered non-instant milk
¼ cup yeast fortified with calcium
¼ cup soy flour or powder
¼ cup wheat germ
1 teaspoon vanilla (not vanillin)

In blender, thoroughly mix eggs, yogurt, calcium gluconate, lecithin, safflower oil, kelp, and magnesium oxide. Add 2 cups skim milk, powdered milk, yeast, soy flour, wheat germ, and vanilla, and mix. Add remaining 2 cups skim milk, plus fruit or fruit juice, carob, honey, additional vanilla, or other flavoring to taste, if desired. Drink two-thirds of a cup six times a day (with each meal and at midmorning, midafternoon, and bedtime).

allow for taste acclimation to juices, a blend of 50 percent apple and 50 percent carrot juice should be taken first. As rapidly as possible, eliminate the apple juice and add other vegetable juices to the carrot juice. This is a way to ease into drinking celery, beet, potato, and other vegetables as juices. Definitely don't drink canned juices, since the heat of canning destroys the vegetable enzymes. Prepare and drink the juice each day to prevent oxidation of the liquid, and eat nothing solid for two days.

Follow the anti-arthritis diet and take the food supplements while you are under treatment with DMSO. Continue on this diet as part of your lifestyle thereafter. And absolutely avoid refined sugar in any form.

DETOXIFICATION

A process of detoxification goes along with the anti-arthritis diet and supplementation program. Each day a coffee enema could be administered. (It's the only useful purpose for coffee.) Cool one cup of brewed (non-instant) coffee to body temperature and introduce it into the rectum with a rectal syringe. Retain the coffee for fifteen to thirty minutes. The caffeine-stimulated secretion of bile is an important part of the detoxification plan, as it helps to restore the alkaline condition of the small intestine.

Continue colonic irrigation with coffee enemas until the bowel movements become regular, twice a day if possible. Part of the arthritic's problem is that he or she does not get rid of toxic products catabolyzed by the body. The bowel habits are irregular. Drinking four to eight glasses of freshly prepared vegetable juices also helps to bring bowel movements back to normal.

THE MANNER COCKTAIL FOR ARTHRITIS

The Manner Clinic utilizes what it calls the Manner Cocktail for the permanent relief of various forms of arthritis including tendinitis, gouty arthritis, bursitis, rheumatoid arthritis, and osteoarthritis; chronic back disorders; and acute sprains and strains. The cocktail consists of a combination of vitamin C, amygdalin, and DMSO. It was developed by Dr. Manner around 1987 to act as a chelating agent, which grabs metallic ions out of the body, and to enhance electron density at the oxygen atom and the steric availability of the oxygen, which increases the packing of the oxygen atoms so that more oxygen is present to nourish the cells.

Being both anti-inflammatory and analgesic (causing the reduction of pain) in its action, the DMSO infusion is exceedingly useful for the correction of arthritis and its many complications. To learn more about the administration of DMSO via the Manner Cocktail, contact the Manner Clinic.

REPORTED ARTHRITIS-DMSO INVESTIGATIONS

In 1989, five Italian physicians investigated the complications and symptoms of rheumatoid arthritis and tested the efficacy of dimethyl sulfoxide on the overall condition. Writing in the journal *Minerva Medica*, the doctors concluded: "In this study we have investigated the role of oral dimethylsulfoxide (DMSO) therapy in two patients with primary amyloidosis (AL) [a form of rheumatoid arthritis] with secondary amyloidosis (AA) to long-standing rheumatoid arthritis. DMSO treatment produced no beneficial effects in the patients with idiopathic [cause unknown] amyloidosis. Instead the patients with secondary amyloidosis experienced a subjective improvement, a decrease of inflammatory activity of the rheumatoid arthritis, and an unequivocal improvement of renal [kidney] function following three to six months of DMSO therapy. No serious side effects of DMSO were observed except for unpleasant breath odour. We conclude that a treatment with oral DMSO may prolong life of patients with secondary amyloidosis."[1]

With acute gouty arthritis in a 1981 Russian study, DMSO was administered for the condition and compared to indomethacin, a drug therapy. The DMSO treatment was more effective for gout.[2]

Favorable effects for juvenile rheumatoid arthritis were reported in a case, in 1984, when DMSO was administered to a girl with secondary amyloidosis as a complication of her arthritis. Dimethyl sulfoxide was applied by topical application to the skin. The young girl's gastrointestinal symptoms and massive proteinuria (protein in the urine) improved. Her decreased left ventricular function of the heart and her kidney's creatinine clearance also improved remarkably. The ten collaborating Japanese physicians on this case came to the conclusion, "The favorable effect of dimethyl sulfoxide in this single patient deserves further study in a controlled trial."[3]

Two Russian orthopedists used DMSO to treat rheumatoid arthritis without complications, as published in their 1981 case report.[4]

Another group of Russian doctors in 1983 investigated DMSO for the treatment of rheumatoid arthritis and compared its effect to colchicine. DMSO was more advantageous and produced no kidney complications.[5]

Ordinarily Still's disease is a chronic arthritis developing in children before the age of sixteen. There are several different forms of arthritis affecting children, and some authorities confine the diagnosis of Still's disease to the following: a disease of childhood marked by arthritis (often involving several joints) with a swinging fever and a transitory red rash. There is often severe illness affecting the entire body and the condition may be complicated by enlargement of the spleen and lymph nodes and inflammation of the pericardium (heart muscle) and iris of the eye. But seven Japanese clinical investigators reported on DMSO usage for a case of Still's disease in a thirty-seven-year-old man with the adult-onset variety. He suffered from severe diarrhea.

The Japanese doctors' viewing of the patient's upper and lower gastrointestinal tract by means of endoscopy revealed swollen mucosa with white patches, erosions, bleeding, and amyloid deposits. As previously defined, amyloid is a glycoprotein, resembling starch, that is deposited in the internal organs in the presence of the pathological condition amyloidosis. Amyloidosis is infiltration of the liver, kidneys, spleen, and other tissues with amyloid. The clinicians took biopsy specimens from the man's bowel.

After they administered three months of therapy with DMSO and prednisolone, improvement in the endoscopic appearance of the patient's gastrointestinal tract was observed. Amyloid deposits in the biopsy specimens were reduced in the stomach and appeared totally negative in the large intestine. Their patient had a successful recovery from the use of DMSO.[6]

The author of *Malpractice* and *Confessions of a Medical Heretic*, Robert S. Mendelsohn, M.D., of Chicago, who before he died was Associate Professor of Preventive Medicine and Community Health in the School of Medicine of the University of Illinois, said in an interview: "From my experience with DMSO seventeen years ago, I believe it has to be approached the same way as any other medicine—with extreme caution. Should it be used for arthritis? I would regard it as any other drug—to be employed when everything else fails. My impression is that once a person begins living right in terms of good nutrition, sufficient exercise, and healthy lifestyle, his arthritis will improve all by itself. You don't have to resort to DMSO just as you don't need Indocin, codeine, Motrin, Butazolidin, gold injections, and other anti-inflammatory arthritis drugs.

"This, despite our seeing very few reports of DMSO side effect—and no fatalities. If I had to rank therapies, I would place DMSO way ahead of the conventional anti-arthritic medicines. It is preferable to any of them. But I would rank DMSO use behind proper diet and good nutrition. . . . I suggest water exercises for crippled arthritics. What happens if you can't do those water exercises? Well, if you're stuck then you go to DMSO.

"My argument is that if the Government is going to prevent you from using DMSO, it should absolutely keep you from using all the other conventional arthritis drugs, which we know have many dangers. We don't know of any dangers with DMSO. Of course," added Dr. Mendelsohn, "this kind of reasoning would put the rheumatologists out of business.

"For all the people who have come to me for relief of arthritis, what have I done? I've taken them off the drugs they've been on; I improve their diet; I start them on the water exercises. It disturbs me that I've not prescribed DMSO; I wonder why this is?

"It's a question many physicians will be putting to themselves in the forthcoming weeks. Thousands of arthritics have been wondering the same thing. When will we be able to get DMSO by prescription or over the counter, as we can with other anti-arthritic medications?"

CHAPTER 8
Adapting DMSO for Foot and Leg Problems

In the spring of 1963 DMSO was still in laboratory research, and not yet adapted for human application. That is the period when Sam Bell of Bloomington, Indiana, now the track coach at Indiana University but then coaching at Oregon State University in Corvallis, Oregon, came in contact with the solvent as a possible treatment for leg and foot problems.

"At that time, I had two athletes who were having leg problems," Mr. Bell told Senator Edward M. Kennedy, who chaired a hearing conducted July 31, 1980, by the Senate Subcommittee on Health and Scientific Research of the Committee on Labor and Human Resources. The hearing was an in-depth look by Senators Howard M. Metzenbaum (D-Ohio), Richard S. Schweiker (R-Penn.), and Orrin G. Hatch (R-Utah) who joined Senator Kennedy on the "Examination of Testing of DMSO and FDA's Role in the Process."

The two athletes Sam Bell described were Morgan Growth and Norman Hoffman, both world-class 800 meter track athletes and both potential scorers in the National Collegiate Athletic Association (NCAA). But Growth had inflammation of the Achilles tendon and Hoffman suffered with a pulled hamstring muscle.

"We had a chronic problem with both of them," Sam Bell continued, "and what we were doing trainingwise was having no effect on them. I had read in the paper some of the things that Dr. Jacob had discovered with DMSO, and I called him at the University of Oregon Medical Center and asked him if I could bring these two athletes up to see him. We went up there to visit with him, and he examined them and gave us some DMSO to use and told us how to use it. We used it topically; that is, we put it on the skin."

The recovery for Morgan Growth's leg tendon was nothing short of remarkable. The Achilles tendon injury, according to Coach Bell, is a chronic injury that hardly ever rights itself when one is really hurt. But that spring, Growth was the NCAA champion in the mile run at the University of New Mexico. And the hamstring problem for Norm Hoffman that kept him away from training was solved completely. Hoffman ended up becoming the 1963 NCAA champion in the 880 meter run.

Coach Bell had a little of the DMSO left over, and that fall, while he was doing some yard work, he sprained an ankle grubbing out a tree stump. It was the renewal of a prior injury from his college football days. "I ended up deciding maybe I ought to experiment with DMSO myself," said Bell, "and I gave myself six treatments over a period of three days. My ankle, because of it being an old injury, always swelled up very badly whenever I sprained it again. Within three days, I had no swelling, no soreness, no discoloration; I could do anything I had been doing on it."

His next experience with the drug came in the fall of 1964. At that time, Bell was running a two-day Olympic trial in track and field at Oregon State University. One of his participants was a young man, Daryll Horn, whom Bell anticipated would win a place on the United States Olympic team. Horn was the number two ranking long jumper and the number two ranking triple jumper in the country. Triple jumping entails a hop, step, and jump in a three-stage take-off, a very difficult feat that takes exceedingly strong legs. Daryll Horn had graduated from Oregon State University in midyear, 1963, and had gone into the air force. He was then allowed on detached duty to train for the Olympic trials. Just prior to those trials he was training at Stanford University in California where the Olympic trials were to take place.

Bell flew to southern California to observe the Olympic trials, but he couldn't find Horn in the training camp there. He asked Peyton Jordan, the coach from Stanford University, where the young athlete was supposed to be. Jordan said, "Well, I hate to tell you this, but he had a massive hamstring pull on Monday, and he is staying at Palo Alto to try to get treatment as long as possible before he comes down here. But there is no way he will be able to compete."

Immediately Bell got on the phone to Daryll Horn in Palo Alto, California, and heard the athlete say, "Coach, I am black and blue from the gluteus [the big butt muscle] to down below my knee. I cannot walk without a limp."

The coach told Horn to "get on an airplane and get down here as fast as you can." Then he phoned Dr. Jacob in Portland, Oregon, and asked him if he could get some DMSO to treat the young man.

"If you can have someone pick it up, I'll supply the DMSO," responded Dr. Jacob.

Bell asked a friend to go to Dr. Jacob's office and carry a supply of the solvent to the Portland airport where he found a stewardess who would take it to the Los Angeles airport. The coach met this airplane and got the DMSO.

Daryll Horn arrived for treatment on the next flight in from Palo Alto, on a Thursday with the Olympic trials scheduled for Saturday afternoon. Bell doused the athlete's injury with DMSO. The odor caused Horn's roommate to change sleeping accommodations. Skin irritation developed on Horn's leg, which they ignored. The immense discoloration of the leg injury started to fade right away and the pain went with it.

"To make a long story short," said Bell, "we practically bathed Daryll in the stuff for two days, and on Saturday afternoon, he missed [making] the Olympic team by a quarter of an inch. On Sunday, we went back and competed again, and we continued to treat him over Saturday night and Sunday morning, and he went back and competed again and he missed the Olympic team in the triple jump by a half-inch. He obviously did not come back to where he was, but the fact that he was even able to compete, I thought was a minor miracle. He competed with no discoloration of the leg; it was totally gone in two days, and the soreness was gone. I think, obviously, the strength was not quite back there, but the fact that he was able to operate at all is an amazing thing."

PUTTING DMSO TO USE IN FOOT CARE MEDICINE

At about the same time Sam Bell was making his attempt to get Daryll Horn accepted as a member of the United States Olympic team, DMSO was intriguing scientists throughout the world. Pharmaceutical companies were beginning to allocate quantities of the drug for research. They solicited participation from proven and respected medical investigators who were willing to enter into clinical trials in their separate specialties. They started to use DMSO for burns, arthritis, skin conditions, musculoskeletal pain of all kinds, and many other conditions. "Soon there were hundreds of publications reporting on 'miraculous cures' with the drug, for everything from ingrown toenails to vascular headaches," said Dr. Jack C. de la Torre, Associate Professor of Neurosurgery and Psychiatry at the University of Miami School of Medicine.

Merck and Company, one of the several pharmaceutical companies considering DMSO as a commercial product, approached various medical organizations to select outstanding members as investigators. The American Podiatry Association (APA) was asked early in 1965 to select doctors of podiatric medicine to participate. I, Morton Walker, D.P.M., had just won the 1964 APA Silver Anniversary Gold Medal for scientific research and writing, the highest award ever presented by the American Podiatry Association. Therefore, Merck and Company executives were directed to me as a candidate for their DMSO research project. The Food and Drug Administration had already approved other clinical investigations that had previously brought me nine additional research, writing, and scientific exhibit awards. I eventually won twenty-two such awards.

Merck and Company offered to pay all costs for the study and record keeping of DMSO treatment on foot and leg problems. During that 1964–1965 period, the drug companies of Merck, Syntex, Squibb, Geigy, Schering, and American Home Products collectively spent $20 million to finance clinical trials. There were 1,500 clinical investigators involved, most of them physicians. In the spring of 1965 when the Merck pharmaceutical company made its grant offer to me, Connecticut podiatrists were not permitted by law to give internal medication, so the drug would only be used on the skin for foot and leg troubles.

The year before this new Merck and Company clinical trial, I had concluded a study for the Armour Pharmaceutical Company on the chymotrypsin (a pancreatic enzyme) product Chymar (whose name has now been changed to Biozyme). For that investigation, I applied the Chymar ointment under an impervious wrapping. It was the first time plastic coverings were used in podiatry for driving a medication into the locally affected inflamed tissues of the feet, for example for corns and calluses. I adapted this technique for the DMSO clinical trial, too, and it worked quite well.

Alternately, I inaugurated a technique of driving in the DMSO, especially for a deep-seated lesion like a painful heel spur, using ultrasound. Instead of the usual ultrasound gel or mineral oil, DMSO was applied as the coupling agent between the ultrasound machine's quartz crystal and the skin. This worked well. I was able to eliminate much of my patient's heel spur inflammation.

These foot and leg studies were conducted over a four-month period starting in 1965. Certain precautions were taken before beginning the studies. Much reading on the subject was done. For two months, only a few podiatric patients received the DMSO treatment. A long memorandum from the pharmaceutical company arrived September 8, 1965, detailing all the benefits of the product, how the doctor should use it, what it's for, how DMSO acts in the body. This was a memorandum sent to every medical researcher in the country who had been certified by the FDA to use DMSO on an experimental basis. A representative of Merck and Company arrived with more DMSO supplies and with report forms for recording patient responses in a full-scale clinical trial.

Unknown to me, a woman in Ireland died from the administration of DMSO on September 9, 1965. This report was not *documented* and, in all probability, she died from other causes simply while using DMSO. But the death produced panic among officials of the FDA and brought great political repercussions for Dr. Stanley Jacob and his co-workers at the University of Oregon. No notification from the pharmaceutical company or the FDA relating to this occurrence arrived, however, and the clinical investigation on DMSO for foot and leg problems continued.

I performed clinical trials on the lower extremity problems of 124 patients. Excellent results came out of the different DMSO applications. Records were kept; objective and subjective observations were reported on the furnished forms; more DMSO supplies were requested.

This podiatric study of DMSO came to an abrupt halt November 10, 1965, when a "Dear Doctor" letter arrived advising that all research on the project must cease. The FDA demanded that the used and unused supplies of DMSO and all records of patients for whom it was administered must immediately be returned to the sponsoring pharmaceutical company. I didn't have to mail these items because a company representative promptly arrived to take everything away—all patient reports, supplies of DMSO, even duplicates of the records. Instructions were given to report any deleterious effects from the product's use, but there were none. No published report ever appeared in the medical literature on this four-month podiatric study of DMSO's adaptation for a variety of foot problems. All the records of clinical trial were confiscated, and what follows are strictly the impressions of this researcher twenty-seven years later. They are based on the patients' personal foot health histories with relation to their individual toe, foot, ankle, or leg problems.

BIG TOE BUNIONS

Bunions are formed from deviation of two adjoining bones, usually at the joint of the big toe and the first metatarsal.

There are two types of bunion. The acute type, or bursitis, is sudden and painful. If it is not given proper attention, the acute bunion may gradually develop into the second type—the chronic bunion, or *hallux valgus*, which is an often painless deformity of the big toe. Sometimes, however, it aches a lot.

The bursitis bunion is an inflammation of a bursa, a sac containing fluid about the consistency of the white of an egg. This bursa acts as a lubricant between the skin and the bones. Continual irritation by external pressure such as an ill-fitting shoe causes the sac to become inflamed, and the condition gets acute and painful—a bursitis.

Hallux valgus is a common affliction that strains the foot and produces an abnormal prominence of the big toe joint. It widens the foot to bring about a loss of balance. Standing and walking become difficult. Arthritis in the foot can occur early in life from this condition.

Osteoarthritis is a frequent consequence of ignoring the big toe bunion. Calcification at the points of stress comes on; joint expansion locks in; the deformity can be accommodated only with bigger shoes.

With DMSO application, the acute stage of bunion, primarily bursitis, improved remarkably. Hallux valgus did not. The impervious wrapping and ultrasound both worked well with DMSO painted onto the inflamed area. The procedure entailed using DMSO and ultrasound as the office treatment and sending the patient home with DMSO under the plastic cover to be held in place with a protective felt padding and supportive strapping for three days.

At the time of this study, no DMSO supply was ever dispensed for application by the patient at home because it was uncertain what the side effects would be. It was kept strictly under my control, and I made the applications in the podiatry office.

Invariably the pain of bunion disappeared by the time the patient returned. No further treatment was needed until the patient brought on a resurgence of the bunion flareup by wearing fashionable but abusive footwear.

HAMMERTOES

The hammertoe, one of the most painful of foot ailments, is marked by contracture of the tendons on the top of the foot. Accompanying this phenomenon is a laxity of the ligaments and angulation of the second and third phalanges, the individual bones of each toe.

Tight shoes compress the feet and constrict the muscles that move the toes so that the muscles waste away. The toe motions become puny and weak. The toe seeks room anywhere it can in an ill-fitting shoe. It curls up and arches until the toenail is nearly vertical. The affected toe may rise, contract, and overlap other toes. Its tip may strike the ground with each step and become flat and squat. A hard corn can form and the nail can split and grow inward. Although any toe may be so affected, the second suffers most often. It is usually longer than the other toes.

The experimental DMSO treatment was the same as with acute bunions—first ultrasound and the drug applied and then a dressing with impervious plastic wrapped over the solvent. A return visit by the patient in three days saw the pain gone from the deformed toe, although the deformity remained. The pain might return a day or two later if nothing was done to permanently correct the malformation.

ARTHRITIS OF THE FEET

Arthritis can affect the joints anywhere in the body, including the feet. Arthritis in the feet results in most instances from mechanical strain, not from infection. It is sometimes associated with knock-knees, bow-legs, flat feet, and weak feet. The condition also contributes to such deformities of the feet as fallen arches, high-arched foot, hammertoes, bunions, and heel spurs.

Although arthritis cannot be cured at this time, the aching distress and discomfort that accompany the disease can be partially relieved. Treatment of arthritis of the feet must be directed both at the general cause and to the relief of local symptoms.

The general treatment of the problem is the responsibility of your family physician, for the entire body and its general breakdown may be involved. Treatment may involve building up your resistance with diet, exercise, relaxation techniques, weight control, and other things that might constitute your lifestyle. Local treatment may include foot rest, heat applications, splinting, traction, physical therapy, and the use of drugs. The specific causes will be looked at, such as mechanical strains, allergic factors, climatic conditions, congenital defects, tumors, infection, injury, toxins, disturbances of the circulation, poor nutrition, and others.

Using DMSO as a local treatment, it's likely you'll be able to help yourself a great deal. The following regimen of care may give relief to a red, hot, swollen arthritic joint, whether in the heel, the ankle, or the big toe. Arthritic toes respond quite well to this procedure:

1. Paint the acutely inflamed joint with a quantity of DMSO in about

70-percent strength or a little higher concentration. Don't go beyond 90 percent because the method of wrapping that follows may bring about a severe skin reaction from the DMSO under the hot wrap.

2. Apply several layers of roller gauze over the entire foot that's inflamed.
3. Rather than painting the skin directly, you might wrap with the gauze first and then saturate it with DMSO.
4. Cover the whole area with rubber sheeting or thin foam rubber.
5. Apply a layer of flannel or felt that has been dipped in hot water and wrung out.
6. Put hot water bottles around the inflamed area or cover it with an electric heating pad wrapped in towels.
7. Hold in the heat by covering all the above with Turkish towels.
8. Elevate the foot and leg in bed to a level with the heart.
9. Continue this treatment for as long as you are comfortable with it, but not longer than sixty minutes for any single application.
10. Reapply the DMSO every four or five hours, as needed.
11. After you've used this treatment for twelve hours (a maximum of three times), remove pads, bottles, gauze, and wash the foot so as to take off any DMSO. Apply a soothing lotion or ointment of the cortisone family, or aloe vera to the treated foot.

Caution: Note that you are using two forms of therapy in this procedure—DMSO with its anti-inflammatory properties, and moist heat with its own inflammation-reducing effect. The heat seems to catalyze the DMSO into even greater effectiveness. But I caution that you can get too much of a DMSO skin reaction—even too much of an anti-inflammation response. Too much of anything is no good. Therefore, I strongly suggest that you take precautions with this treatment, at least the first few times you use it. Keep checking the condition of your arthritic joint and the skin over it. Don't allow skin irritation to set in. Take your body temperature; if you become at all feverish, discontinue the procedure. Remove the wrappings as described in step eleven and soothe the foot. This is a highly powerful way to rid the involved foot of an arthritic inflammation.

In practice, in 1965, this method was used with success, but it was administered by a doctor of podiatric medicine who knew the sort of reactions to avoid. The pain, swelling, and other signs of inflammation disappeared from a patient's feet in the foot care office while the patient occupied a small treatment room. He or she went home without discomfort, and the relief lasted several days.

HARD AND SOFT CORNS

About 40 percent of all persons who visit a podiatrist do so initially because of hard and soft corn problems, and women comprise 80 percent of these people.

Hard corns are growths of horny skin, generally on the top of the toes. Soft corns grow between the toes. Both types can be easily distinguished from the normal tissue surrounding them. Within a hard or soft corn is a central radix, or eye, of hard gray skin, and around the center is a painful inflamed ring of skin and flesh. The ring is raised and yellow. Pain usually is the main symptom.

The corns come from friction and pressure arising from an underlying prominence of bone. The sharp edge on the toe bone rubs the skin from inside and sometimes wrong-fitting shoes rub the skin from the outside. The skin eventually dies and builds up layer after layer to create the corn. Irritation and pain increase as the corn grows.

People suffering from corns can be relieved of their problem either temporarily or permanently. Nobody has to feel the agony of hard corns. Temporary relief does nothing to prevent the corns from growing again at the same place. It is palliative.

Painting DMSO on corns was just such a temporary measure. It was done after the corn was shaved to remove the horny skin causing discomfort. No padding with moleskin was necessary after palliative corn removal if DMSO application followed the procedure; however, the corn soon returned without permanent removal of the underlying bony prominence.

CALLUSES

Calluses are thickened masses of skin that form on the weight-bearing surfaces of the feet. They come from constant friction and pressure. The pathological callus such as one developed on the ball of the foot is not healthy.

This kind of plantar callus is surrounded by an inflamed red rim and has fluid permeating the underlying tissue. It is often swollen, hot, and painful and frequently appears as a hard, dry, hornlike mass of yellowish or grayish skin. It may be thick in the center and gradually taper at the sides. Within its center could be a deep, hard, gray central area that seems like a pebble when removed.

Because the thickened skin of calluses loses its elasticity, the skin no longer stretches to normal length across the ball of the foot when the feet are flexed. These calluses seem to "burn."

Sometimes corrective treatment means redistributing the weight on the foot with supportive orthotic devices worn in the shoes. Exercises may be prescribed. Footgear might be changed. Or surgical correction of the involved metatarsal bone and the associated contraction of the toes may be required. Most of the time the person with calluses goes to have them pared away. If DMSO is put on after such paring, no moleskin padding is required to rid the area of tenderness. However, DMSO does not penetrate the hornlike skin without such removal first.

PLANTAR WARTS

Plantar warts grow on the sole of the foot as raised lumps of flesh. They are benign tumor-like growths that are well supplied with blood vessels and nerves. You may mistake them for corns or calluses because they are covered with callus tissue and because they hurt.

The plantar wart is pearly white, soft and spongy, and has tiny spots, black, brown, or red, in its center. These spots are the blood vessels. Walking flattens the wart so that it remains thickened and rough in texture. Varying in size from a pinhead to a silver quarter, it may grow either singularly or in clusters. It hurts severely when pinched.

Injury to the plantar of the foot allows entrance of a virus into the skin that may cause the plantar wart to grow. In fact, there are wart seasons, those times in the summer when people walk barefoot and bruise the bottoms of their feet.

A variety of techniques to get rid of plantar warts exists. DMSO application is not one of them. All it does is take away plantar wart pain after the overlying hard skin layer is shaved. If this is done and a plastic wrap put on over DMSO, the wart macerates, softens, and possibly may go away on its own.

INGROWN TOENAILS

With ingrown toenails, the lateral edges of a nail penetrate the skin and cut into the flesh of the toe. Unless soon corrected, severe complications can result.

The complications of inflammation, infection, ulceration, and gangrene may follow one another progressively. Anyone who suffers from ingrown toenails seldom is able to endure the pain and usually seeks aid before the more serious complications develop. Teenagers seem to be especially susceptible, perhaps because they tend to disregard the early warnings that adults will heed.

Injudicious cutting of toenails is the most frequent cause. At first, inflammation appears, then in turn discoloration, a mild swelling, and some escape of fluid. Pus forms, redness increases, and the toe balloons with pain if these preliminary signs are ignored. A bloody mass of material called "proud flesh" will arise at the edge of the nail between the nail plate and the nail groove.

If treatment has not been given by now, a dangerous infection may spread along the whole toe, and red streaks will eventually appear along the top of the foot. This needn't occur when treatment is swift, painless, and permanent.

DMSO relieves the beginning symptoms of ingrown toenails merely by placing a drop on the inflamed area. But this may not be the best procedure because of the other progressive symptoms leading to infection.

CLUB NAILS

Older people sometimes have thick, ugly, deformed toenails, a condition that may be symptomatic of a systemic disease or chronic injury such as jogging in poorly fitting running shoes. Injury often causes the toenails to look discolored, elongated, and thickened.

Overgrown toenails are known as club nails. They may become extremely hard and curl under the toes, to give the shape of a grotesque ram's horn. Reduction of these nails does not have to be painful. In fact, it's best to keep a ram's horn-like toenail cut as short as possible so as to avoid providing surrounding parasitic fungi a nesting place in which to grow.

The nails are first rubbed with castor oil or warm olive oil combined with 90 percent DMSO. This softens and reduces sensitivity of the nails at their roots. Then they are cut with strong nail clippers. Smoothing down the rough edges is required so that hosiery won't be snagged. Besides, this gives the overly thick nail a more pleasing appearance.

However, the main purpose in the reduction of overgrown nails is to remove pressure on the nail grooves and thus eliminate the source of discomfort. Reduction also leaves more space in the shoe in which the toe may move. More room in the shoe may also relieve pressure and prevent corns from forming on adjacent toes.

After the above procedure is completed, the flattened nails may be painted with a mixture of DMSO and oil again. This gives a prolonged effect of comfort and brings the formerly compressed tissues underneath back to a more normal state.

Thereafter, to prevent overgrowing such as the club nail condition described here, observe the following simple procedures:

- When you cut your toenails, cut them short, but cut them square— straight across.
- Use toenail clippers. Do not, in any case, round the nails.
- After cutting, place one drop of DMSO in a medium strength onto the cut end.

There is little in the human anatomy that does not serve a specific purpose. Just as the hair on the head has its function, so the toenails have theirs—in this case, to protect the bones and the nerves of the toes. Yet because we wear shoes, the toenails, instead of protecting the toes, can be a potential source of annoyance. However, we can insure ourselves against the problems they may cause by caring for them properly.

FUNGUS TOENAILS

Infections of the toenails caused by a fungus are among the most frequently seen nail afflictions. One out of every four persons over the age of thirty who visit podiatrists has such a nail malady.

Fungus toenails are caused by parasites such as yeasts, molds, or fungi, all of which grow as ringworm. These parasites are prevalent in shoes, which, because they are the only item of clothing that is never thoroughly cleaned inside, are a constant source of infection and reinfection.

Fungus toenails appear dry, lusterless, scaly, and streaked; they are raised from the nail bed; and they have a grayish-yellowish-brownish worm-eaten look. Part or all of the nail may be affected because, as the infection progresses, it works back toward the nail root. The average person pays no attention to the nail's crumpled appearance because it is painless. But the infected nails are a source of athlete's foot.

In treating fungus toenails, a podiatrist removes the crusted, powdery substance that forms, and files the nail thin. He may prescribe the oral antibiotic griseofulvin, ionize the area with copper sulfate, or apply various liquid and ointment fungicides. In many cases the nails are removed entirely, either temporarily or permanently, depending on the severity of the problem. If the nail is temporarily removed, the doctor directs his treatment to the nail bed and to the growth center from which the new nail will grow uninfected with fungus. This is where DMSO works effectively.

A paste is made from 30 cc of the 90 percent liquid solvent, with two 250 mg microsize griseofulvin tablets. Spread the paste into the nail matrix area after healing of the nail bed has taken place. Hold the DMSO paste in position with an adhesive strip and treat the toenails in the same way every day. Newly formed uninfected toenails should appear from under the flesh in a couple of months following surgery. Keep putting on the paste for the entire time it takes for the whole toenail to grow over the nail bed—about six months.

Other liquid fungicides may be mixed with DMSO and painted onto the healed nail bed. Form a puddle under the flap of flesh overiding the toenail growth center. As the nail grows out it will be in continuous touch with the penetrating fungicide, particularly if a piece of plastic is taped over the toe. The DMSO is itself fungistatic, so you are treating the problem with two remedies at once.

ATHLETE'S FOOT

The medical name for athlete's foot, *tinea pedis*, best describes it and its cause. *Tinea* means "fungus" and *pedis*, "of the foot." But please realize that "athlete's foot" describes the set of symptoms and not the main cause.

Fungus by itself does not create the foot disease. Because it is a parasite, fungus must have the proper medium in which to thrive. The skin of the foot, encased in a hot shoe, with the heat incubating fungus growth, is that superb medium. Much as a toadstool lives and grows in topsoil, the fungus lives and grows on dead skin, such as the dead skin of corns and calluses. It is present on the feet of hundreds of thousands of people, men more commonly than women, because women's shoes are more open and allow the dispersion of the heat generated in walking.

Once a person has been infected, the symptoms show quickly as scaling between the toes or along the borders of the heels and the longitudinal arches. There is itching and maceration with wrinkling and peeling skin. The sure sign of athlete's foot is tiny blisters that appear in groups that may break open, leaving circular, shiny, red areas underneath.

The symptoms are known to recur from warm season to warm season in 80 percent of cases; it is chronic in four out of five infected persons. Still, there is excellent treatment available in the form of antifungal remedies applied to the feet with DMSO as the carrying vehicle. This solvent penetrates the upper skin layers and sends the antifungal agent deep into the tissue to kill any fungus on top of or within the skin. Additionally, DMSO is itself a fungistatic substance that stops athlete's foot symptoms by discouraging growth of the pesky parasite.

To help yourself get rid of athlete's foot, the procedure followed by health professionals is to dress the infected skin with the suitable athlete's foot remedy for the type of symptoms you're treating: a cream for sore, exposed skin surfaces; an ointment for thickened, scaling areas; a liquid for unbroken blisters. Then, cover this remedy with the matching form of DMSO: cream, gel, or liquid. Use not less than a 70-percent strength of DMSO for more effective penetrating power. The condition should disappear in a short time and possibly not recur, especially if you keep this remedy at hand.

FOOT ODOR

Foot odor, one of the most annoying problems, although it is neither painful nor infectious, is known scientifically as *bromidrosis.*

Bromidrosis is not necessarily due to lack of cleanliness. While proper foot hygiene will help, foot odor is, genuinely, a physiological problem. Those who suffer from it are subject to humiliating social situations. The main cause is a functional disturbance in the nervous system. More than washing the feet is needed to bring relief and to eliminate the annoyance.

The symptoms of bromidrosis are, besides the obvious smell, a sogginess of the skin between the toes and tenderness of the flesh of the foot. There may be tiny blisters on the balls of the feet or on the heels.

Foot odor does not always yield quickly to treatment. However, there are methods that will diminish the problem and maybe eliminate it altogether.

Painting the soles of the feet with 50 percent DMSO is possibly one of them. Although it may seem you are merely substituting one bad smell for another, the DMSO odor will go away in a day or two leaving the feet free of their own bad odor—at least for a time. The longer you keep the DMSO on, the longer the foot odor stays away.

As an aside, I do advise that many people find dramatic relief from "smelly feet" by eliminating sugar from the diet, taking adequate amounts of B complex vitamins, and taking a zinc supplement.

DANCER'S FOOT

Dancer's foot is an inflammation and, in severe cases, a displacement or fracture of the two small bones located beneath the head of the first metatarsal. As you would suspect, it most frequently affects people who dance a lot.

The sesamoid bones are located in tendons that run beneath the big toe joint. Their function is to lessen the friction as the tendons move. Unusual stress can injure these two small bones.

Dancing places an unusual weight on the sesamoids and damage can occur. Inflammation and pain jeopardize the dancer's ability to perform. If he or she ignores the pain, the small, tender sesamoid bones may fracture or be displaced. It can happen to anyone and not just to dancers.

In treating this foot problem, a diagnosis is mandatory. Then, appropriate padding of the joint is called for after physical therapy measures reduce the inflammation. DMSO with ultrasound proved excellent as the particular form of physical therapy. It took inflammation out of the dancer's foot condition right away. The pad applied then is placed on the foot, in the shoe, or as part of an orthotic to shield the sesamoids from undue stress.

METATARSALGIA

Metatarsalgia, or Morton's toe, is a sudden sharp, stabbing pain felt in the toes. Morton's toe comes on from an inflammation of the nerve between the third and fourth metatarsal bones that produces an agonizing feeling. Runners are sometimes the victims of this neuralgic pain.

Metatarsalgia is caused by the compression of a small toe nerve between two displaced metatarsal bones. Inflammation occurs when the head of one displaced metatarsal presses against another and catches the nerve between them. With every step the nerve is rubbed, pressed, and irritated. Consequently, the involved nerve becomes enlarged with a sheath of scar tissue that forms to protect it. The tissue enlarges into a neuroma that must eventually be removed surgically to get total relief of the pain.

The podiatrist may bring relief of Morton's toe using techniques other than neuroma surgery. This can be done with injections of a local anesthetic mixed with DMSO into the foot. A pad may be placed in the shoe to spread the metatarsal heads away from each other. Or, orthotic appliances may be worn by the patient. The podiatrist takes the precaution of injecting very slowly, because intramuscular injections may produce pain, though the local anesthetic tends to disguise it. Good technique will avoid discomfort for the patient.

FALLEN ARCHES

So-called "fallen arches" really are weakened feet that are so strained they have developed symptoms.

In the classic case of fallen arches, nearly all the bones of the foot change position. The heel bone rolls inward, the ankle drops, the shin becomes more prominent, the cuboid bone is forced outward, and both the big toe and the fifth toe rise. The other bones sink, and the inner longitudinal arch "falls."

The victims feel pain and burning in the foot and tiredness and aching pain in the legs. They cannot stand or walk for any length of time. Painful calluses may grow on the ball of the foot because the front metatarsal arch falls, as well.

Check yourself for fallen arches by looking for a "flatness" of your feet. Or, stand before a mirror and observe the backs of your feet. Notice whether the heel tendons bow inward toward each other. This is *Helbing's sign.*

Relief from the discomfort of fallen arches comes from treatment with a variety of devices designed by the podiatry profession. The podiatrist may restore normal function to damaged muscles and ligaments in three steps: (1) physical therapy using DMSO and ultrasound to reduce the inflammation, (2) application of a corrective strapping, and (3) making a pair of orthotics for the weakened feet. The length of time you have the trouble and its severity determine how effective DMSO three-step treatment will be. Realize that if nothing is done to manage the fallen arches, there will be periodic episodes of pain as the symptoms appear, are treated and disappear, and appear again.

DMSO seems highly efficacious for acute foot problems but hardly effective for chronic foot problems, except for chronic calcaneal spur inflammation.

HEEL SPURS

On the heel bone, the *calcaneus,* a spurlike growth of calcium, sometimes forms where the muscles and ligaments of the foot are attached. One or more spurs grow on the heel bone, but are padded by the flesh of the foot, so that the spur may take years to become a problem.

The heel spur hurts when you place your weight on the bone. Anyone may be affected. Women are as likely to suffer from it as men. It is seen most often in persons past forty, and the condition may be associated with arthritis or poor circulation.

The underlying cause is chronic foot strain brought on by weak feet, prolonged standing, improper footgear, or structural misalignment of the feet. In each case, the feet are inadequate to the tasks they must perform and strain brings on physiological change with overgrowth of calcification.

The pain comes actually not from the spur point but from the inflammation around the muscles where they are attached to the bone. It is most severe when you start to walk after a rest.

For full relief of painful heel spurs, the doctor will diagnose and analyze the problem and recommend a course of treatment. It should include ultrasound and DMSO employed daily to take out the deep-seated pain of inflammation. The DMSO impervious wrap is also excellent to strap onto the heel to pull out the painful inflammation.

ANKLE SPRAINS

The sprained ankle, a common injury, is the result of a violent twisting of the foot. You may sprain an ankle quite casually as you stroll along the street. You may sprain it when you step upon an uneven surface, like a rock or a curbstone, when you catch a high heel in a grating, or when you jump from any height. The more active you are, the greater the possibility that you will sprain your ankle.

Since a sprain occurs if the foot is twisted, it is most likely to happen when the foot is somehow off balance. When the weight of the body comes down on the foot, instead of being transmitted directly to the ground, it is caught on only one side of the foot. The strain placed on the ligaments when the foot is off balance and the weight suddenly thrust upon it will be greater than the ligaments can withstand. Consequently, the ligaments that connect the anklebone and the shinbone tear. The more violently the ankle is twisted, the greater the damage and pain.

Immediately after the sprain, the signs and symptoms of injury appear. Placing any weight directly on the injured foot may cause pain. If the sprain is slight, the ankle becomes tender and sensitive. If the sprain is severe, the ankle may become hot, swollen, tender, and so painful that you cannot walk. The ankle becomes discolored, sometimes red, sometimes blue. As the swelling increases, it is accompanied by throbbing.

Emergency care for a sprained ankle can begin even before you get to a doctor. First, take weight off the ankle. Sit down. When a sprain is truly severe, this suggestion is scarcely necessary, for in such cases walking will cause considerable pain. But you can get some comfort within a few minutes by dosing the torn ligaments or pulled muscles with 90 percent DMSO. You may feel some burning or see redness appear, but the pain of inflammation will go out of the ankle.

Still, don't bear weight on the ankle. The seriousness of the injury cannot always be determined immediately, for the symptoms don't appear all at once. The sprain may seem to be only a temporary impediment, especially with the swift application of topical DMSO, but using the ankle may easily increase the damage. Do not take the risk.

The DMSO will reduce the swelling or prevent it from coming up altogether. Devise a proper support for the ankle by wrapping gauze over the DMSO-moistened skin, covering with impervious plastic kitchen wrap, and taping with one-inch strips of adhesive strapping over everything. Eliminating the pain, remember, is not healing the sprain; support is mandatory to hold the torn ligaments against the leg bone so that they don't move much. Change the strapping every four days, wash the skin each time, recoat with DMSO, and keep up this procedure until there is no more pain from the direct pressure of palpation with your fingers.

The majority of sufferers of foot and leg problems, instead of seeking professional care, turn to the many gadgets, special materials, and patent medicines that are widely promoted as cures. Most of these products are, unfortunately, ineffective; some must have been invented in the offices of the advertising agencies that promote them. Others are "family recipes" that have been handed down from generation to generation, given new names, packaged artfully, and marketed at high prices.

The money you spend for foot gadgets often is utterly wasted. Still, the public goes from one "remedy" to another in its never-ending search for relief.

There are no panaceas. The only truly effective products for use on the feet are those that have been tested and proved in laboratories, in clinics, and in doctors' offices. Yet the one medication that seems to be most applicable to foot and leg problems—as close to a panacea as we can come—is DMSO. It is useful for a broad range of lower limb difficulties and should be considered as an excellent emergency remedy and follow-up therapy for the many troubles that plague our feet.

CHAPTER 9

Using DMSO in Head and Spinal Cord Injuries

Clara M. Fox of Toutle, Washington, was stunned September 15, 1979, to learn that her son Bill had a near-fatal injury that left the young man completely paralyzed. Through a series of hospital transfers during the first six hours, William J. Shaal was taken to the University of Oregon Health and Science Center in Portland after his devastating accident. It was a lucky move because DMSO is a therapeutic ingredient used in this institution's surgical intensive care unit. George Greccos, M.D., the physician attending Bill Shaal's case, made intravenous infusion with the experimental drug an integral part of his treatment during the first ten days.

Bill had a broken neck; he was paralyzed from the site of injury downward. He couldn't willfully urinate, defecate, move any limbs, talk, eat, or perform any other kind of voluntary function. With his head cleanly shaven, ugly but necessary steel tongs were drilled into his skull to keep the spinal column immobilized. Thin ropes and pulleys with weights attached stretched his neck at the crucial point, in order for it to come back into place and possibly heal. He remained in traction for forty-five days after coming out of intensive care where he had teetered between life and death for four days. The youth was eventually hospitalized for over six months.

Spinal cord injuries are extremely serious, and lacerations or cuts across the cord inevitably leave the accident victim permanently without function. An acute transverse cord lesion causes immediate flaccid paralysis and loss of all sensation and function of the autonomic system below the level of injury. The flaccid paralysis gradually changes over hours or days to spastic paraplegia due to exaggeration of the normal stretch reflex. The limbs exhibit spontaneous jumps or spasms. Later, if the spinal cord in the lumbosacral region is not entirely severed, extensor or flexor muscle spasms appear, and deep tendon reflexes and autonomic reflexes return very gradually.

Depending on how complete the trauma to the cord is, there may be only partial motor and sensory nerve loss. Voluntary movement could return but it is disordered; sensory loss is determined by which portion of the spinal tract is affected. The lost or impaired senses may include the sense of posture, vibration, light touch or pain, temperature, and deep touch. A half-cut through the cord results in spastic paralysis, loss of postural sense on the side cut through, and loss of pain and heat sense on the opposite side.

With an injury such as that sustained by young Bill, the severed nerve processes in the cord cannot recover and damage often becomes permanent. Still, if there is any movement or sensation during the first week after the injury, the signs are favorable for some recovery. Any dysfunction remaining after six months is likely to remain permanent.

Severe cord injury above the fifth cervical vertebra is usually fatal. Bill's was at that point. Certainly there is motor and sensory loss, and the reflex arcs that control the bladder, sexual activity in men, and bowel function are destroyed.

While DMSO works effectively for healing spinal cord lesions when administered intravenously within ninety minutes of the injury, Bill Shaal did not get the DMSO until seven hours later. Yet, after several days he began to have distinct feelings in his shoulders and arms, then in his upper chest to just below the nipples. His family was overjoyed to see that his senses were returning, Clara Fox said, ". . . and before he was taken off the drug, he was even beginning to experience feelings and sensations in his bladder and kidneys, asking for his urinal time and again, and in each case, actually urinating in it. Of course you can imagine the excitement that came with each new discovery."

This was phenomenal, because Bill's problem was so serious that Dr. Greccos, when he met the family coming into the hospital the first time, showed them the patient's X-rays and explained that their son might not live. He said most of the reason Bill had even made it that far was due to his excellent physical and mental condition. The physician added candidly that if Bill did live, he would undoubtedly be paralyzed for the remainder of his life, from the site of injury in his neck on down.

During the course of the first two weeks, the patient fought off three bouts of pneumonia and a very bad urinary tract infection. It is not uncommon for victims of cervical cord damage to have respiratory difficulties and bladder problems. The family members, the patient, and the doctor realized, however, that DMSO had literally saved the young man's life by drawing the fluid and pressure from his spinal cord and head while slowly restoring feeling in his body. Without intravenous infusion of the drug, he would have died.

Much of the cartilage in the patient's neck had disintegrated. Bill needed an operation to remedy this, and it was performed five weeks after the hospital staff had taken him off DMSO. The surgical procedure involved implanting two stainless steel surgical rods in the back of his neck, fused together with some bone and muscle taken from his left hip. The operation was definitely successful.

A physical therapy program had been incorporated as part of the rehabilitative process, but postoperative pain prevented the patient from participating in it. He needed more fervor in exercising but couldn't find it in himself. As the days rolled by, he slowly deteriorated, which the young man and his mother traced to the need for reintroducing DMSO intravenous treatments. The only thing the hospital staff allowed was some topical applications of the drug to the painful areas in his neck, shoulders, arms, and other parts of his body. DMSO on the skin did minimize the pain.

Then some family members began to notice smooth and fluid motions in Bill's legs when they applied the solvent. His mother described these motions to the hospital staff, but her descriptions were dismissed as probably the spontaneous jumps or spasms of paralysis from hemisection of the cord. The nurses and medical students in this teaching hospital regarded the motions as simply natural leg spasms that occur from time to time.

"Then one day, one of his legs made such a motion while Dr. Greccos was standing by talking to him. The doctor came out of Bill's room with a look quite close to awe and wonderment, and flatly stated that now he realized what we were talking about, and instantly agreed that this indeed was not a regular spasm, but something quite different on which to speculate in the coming weeks," said his mother. "For close to three months after they took Bill off the DMSO, we fought daily to have the intravenous procedure continued, without much luck. But we finally got our point across shortly after the Christmas holidays, and they did agree, but with certain stipulations."

The medical staff wanted to move the patient across the city for a series of neurological tests run on special equipment at Good Samaritan Hospital. If these tests indicated any hope of noticeable improvement to which they could credit DMSO, then they would put him back on the drug twice a week for a number of weeks. After that, he would be returned to Good Samaritan for another series of the same tests and reevaluated. If there were not significant changes, then the IV DMSO would be discontinued.

"From that time on," reported Mrs. Fox, "Bill quickly and steadily improved, to the point where he could now tolerate maximum occupational and physical therapy for three to five hours per day without any pain; just sheer exhaustion from working himself so hard. He jumped from lifting two-and-a-half pounds of weights on his right arm and wrist, to between fifty to sixty pounds; and from one-and-a-half with his left arm and wrist to between thirty-five and forty. By being able to accomplish this, he has worked back his triceps [muscle] in the right arm, which up to then had been gone; and I might add, a very good biceps muscle of which he is extremely proud, and ready to take on anyone in a good arm wrestling match. And slowly but surely, the left triceps is coming around, and we are increasingly confident that before long, he will also have all of that back."

On March 13, 1980, Bill was taken back to Good Samaritan Hospital to have the earlier tests rerun and reevaluated. The results were nothing short of amazing. All readings in the prior tests indicated his dramatic improvement. Additionally, the patient showed that he had nerve sensory motions in his right foot. The patient was being restored to near what he had once been.

He was permanently dismissed from the hospital. Bill came home able to feed himself, brush his teeth, shave, comb his hair, dress, and bathe himself.

Where six months before he was more dead than alive and the family prepared for his lifetime of complete paralysis, now the young man was able to operate his manual wheelchair aptly by himself. Even a month before, he couldn't manipulate the wheelchair alone. But DMSO intravenous injections had changed all that.

"During the last six months, I have spent many hours in Dr. Jacob's clinic with his beautiful and caring staff, watching miracle after miracle happen right in front of my eyes," wrote Clara M. Fox to Claude Pepper, then Chairman of the House of Representatives Select Committee on Aging. "I have seen people who have been totally paralyzed for twenty years or more being treated and starting to move. The wonder in their eyes is indeed a sight to behold. I have witnessed the awe in the eyes and actions of a young couple whose child is being treated for Down's syndrome, and listened with rapt attention as they relate how far that child has come from death's door to today. I have sent or personally brought people with various illnesses or pains to Dr. Jacob's clinic and seen them smile with utmost satisfaction at having been cured or helped after years of discomfort and pain. And then I have sat back and watched Dr. Jacob absolutely ecstatic after another successful case of treatment. How very proud and happy he is to be able to help this human race of ours.

"I have also done a lot of reading and research into the full and real story of this remarkable drug, and I can only summarize with all my hopes and prayers, along with millions of others, that this humble man can see all his work and dreams materialize into that final success of having DMSO returned to the market by the Federal Drug Administration, so that all Americans might have the chance to be helped or saved through all those efforts. I urge everyone connected with this possibility to please check carefully all the facts, and help to answer these prayers."

DMSO RESEARCH INTO REVERSING
NEUROLOGICAL DISORDERS

Laboratory experiments are continuing with DMSO used to treat simulated trauma created in the spinal cords of monkeys. Under ideal conditions, the external factors and reproducibility of the monkey injuries are closely controlled, and "the effects of DMSO have been often dramatic, sometimes unusual, and seldom without effect," says Jack C. de la Torre, Sc.D., M.D., Chief of the Department of Neurosurgery, University of Miami School of Medicine, Miami, Florida. He was interviewed at the semi-annual meeting of the DMSO Society of Florida, Inc., held in Sarasota, Florida, in November 1980. "The important question facing our research at the present time is not so much whether DMSO works, since this has been repeatedly shown in our laboratory and those of others, but . . . how does it work?"

Dr. de la Torre's experience with DMSO currently spans twenty-four years, and includes both basic and clinical research. He has been experimenting with head and spinal cord injuries, stroke, burns, urine excretion, respiratory stimulation, brain swelling, and cellular mechanisms. He uses seven different species of animals, including human beings. He has discovered that DMSO exerts a positive effect on a number of life-threatening conditions, including head and spinal cord trauma, cerebral embolism, and respiratory distress.

Neurological head and spinal cord injuries and stroke are complex medical problems. Nevertheless, DMSO's wide range of action makes it useful in many of these cases. Through a combination of increased diffusion of fluids across body membranes and dehydration, the solvent relieves the damaging swelling and pressure that often accompany head and spinal injury. This relief comes about by the substance crossing both the skin barrier and the blood-brain barrier. The blood-brain barrier is a protective mechanism that exists between circulating blood and the brain, which limits the number of molecules reaching the brain. It prevents certain foreign proteins, natural body proteins, and other substances from entering, some of which may be toxic to nervous tissue.

"At first we thought that this property of DMSO might be a disadvantage," says Dr. de la Torre, "because we assumed that once it penetrated the barrier, it would simply accumulate in the nervous tissue and cause more swelling. What it does in fact is enter the tissue, pick up water madly, and then rush it out of the system, relieving the pressure."

The ability of DMSO to rapidly cross skin and blood-brain barriers enables it to assist in the penetration of other drugs, as was pointed out earlier. "For example, some tumors in the brain must be treated with chemotherapy injections. Huge quantities have to be injected before the drug begins to work, and at that point the toxicity of the drug may kill the patient," said de la Torre. "If you have a drug, such as DMSO, that can transport the anti-cancer agent into the tumor and the immediately surrounding area, you can use decreasing concentrations of the chemotherapy agent."

Because DMSO can penetrate skin barriers with ease, but not damage cells, DMSO is in a class by itself as a new healing principle. Furthermore, it protects the cells from mechanical damage.

Ramon Lim, M.D., Associate Professor of Neurosurgery and Research Associate in Biochemistry at the University of Chicago School of Medicine, has conducted some experiments using DMSO with glial cells. Glial cells comprise the supporting tissue of the brain and spinal cord. Dr. Lim prepares cultures of glial cells and DMSO, which he then subjects to sound vibrations. DMSO prevents cellular membranes from breaking under the vibrations, preserving the contents of each cell. The saclike lysosomes contained within cells, for example, would release enzymes harmful to other cell systems if they escaped the confines of their parent cells, and thus aggravate swelling and pressure. With DMSO instilled within the cells, this enzyme release by lysosomes doesn't take place, as shown by Dr. Lim's experiments on the glial cells.

Much of the permanent neurological damage in head injury and stroke is caused by a reduction of blood flow into the brain. An interrupted blood flow results in an inadequate supply of oxygen and nutrients to brain tissue. DMSO permits better blood flow by lessening platelet adhesiveness and aggregation and clot formation. Ordinarily, these are conditions that can clog the veins and arteries.

DMSO stimulates the release of a prostaglandin that increases blood vessel diameter. It also inhibits the release of another prostaglandin that constricts vessels and reduces blood flow.

Dr. de la Torre stresses that spinal cord injury patients who are candidates for DMSO treatment have to meet two criteria. First, the accident victim's injury must be recent, for if it is more than a few hours old, the pathologic consequences will have been well established. It won't be reversible by any means. "In our DMSO research experience, one-and-a-half hours has been the limit," says the neurosurgeon. "We do not know how long this limit can successfully be extended, because it depends upon the site and extent of the lesion."

The second criterion for a patient is that he has to have so serious a spinal cord injury that conventional treatment would be of no use, and spontaneous recovery would be impossible. "Many patients arrive with a loss of sensory sensation, and even a loss of motor ability, and yet they recover, sometimes without treatment," de la Torre says. "If DMSO is administered to such patients, there is no way to determine whether their recovery is spontaneous or due to the action of the drug."

How does a doctor isolate the patients who will not recover with conventional therapy? "We have a test, called the somatosensory evoked response," he says, "which measures activity at the somatosensory cortex in the brain when a stimulus is applied to a peripheral nerve. If there is permanent damage to the spinal cord, no activity will be recorded. From our experience with laboratory animals, we believe patients with no response will probably not recover motor function. By reversing this non-recording of activity in the brain with DMSO, we know we have done something."

THE EMERGENCY THERAPEUTIC PRINCIPLE

DMSO has been referred to as a "therapeutic principle" by its co-discoverers. It is a drug that is useful in a number of diseases that have no common denominator. "I think this comment refers to the fact that there has been very little exploration of the drug as a pharmacotherapeutic agent," says de la Torre. "The more we study it, perhaps the more we will discover about its potential application in a number of disorders, used both alone and in combination with other drugs."

He believes that DMSO is establishing its therapeutic benefit, without toxicity, in a large number of serious health problems. He thinks it should be carried in ambulances and paramedical units as an emergency therapeutic tool. "I think that this would be almost mandatory," says de la Torre, "especially if we establish that these severe kinds of injuries to the spine and the brain become permanent within four hours. Using some established criteria to evaluate the injury, a paramedic would apply or not apply DMSO, depending on each individual case. If we can establish that it does no harm in any condition, then it might be injected as a prophylactic drug, even for an injury that is considered permanent at that moment."

The neurosurgeon and his former colleagues at the Division of Neurosurgery, the University of Chicago Hospital, Drs. John F. Mullen, K. Kajihara, and Henry Kawanaga, saw some startling results from their own work with the drug, and reported this at scientific meetings. "We always played down the effects of DMSO," says de la Torre, "because the drug had had a miraculous label attached to it. Doctors tended to elbow each other at meetings and giggle, implying 'how can anything be that good?'"

Over time, the pharmacologic versatility of DMSO finally has been confirmed among numbers of clinicians who have experimented with it privately. "I do not see many doctors giggling anymore; they are beginning to suspect that there is something to this after all," says de la Torre. "I think that when more people learn to accept DMSO not as a miracle drug, but as a drug with many potential uses, perhaps they will be stimulated to go to their laboratories and begin to do some of this work." More research is needed, for research is what the FDA demands before DMSO can be released as an approved drug for a larger number of applications.

ANIMAL EXPERIMENTS USING DMSO IN BRAIN EMBOLISM

Occlusive infarction of the brain occurs when there is death of brain tissue from a cutoff of the blood supply. The blood that brings oxygen and nutrients may be blocked by a blood clot called a *thrombus* or by a plug of clotted blood or foreign materials called an *embolus*.

To study the action of DMSO on the gross manifestations of such occlusive brain infarctions, twenty normal rhesus monkeys of either sex were used in a laboratory study by medical scientists from the University of Chicago School of Medicine and the Eastern Virginia Medical School who pooled their resources and talents.[1]

Symptoms of brain infarction can be simulated in monkeys by injecting them with air to cause a cerebral air embolism. They will go into convulsions, experience sensory changes, show eye motor deficits, and have paralysis and respiratory disturbances.[2] This should not be considered cruelty since these monkeys are raised for the specific purpose of laboratory research. They live an exceedingly joyful life until they enter the scientific methodology. Their contributions extend the health and life span of mankind.

Members of the monkey group, in one experiment, had their middle cerebral arteries compressed by a small Mayfield clip.[3] The clip remained in place for seventeen hours. DMSO treatment began the fourth hour following this arterial occlusion and continued once a day for four days. Monkeys that survived this procedure were sacrificed seven days following the occlusion. During the entire experiment, the animals were monitored with quantities of laboratory and clinical tests that told a great deal about brain embolism.

In humans, brain emboli can come from fatty plaques in the large arteries that supply the brain. They also can be pieces that break off from thrombi in damaged hearts. They may arise from an accumulation of platelets, fibrin, and cholesterol on the surface of ulcerated plaques in hardening of the arteries; from vegetations on the heart valves in bacterial endocarditis; from mural thrombi in rheumatic heart disease or following heart attack; or from clots following open heart surgery. Brain emboli can also hit underwater divers suffering from decompression sickness. If the blood supply is blocked by one of these emboli for more than a few minutes, death in a portion of the brain results and neurologic damage is permanent.

Acute stroke is another manifestation of blood supply blockage to the brain. Such cerebrovascular disease is the commonest cause of neurologic disability in Western countries. Most of the time it comes from hardening of the arteries, high blood pressure, or a combination of both. Stroke hits abruptly with symptoms and signs reflecting the area of brain that is damaged. Occlusion of either the internal carotid artery or the middle cerebral artery, as was done to the monkeys, can produce a severe set of neurologic abnormalities, almost like those displayed by the monkeys.

DMSO prevents or reverses the pathologic sequence that results from cerebrovascular insufficiency, which finally brings on a localized area of brain death from an embolus. The drug just has to get to the site of injury fast enough.[4]

DMSO stimulates prostaglandin synthesis, which arrests or reverses the potential pathological damage seen following brain infarction.[5,6,7] The prostaglandins (PGs) are a group of cyclical fatty acids that possess diverse and potent biologic activities that affect cell function in every organ system. PGs have sedative, tranquilizing, and anticonvulsive effects on the central nervous system.[8,9]

DMSO increases the oxygen available to the brain tissue through vasodilatation of other blood vessels besides the one blocked by an embolus.[10,11]

DMSO also helps in the release of energy and allows the ischemic tissue sufficient time to reach a hemostatic balance and reverse or prevent further damage to central nervous system cells.[12]

Other experiments on dogs revealed that the DMSO-treated animals did significantly better than untreated control animals when they underwent experimental acute spinal cord injury. An animal's recovery rate was related to the initial dose of DMSO given and to the time interval that elapsed after injury before the drug was given. High doses and earlier treatment resulted in much faster recovery.[13]

When forty rhesus monkeys were subjected to acute experimental head injury by compressing the brain with an extradural balloon, a variety of symptoms developed. When DMSO was given to these animals, fewer died, and neurological defects in the surviving animals were less evident in DMSO-treated monkeys when compared with control animals.[14]

The scientists doing these experiments are studying the effect of DMSO on severe head trauma such as brain compression.

Serious head injury from gunshot wounds could result in brain compression. "We do not have any drugs to adequately treat most severe head injuries," says de la Torre, "and we have high hopes that DMSO may be able to fill this gap, at least until we learn more about the pathology that is involved in these injuries."

SUMMARIZING THE KNOWLEDGE OF DMSO USE
FOR THE CENTRAL NERVOUS SYSTEM

In his March 1980 appearance before the House Select Committee on Aging, Dr. de la Torre crystallized his experimental work with DMSO.

The questions he answered summarized nearly everything currently known about adapting the drug to central nervous system disorders.

Over the years thousands of laboratory animals have been used in dozens of experiments to accumulate sufficient knowledge before employing the solvent to humans. The de la Torre group alone has included DMSO therapy for more than 500 animals, four different animal species, and various models of neurological trauma, dating from early 1971 when head and spinal injuries were being explored. The following information comes from the neurosurgeon's testimony:

In the injured animal, there is an improvement in cortical flow within thirty minutes from giving DMSO, even after cortisone has stopped being secreted. Cortisone is a natural body substance that helps the experimental model fight off the effects of head trauma.

By infusing DMSO, there is an increase in the carotid artery blood flow to the brain, as well. The carotid arteries are two brain vessels that bring oxygen and nutrition to where they are needed. This circulatory mechanism will shut down from the trauma and constitute a kind of brain death by itself without the DMSO infusion. DMSO-treated animals respond much better than those animals that are given something else.

DMSO also appears to restore the subject's electroencephalogram. In these model injuries, the animals are brought to a point where the electroencephalogram reading becomes flat, just preceding brain death and eventual death of the animal. Ten minutes after the injection of DMSO, the electroencephalogram returns and the brain becomes active in its own healing and thinking.

Elevated blood pressure is stabilized in these experimental animals treated with DMSO. This is important because following head injury or spinal cord injury there is always an increase in blood pressure in both animals and humans. If the elevated pressure is not controlled, it may lead to death.

There is an increase in the respiratory pattern of the injured models with using DMSO. The animals appear to breathe deeper and faster, a desirable effect because in many brain-injured patients, respiration becomes too shallow and may eventually stop.

In urine output, DMSO produces a diuretic effect and increases the body's excretion by five times compared to other drugs.

After the intravenous administration of DMSO, there is an elevation in the amount of spinal cord blood flow to the region of trauma. One of the first things that happens after spinal cord trauma is that a reduction of oxygen and blood flow sets in, inasmuch as the blood vessels constrict or shut down and prevent the spilling of necessary enzymes and other materials into the tissue. Without some treatment, the tissue then swells. Eventually this leads to paralysis. In cerebral stroke, the animal will either become comatose or lethargic or die. With DMSO infusion immediately after injury, all of this is prevented.

Water accumulates in the brain as a result of trauma, because the damage breaks down many of the cells. They spill their contents into the tissue, increasing water content and thus pressure in the brain. This fluid buildup in the cranium, which is nothing more than a bony box, will eventually compress vital centers at the bottom of the brain and lead to death. But medical scientists have observed that treatment with DMSO brings about significant reduction of intracranial pressure. "If DMSO were effective only for decreasing intracranial pressure," de la Torre points out, "it will still be a very useful drug. . . . It picks up water, carries it to blood vessels, and then removes it from the brain. So it really dries out the brain, in a sense."

In the same way, an accumulation of blood that is compressing the tissue in an area critical to survival may cause irreversible brain damage, but DMSO will carry even this nontoxic blood away. Experiments performed in 1992 at the University of Health Sciences–The Chicago Medical School have achieved reduction of the spilled blood, but the investigators cannot explain how the injected DMSO does this. They theorize that the perfusion of blood vessels in other areas of the brain takes over the function of the damaged blood vessels by the action of the DMSO.

DMSO tends to protect nerve cells from the actual physical disruption that occurs following injury. It provides better protection than other treatments. Scientists have verified this by observations with the electron microscope and the light microscope. Thus, DMSO prevents the paralysis that may ensue following trauma; it prevents or reverses many of the pathologic signs that are usually present in brain trauma; it alters the severe effects seen after an embolic brain stroke. These are benefits that will eventually affect more than half a million Americans each year.

POTENTIAL IN TREATING MYASTHENIA GRAVIS AND OTHER DISORDERS

Along with showing DMSO's great effectiveness in treating central nervous system injuries, de la Torre projects how it will open possibilities for the treatment of other neurological disorders that affect brain swelling. For example, the substance is already finding use in treating the consequences of the removal of a brain tumor, where swelling of the tissue develops after the tumor excision.

In children, there is Reye's syndrome, where an acute increase in intracranial pressure occurs from the invasion of a suspected viral agent. Surgery or drug therapy is often ineffective in Reye's syndrome, but DMSO may do the job of relieving the pressure on the child's brain.

Ordinarily, antibodies protect people against disease. In myasthenia gravis, however, abnormal antibodies hamper the transmission of nerve signals to the muscles and thus produce the weakness symptomatic of the disease. Myasthenia gravis, a rarity, affects about one out of 20,000 people. It is characterized by sporadic muscular fatigability and weakness, occurring chiefly in muscles innervated by cranial nerves, and characteristically improved by cholinesterase-inhibiting drugs. The causative defect is believed to be located at the neuromuscular junction and to be related to an impairment of acetylcholine's ability to induce muscle contraction. DMSO, a cholinesterase inhibitor, has markedly reduced the abnormal antibodies characteristic of myasthenia gravis.

Animal experiments at Johns Hopkins University made use of DMSO simply as a solvent to increase absorption of an immunosuppressive drug called frentizole, which researchers were testing. Their object was to use frentizole to reduce antibodies in rats that had been treated to give them a disorder much like myasthenia gravis. The experimental treatment worked, but it proved to be the solvent, not the immunosuppressive drug, that was doing the work.

In January 1981, reporting in the British scientific journal *Nature,* the scientists Alan Pestronk, M.D., and Daniel B. Drachman, M.D., stated their intent to test DMSO in human beings, because they knew of no current treatment that diminishes circulating antibodies as quickly, safely, and effectively as DMSO did in the experiments. The scientists stressed that their observations were made in only one set of experiments with one species, however. They do not know whether the same effect would occur in humans or whether DMSO would have any value against the disease. This remains to be seen.

Dr. Pestronk and Dr. Drachman said their discovery might have important implications for treating not only myasthenia gravis but also other diseases in which the body's immunological defenses turn against some of the body's own cells or tissues. Such disorders are called autoimmune diseases. Several other serious diseases, including rheumatoid arthritis, involve autoimmune factors.[15]

TREATMENT OF INTRACRANIAL HYPERTENSION

Writing in the June 1984 issue of the journal *Neurosurgery*, three neu-rologists described their application of DMSO for the reduction or elimination of intracranial hypertension (high blood pressure within the skull's chamber) from head injury. They discussed their experience in six patients, two who had received a bolus administration (an intra-venous "push" injection) of 10 percent dimethyl sulfoxide and four who had received a 20-percent solution titrated (measured by counting drops) against the intracranial pressure (ICP).

Five of the patients in this series suffered from severe head injury, and one had a cortical venous thrombosis (blood clot of a vein in the cerebral cortex) associated with pregnancy. The first two patients were treated with a rapid infusion of a 10-percent solution of DMSO. Initially, the ICP was satisfactorily controlled using this method. Over time, however, fluid overload, severe electrolyte disturbances, and an ultimate loss of ICP control occurred. In subsequent patients, a 20-percent solution titrated against the ICP was used. Although ICP control was better achieved using this method of administration, problems with fluid management and electrolytes occurred again despite a high level of vigilance on the part of the three clinicians.

In addition, because of the solvent properties of DMSO and its propensity over time to dissolve (reduce the potency or concentration of) most standard intravenous infusion systems, mechanical difficulties in its administration were encountered in all six patients. In their clinical journal report, the doctors wrote, "The mechanism of action of DMSO is not well understood. It differs from the barbiturates, but acts too rapidly to function solely as a diuretic. The drug is extremely complex to use, and difficulties with its administration may make its risks ultimately greater than its potential benefits. Until more laboratory data are available concerning its use and better delivery systems are devel-oped, neurosurgeons are cautioned against treating intracranial hyper-tension with DMSO."[16]

MULTIPLE SCLEROSIS SUCCESSFULLY TREATED

DMSO finds use in the treatment of multiple sclerosis, in Russia, as revealed by a 1984 clinical journal report. Thirty-four patients with multiple sclerosis were treated with the Russian branded product named Dimexide (dimethyl sulfoxide). The use of the drug was found

to be desirable, since it had a positive effect on immunity and antialler-
gic and reparative action on the injured tissues. The treatment proved
most effective in patients with a remitting course of the disease. In
patients with a rapidly progressive course, the improvement was unstable. No side effects were observed. The beneficial therapeutic effect
of dimexide may be explained by remyelinization (new growth of nerve
sheaths), a reduction in the edema (swelling), and neurodynamic improvement (improved movement of nerve impulses).[17]

NO DMSO TOXICITY IN CENTRAL NERVOUS SYSTEM TREATMENT

In all of his group's studies, Dr. de la Torre found no significant toxicity
involved with the drug, even with high intravenous doses. He explained, "We took a series of rhesus monkeys that are phylogenetically
very close to man, and injected high doses of DMSO intravenously for
nine days. Before and after, we tested these monkeys for their serum
chemistries, their cardiovascular responses, their neurological signs,
and their ophthalmological changes, if there were any.

"Following the toxicity studies, which took eighteen weeks, we
concluded that there were no significant changes in the serum chemistry at any time during the observation period. These changes were
compared to a control series of animals.

"There were no changes in the urine, and there were no neurological
changes. There were no changes in the cardiovascular responses. There
were no ocular changes. We were curious to see if there might have been
some changes in the refraction or translucency of the lens, since some years
previously this had been reported to have been a problem in rabbits.

"One of the ophthalmologists reviewed these animals before and after
DMSO, not knowing which animals had received the drug, and it was
concluded that there were no changes at all in the eyes of these animals.

"Then following the experiments, the animals were autopsied and
the tissues examined histologically. No pathologic changes in the his-
tology were found.

"So, our conclusion, then, is that DMSO, at least as far as these events
were concerned, is an effective and relatively nontoxic drug as used
intravenously.

"Our results in spinal cord injury, brain trauma, and stroke have been
confirmed by at least three different groups of investigators in other parts
of the country for each project," Dr. de la Torre said. "We feel that DMSO
is a highly effective drug in central nervous system injuries."

CHAPTER 10
DMSO Therapy for Mental Disabilities

Melody Clark had her first psychomotor evaluation when she was six months old. Her parents, Mr. and Mrs. Dale Clark of Wenatchee, Washington, learned that Melody would be so severely retarded that in all likelihood she would never progress mentally beyond the age of six. She was born with an extra chromosome 21—a total of forty-seven chromosomes instead of the normal human forty-six—making her a victim of Down's syndrome or trisomy 21.

Patients with Down's syndrome are labeled trisomic mongoloids, because of certain characteristics peculiar to an individual with three of a particular chromosome rather than the normal pair of homologous chromosomes. Typically, the affected child is born to an older mother, although the condition may also occur in babies of mothers of any age. The overall incidence is about 1 in 700 live births, but there is marked variability depending on the mother's age. In the early child-bearing years, the incidence is about 1 in 2,000 live births; for mothers over age forty, it rises to about 45 in 1,000 live births. Close to 50 percent of infants with Down's syndrome are born to mothers over thirty-five years of age.

The babies tend to be placid, rarely cry, and demonstrate lack of muscular tone. Their physical and mental development is retarded; the mean intelligence quotient (IQ) is about 50. Facial characteristics differ from the normal: an unusually small head, flattened at the rear, and disproportionately short; slanted eyes with folds of skin extending from the root of the nose to the inner termination of the eyebrow are present. Gray to white spots resembling grains of salt clustering around the periphery of the iris are usually visible in the period just after birth and disappear during the first twelve months of life. The bridge of the nose is flattened, and the baby's mouth is often held open by a large, protruding tongue that is furrowed and lacks the central fissure.

The hands of such children are short and broad, with a single palmar crease ("simian crease"). Their fingers appear short with incurvature of the fifth finger, which often has only two phalanges. The feet have a wide gap between the first and second toes, and a furrow on the foot sole extends backward. X-rays of the children's hips disclose decreased acetabular and iliac angles, and prior to the availability of chromosome analysis this was a major finding in confirming the diagnosis.

Congenital heart disease is found in about 35 percent of Down's syndrome patients. Thus, life expectancy is decreased by the threat of heart disease and by susceptibility to acute leukemia. However, many youngsters without a major heart defect survive to adulthood but not to old age.

When Melody Clark was eleven months old, her parents placed her on DMSO therapy under the supervision of Dr. Stanley Jacob. At that time, she couldn't stand because her legs were just like a rag doll's. She could not roll from her back to her abdomen. Her eyes were constantly out of focus; she was almost unable to see. By age eight, Melody had progressed from a severely retarded child to one who was only mildly retarded—a circumstance that is highly unusual for this heretofore irreversible condition.

After seven years of treatment with DMSO, Melody ran, jumped, turned somersaults, and played on a trampoline. She was on a second grade level at school and excelled in arithmetic. She had an excellent grasp of mathematical problems and was a good reader and a fine speller. She had worked her way up from a class for "trainables" to a special education class for educable children. She attended Sunday school with normal children and also enjoyed camp with normal children during the summer of 1980. Equally important is that Melody was quite popular with her classmates—she was very social-minded.

Not only did she advance mentally, but the DMSO therapy brought about actual physical changes. Her features altered. Melody was born with an extremely high roof in her mouth, and now it is within the normal range. Her dentist, David K. Priebe, D.D.S., of the Eye and Ear Hospital, Wenatchee, Washington, testified to this change. Dr. Priebe wrote:

> For the record I'd like to share some observations about Melody Clark's oral development. Melody has been a regular patient under my care since 11 August, 1976.
>
> I have been paying particular attention to tooth size and

nature of dorsal tongue mucosa, all of which have altered developmental patterns in Down's syndrome children.

It is my clinical impression that this patient seems to be significantly more normal in every aspect of the above compared with other Down's syndrome children of similar age. Palate development, while high, has lowered considerably during the time she has been with me. Arch development and particularly tongue development seem to be becoming within the range of normalcy.

Behaviorly, Melody has demonstrated that she can handle the stress of dental treatment as well as children not having Down's syndrome.

Progress reports on Melody's functional development in the classroom showed her able "to read fluently from storybook to teacher and independently complete comprehension questions on take home," said Rose M. Mullan, a special education teacher at the Wenatchee Sterling Middle School. The girl was "able to compute two-digit, one-column addition and subtraction facts from dictated story problems."

When Melody was not yet seven, she could also speak in complete sentences. Ms. Mullan said, "The first response in a complete sentence was made in November 1979. When told at recess that all the balls were being used, Melody responded, 'Denise will share with me.'" Then, she was able to respond to personal data and give her full name, age, address, city, state, birthday, phone number, and parents' names and was able to name in order the days of the week and the seasons of the year.

She was accepted by her peers on her personal merit. "Melody socializes with her peers at recess and in the classroom," noted Ms. Mullan. "She participates in classroom games and shares classroom responsibilities. Melody is very conscientious in completing her school assignments, and she is proud of her academic accomplishments."

Another of Melody's teachers, Marion A. Kennedy, commenting on the girl's writing ability, said: "Melody can group letters into words and generally maintains her letters within the boundary of primary paper. She copies directly from the chalkboard and many sight words she simply reads and then writes on her paper. (As opposed to having to copy letter for letter, she spells.) She always reads her 'boardwork' independently prior to copying it. . . . There is no question that Melody has made great strides in every area of academic and social and physical development this year. The progress is quite remarkable."

"All of this progress is because of DMSO," said Melody's mother, "so I'm sure you realize why I would like to see this drug made available for suffering people. It certainly offers parents like us a lot of hope."

The little girl is unique in the progress she made. No scientist quite understands how DMSO worked to make changes in her—and in other children with Down's syndrome—but that the drug did is undeniable. Don Bonker, a Congressman from Washington state who is one of the members of the House Select Committee on Aging, told Dr. Jacob and all those assembled in the hearing room the day DMSO was discussed, "Today Melody is a miracle child for the entire community. She walks, runs, talks, reads, spells well, her teeth are developing almost normally. Her tongue does not protrude."

"Are you familiar with this case?" Mr. Bonker asked Dr. Jacob. "Today our office has received three phone calls from a community in the state of Washington regarding Melody Clark, this eight-year-old child who has what is known as Down's syndrome. At eleven months she was typically unable to stand or walk, had protruding tongue and all the other symptoms. Her parents heard of Dr. Stanley Jacob and went to Portland to try DMSO on her."

Dr. Jacob knew her well—she was one of hundreds of trisomic (Down's syndrome) children who had some of their abnormalities partially reversed with DMSO therapy.

OTHER DOWN'S SYNDROME EXAMPLES RESPONDING TO DMSO

Bronwyn Nash of Rock Island, Washington, was another trisomy 21, the form of Down's syndrome with the greatest number of problems. She had been treated with DMSO since the age of ten months. When I investigated Bronwyn's case she was twenty-eight months old and improving steadily.

The girl had been very slow to gain weight. Her pediatrician had done several tests to see if there was a medical reason but none was discovered. She was a frail, tiny baby.

It was right after she was put on DMSO for treating her Down's syndrome that Bronwyn's weight started to go up. Dorothy Nash, her mother, described how the baby progressed: "She seemed to have more interest in food and ate a little more but was basically nursing until she was a year old, so we're convinced the DMSO helped her. We and other people around us noticed an increased awareness of people and objects around Bronwyn. She started taking a real interest in reaching out and touching things."

At eighteen months Bronwyn crawled, sat up, and pulled herself to a standing position. She got into her mother's cupboards, started to feed herself, and held her water glass well. She became an alert, cheerful little girl much enjoyed and well loved by the Nash family.

Mrs. Nash said, "We are so pleased to have Bronwyn on DMSO and hope it will be available to others soon."

From Santiago, Chile, Nicholas Weinstein, M.D., supplied the DMSO aminoacid compound used for the Down's syndrome treatment of young Billy King in the United States. The child was suffering from trisomy 21 and had been treated for eight years with traditional therapies, without any improvement. Then, for over two years he was given DMSO therapy with an imported drug product. By the time he was ten years old, the boy had experienced no unfavorable side effects and improvement was definitely observed. His mother, Betty Lou King, reported, "Billy has grown from a size five to a fifteen and has now complete control of his bladder and bowels. He has gained a large vocabulary. His mongoloid looks are diminishing." The photographic comparison of changes in Billy King for just one year are striking. He looks normal now whereas before the boy possessed the facial characteristics of obvious Down's syndrome.

DMSO AMINOACID THERAPY FOR TRISOMIC CHILDREN

Medical teams working in clinical and pharmacological research from Canada, the United States, Mexico, Argentina, and Chile use DMSO aminoacid therapy in an ongoing search for new means to fight mental retardation. The combination of ingredients is not yet approved by the Federal Food and Drug Administration and any physician who employs the compound in this country risks a lot personally and professionally. Parents don't risk much because the medicine has been proved safe after years of clinical trials—and the parents have hardly any other hope of restoring their trisomy children to near normality.

An experiment was carried out with a group of 18 children suffering from trisomy 21. While they showed marked differences on an intellectual level, they were pathogenically homogeneous, as they all had the typical symptoms. The results obtained with this experimental group were checked against those of a control group of 91 children of similar physical and mental ages who had Down's syndrome.

Chief of research was Lydia F. De Coriat, M.D., Assistant Head of the Neurological Service of the Municipal Pediatric Hospital, Buenos Aires, Argentina, who is also President of the Argentine Association for the Scientific Study of Mental Retardation. Dr. De Coriat used an evaluation technique on the children that covered four levels:

1. Impression of the child's parents regarding behavior at home, degree of integration and language organization, and general deportment.
2. The personal impression of the physician regarding clinical changes in the patient including his or her general aspect, muscular tone, psychomotor activity, appearance, and expression.
3. A psychological evaluation made by comparing the IQ in repeated psychometric tests.
4. An evaluation of side effects, laboratory assays, and other supplementary tests for the medication.

For psychometric control of the development of the Down's syndrome babies, the Gesell test for child development was used.[1] The Therman-Merril test was used for older subjects. The neurological maturity of the 109 children of both sexes, aged between two months and five years, was recorded. They had been subjected to early stimulation since babyhood.

Each child was studied and examined for six consecutive months. Only the 18 children of the group received treatment with DMSO aminoacid therapy. It included the intramuscular injection into each child of five series of twelve ampoules of the DMSO aminoacid compound every other day. Additionally, the rhythm of stimulation and specialized learning for all babies and children were maintained at previously determined levels. The diet was kept at an optimum, and psychopharmacological and aminoacid oral treatments were continued where necessary. The 91 children in the control group received only "basic treatment," no DMSO aminoacid therapy. The injections for Down's syndrome children in the experiment were supplemented by daily oral administration of one to three capsules containing the DMSO compound for 180 days.

Analysis of the results demonstrated "a tendency towards accelerated maturity in the children treated, with marked progress in language integration; this could be established in statistically significant degrees in the children treated, reported Dr. De Coriat. "The side effects observed were minimal and did not make it necessary to suspend treatment, save in the case of one child, with a probable allergic exanthema." (Exanthema is a skin eruption.)

The researchers considered the results of this experiment positive and pointed to the DMSO aminoacid therapy as a useful addition to conventional treatments of Down's syndrome.

THE DMSO AMINOACID FORMULA

The DMSO aminoacid therapy used in this research is commercially available under the name "Akron" in Argentina and "Merinex" in Chile. The amino acids in these products are agents for the resupply of the nervous cells and are considered indispensable for the biochemical process that controls the cerebral metabolism. The products have been used for the treatment of depressive neurosis, anxiety, psychic disorders connected with menopause, apathy and fatigue of geriatrics, and poor intellectual performance in children. With assistance from DMSO, the amino acids penetrate the brain and activate the neuronal function, which is suppressed in many syndromes of mental retardation. The earlier this DMSO therapy is begun, the greater the possibility of achieving patient improvement, since the neuronal change is then in full development.

Neurologists and pediatricians in various Latin American and European countries have taken advantage of the Chilean and Argentine investigations and now use the products in mentally retarded and mentally deficient patients. The amino acids comprising the DMSO formula are gamma-aminobutyric acid (GABA), gamma-amino-beta-hydroxybutyric acid (GABOB), and acetylglutamine. Five milliliter ampoules are supplied for intramuscular injection, and there are capsules manufactured for oral administration. Dosage is determined by body weight of the child, as follows:

Up to 8 kg = ¼ ampoule (1.25 cc)
8 kg to 12 kg = ½ ampoule (2.50 cc)
More than 12 kg = 1 ampoule (5.00 cc)

The treatment program with Merinex or Akron involves one intramuscular injection every other day and swallowing two or three capsules daily during the entire regimen. Injections are suspended every 40 days for a rest period of one month, during which time only capsules are administered. The program must last at least one year, in the course of which five series of twenty injections each and two or three capsules per day according to the patient's body weight are administered.

Since mental retardation associated with syndromes of autosomal aberrations (Down's syndrome) is a very difficult medical problem, the manufacturers recommend that after completing the one-year treatment, the patient be given a rest of two months and then the treatment resume. The pharmaceutical researchers involved with DMSO aminoacid therapy seem unable to entirely explain how it actually works to alter complications connected with the patient's extra chromosome. All they know is what they've observed in one clinical trial after another.

MORE THERAPEUTIC STUDIES ON SEVERE
MENTAL RETARDATION

In a paper presented at the third international conference on dimethyl sulfoxide held in New York City under the auspices of the New York Academy of Sciences, five prominent physicians, representing the disciplines of neuropsychiatry, pediatrics, and genetics, from universities and hospitals in Chile, told of another study of DMSO aminoacid therapy in severe mental retardation.[2]

They took a group of fifty-five children with trisomy 21 and divided them into twenty-four patients as controls and thirty-one patients who received treatment. Examinations were conducted by a team of additional specialists, including several pediatricians, a neurologist, a psychologist, a cardiologist, and an ophthalmologist, before the test began and every six months during it, with the exception of the pediatricians, who performed monthly examinations.

All the patients—controls and experimentees—were separated into two age groups. Group One was twenty-eight children less than three-and-a-half years old, and Group Two was twenty-seven children whose ages varied from three-and-a-half to fourteen. The DMSO aminoacid therapy was administered by intramuscular injections with different time rhythms in each group.

Children in Group One were given injections every other day in a series of 90 days alternating with a month's rest. All received a minimum of three series. The dosage was adjusted to their body weight.

Children in Group Two received daily intramuscular injections of 5 cc each over 20 days alternating with pauses of 20 days. During the entire period they were given the same amino acids in the form of one or two capsules per day but without DMSO as an ingredient of the capsule. The total treatment for this second group consisted of five series of 20 injections each—in all 100 injections of 5 cc each over thirty weeks.

The psychometric determinations in children of Group One were performed according to the Gesell test, calculating the development quotient, which is the relationship of motor development, language, and social adaptation according to the child's chronological age. Neurological development was determined by observing the sense organs, coordination, muscle tone, and sphincter control. For the older Group Two, psychometric measurements were performed with special tests such as the Binet-Kulman test. Every 40 days the IQ was computed according to the Gesell, Wieneland, and Binet tests. Additionally, laboratory tests were carried out, including those for red corpuscles, hemoglobin, hematocrit, white corpuscles, sedimentation, urine, hepatic function, amino acids in the blood, amino acids in the urine, and others. Finally, photographs were taken before, during, and after treatment to capture the psychic state and preponderant physical features of the child and any noticeable changes.

The evaluation of results took into account the development quotient and the IQ. If the increase represented more than ten points, this was considered significant clinical improvement. Analyses were made of the motor area, the adaptive area, the language area for the utilization and comprehension of verbal communication, and the social area.

Comparison of the psychometric and motor changes observed in children treated in Group One, under three-and-a-half-years old, with those of the control group reveals the following differences:

- To start with, the controls and the treated children had a mean average *motor index* of fifty-six; after one year the controls' motor index rose to fifty-eight but the DMSO aminoacid treated children's motor index rose to seventy-two, except for six cases where there was really no significant variation.

- In the *area of adaptation,* the averages of the controls were fifty-two at the beginning and forty-nine at the end of the observation. The adaptation averages of the treated group were fifty before and sixty-six after the series of DMSO aminoacid injections.

- Averages in the *language area* for control cases showed fifty-six before and fifty-four after the observation period. The treated patients started with a language area average of fifty-two and ended with an average of fifty-eight, four of them improving by more than ten points.

- In controls, the initial average in their *social area* was forty-five, which rose to fifty a year later. The treated group started with a social average of forty and at the end of the treatment this rose to sixty-four. The mimetic capacity and expression of those treated improved noticeably; their environmental contact was also noteworthy, reported the researchers.

In children of Group Two who were older than three-and-a-half years, the following results were obtained:

- Stagnation was observed in the *motor area* of the controls. Their averages were thirty-four before the test began and thirty-six a year later, when it ended. On the other hand, the initial motor area average of thirty-eight for the DMSO-treated group rose to forty-nine by the conclusion of the clinical trials.
- In the *language area*, the controls were also stagnant, but the use of speech improved in the treated group by sixteen points. In six of the sixteen treated children comprehension improved, too.
- No significant variation was seen in the control group for *graphic age*. In the group treated with DMSO therapy, their initial graphic age average of twenty-four points rose to thirty-nine, which was a significant improvement.

At the beginning of the observation the control group showed an average intelligence quotient of thirty-four and a year later this mean average had dipped to thirty-three. The treated group indicated an average IQ of twenty-nine, which had shot up to forty by the time the treatment program ended. Besides these favorable changes, this older treated group showed other improvements in statics, motor coordination, and muscle tone. Two treated children achieved sphincter control during this test period of one year.

No serious side effects in the laboratory examinations were reported. Nor were any seen in the periodic clinical examinations.

Manuel Aspillaga, M.D., Associate Professor of Pediatrics and Director of the Department of Genetics at the University of Chile, Calvo MacKenna Children's Hospital, led the research team consisting of pediatrician Mila Sanchez, M.D., geneticist Isabel Avendano, M.D., neuropsychiatrist Lucila Capdeville, M.D., and geneticist Chislaine Morizon, M.D., who were with the same institution. These five pioneering physicians stated: "It seems to us that DMSO aminoacid therapy in trisomic children and children with severe mental retardation offers an evident advance in the therapy of this syndrome. Fundamentally, it can be observed that children aged less than three-and-a-half years react in the psychic sphere with greater receptiveness to stimulation, showing a major interest in their environment; there is an increase in their activity, and muscular tonus. A notable improvement is also noted in the adaptive and social phase. Besides, muscular coordination and statics also show a significant improvement.

"We have not observed a correlation between the physical signs and the development coefficient. *We are of the opinion that the progress must be credited to the treatment,*" the five physicians emphasized. "At the moment we dare not make a prognosis relative to future intellectual levels. However, if the parameters approach normality with this treatment, this is already a positive result and may well be the starting point for future progress with this therapy.

"In some of our patients treated later, not related with this work, we administered higher doses, obtaining up to this moment more favorable results," said the researchers. "Finally, we wish to emphasize the fact that, although we have not yet arrived at the ideal treatment, we have reached a new important stage on our road in this difficult medical field, where no progress had been made in the course of various decades."

In another report to the New York Academy of Sciences, Ana Giller, M.D., children's neuropsychiatrist at the Pirovano Hospital of Buenos Aires, and Maria E.M. de Bernadow, M.D., Head of the Laboratory of Genetics, National Department of Students' Health of Argentina, presented a group of twenty-six mentally retarded children ranging in age from seven to twenty. Thirteen had received DMSO aminoacid therapy by mouth and by intramuscular injection. The other thirteen served as controls and underwent only conventional treatment.

The treated children received 5 cc of Merinex, the DMSO-aminoacid product, intramuscularly three times a week in a series of twenty injections, alternating with rest periods of 16 days between each series. During the intervals aminoacid capsules without DMSO were orally administered in dosages of one to two per day.

Each patient was examined before and after 180 days of treatment. The IQ and psychometric profiles were determined by a number of standards applied in psychology such as the Binet-Simon test, standardized by Kuhlman, and the Wics and Therman-Merril test. The age of maturity and organic lesions were determined by the Bender test. The doctors reconciled the following parameters and evaluated them:

1. Visomanual coordination
2. Dynamic coordination
3. Postural control
4. Control of the body itself
5. Perceptive coordination
6. Language age
7. Dynamic coordination of the hands
8. General dynamic coordination
9. Static coordination
10. Speed
11. Space organization
12. Temporal structure

Upon analyzing the mean of variation of the estimated mental age from these twelve tests practiced on the control group within the 100 day period, in comparison with that obtained by the treated group, a definite difference emerged. There was a significant improvement in the psychometric profile of the children treated with DMSO aminoacid therapy. It contrasted with the static state of the control group where the variation was practically non-existent when the conventional approach was used.

None of the children treated with the experimental compound showed any signs of toxicity or intolerance.[3]

THE NEW TREATMENT FOR LEARNING DISABILITIES

For the last three decades learning disorders have been viewed primarily from the perspective of special education problems. During early investigations into the causes of "brain-injured" children, a variety of labels have been leveled at these youngsters. The more common names for their behavioral characteristics include brain injury, brain damage, minimal brain damage, minimal brain dysfunction, hyperkinesis, perceptual defects, dyslexia, hyperactivity, and many more. Still, no single cause has conclusively been found, and treatment has differed with the training and course of study of the diagnosing doctor, depending on whether the doctor is a neurologist, psychologist, psychiatrist, internist, educator, or nutritionist.

But positive neurological findings have been reported in up to 85 percent of the children with learning disabilities. In one study, 97 percent of the patients showed evidence of brain dysfunction. In another study, a genetic component was considered the cause and, in fact, at least five times more boys than girls have learning disorders, which suggests that some are genetically sex-linked. Of the 51.5 million school-aged children in the United States, an estimated 10 percent have some type of learning disability.

The therapy for these disorders may be pharmacological, nutritional, or environmental. Pharmacologically, learning disorders that are, in general, considered brain damage are treated with cell-building substances such as amino acids, phosphates, and potassium. They are administered in combination with "carrying" solvents such as DMSO so as to actively interfere with the language disorder, which may have a bearing on the recovery and/or development of speech. The addition of amino acids to DMSO develops and activates the functional activity of the brain.

A clinical research project was conducted by the Department of Abandoned Children of the National Health Service of Chile, in 1969, under the direction of the department head, Carlos Nassar, M.D. On a total of forty-four children of school age with learning and developmental problems caused by low intellectual capacity, Dr. Nassar used DMSO aminoacid therapy (Merinex) by injection and by mouth.

The personal histories of the children showed high percentages of retardation in learning to walk, speak, in psychomotor development, and other actions. They had unmotivated aggressiveness, rebellion and irritability, convulsive attacks, and convulsive pathologies of the brain. Intellectual examinations before the experimental trials indicated that they had IQs of between thirty to eighty-five. This IQ examination was repeated at three, six, and ten months during the course of treatment with DMSO aminoacid therapy.

A series of twenty intramuscular DMSO aminoacid injections, alternating with the oral administration of capsules, proceeded. Almost all the children were treated during periods ranging from six to ten months, except for six children in which treatment was extended a year.

In contrast with the poor results obtained using other methods of therapy, the progress in mental capacity observed by Dr. Nassar for these DMSO-treated children was extraordinary. He accomplished a heightened capacity for learning in them in a relatively short time. More than 70 percent were classified "favorable" responses. He saw an "increase of the IQ, an evident and accelerated progress in basic achievements, an overall improvement of intellectual capacity, evident progress in reading, writing, and mathematics, better coordination of movements and improved manual skill, and a decrease of behavioral problems." The doctor also saw his patients gain better psychomotor control, and observed the elimination of anger for no reason, a general reduction of irritability, and a lessening of disobedience.

Nassar stated unequivocally, "When analyzing the cases treated and evaluating the clinical and psychometric tests, which were performed with the greatest care and conscientiousness, we can conclude that Merinex is undoubtedly beneficial and useful in the treatment of oligo-phrenic [mentally deficient] children; an increase in their intellectual faculties and progress in basic achievements were registered in a high percentage of the cases. During the clinical research, we observed that the treatment not only increased the IQ but also has a beneficial influence on behavior problems, improves psychomotor coordination, and eliminates irritability, nervous erethism [abnormal excitement], unmotivated aggressiveness, and rebelliousness."

Additional investigations supported the Nassar study. For instance, at the Department of Psychiatry, the University of Chile, neuropsychiatrist Azael Paz, M.D., did research on fifty learning disabled children between the ages of five and fifteen. They did not suffer from organic brain trouble, brain paralysis, congenital brain damage, epilepsy, or pseudoneurotic mental retardation. Their problems were only language disorders.

DMSO aminoacid therapy (Merinex) was administered to a part of the group—thirty patients—exclusively by mouth, in dosages of two or three capsules a day during a period of six months. In the other twenty children injection treatment was given intramuscularly, with 5 cc doses of three ampoules per week, until twenty injections, alternat-ing with a rest period of fifteen days, were completed. The injections were then resumed with the same time rhythm and duration as the first cycle until an average of six months of treatment was reached. During the rest periods, the DMSO aminoacid oral treatment was also given in daily doses of two or three capsules, according to the age of the child.

Dr. Paz reported that there are excellent possibilities for stimulating and accentuating the development, the psychic evolution, and learning of children with the help of this therapy, which activates and stimulates the energetic oxidative metabolism of the brain. The neuropsychiatrist noted a gradual development of the faculty of greater awareness, changes and progress in the moral attitude of the child, the unfolding of the personality, the dawning of self-criticism, and the satisfaction of establishing his own personal identity.

The favorable results reported in this clinical study of DMSO for learning disabilities were summed up by the researcher in the following way:

1. Disappearance of mental lethargy.
2. Evidence of sensorial reactions.

3. Disappearance of automatic movements.
4. Disappearance of inertia, passivity, and negativity.
5. Growing interest and initiative in tasks and activities.
6. Improvement of the physiognomic expression (use of facial features to reveal character) and of the spoken language.
7. Lucid activity, group contact, and disappearance of unprovoked aggressiveness.
8. Losing shyness and developing self-esteem.
9. Successful training to carry out chores, to shop, eat, and dress without help, etc.
10. Learning to read and write and to do homework.

Paz concluded: "The therapy with Merinex, injections and capsules, has led to a rapid biopsychological development and to the evolution of the intellectual faculties of the children, making them capable for school learning." The therapeutic response was quicker and more efficacious in the group subject to treatment with injections and capsules than in the group treated exclusively with capsules alone.

Added to this extensive and convincing South American study, physicians in Spain confirmed, in late 1982, that children victimized by Down's syndrome undergo a positive social adjustment when they are administered DMSO.[4]

REVERSING SENILE DEMENTIA AND OTHER FORMS OF PSYCHO-ORGANIC DECAY

In the brain of a young healthy adult, there are about 12 billion neurons, the cells that send nerve impulses through the body. As part of the aging process each day, the brain loses about 100,000 neurons. They get used up and die and psycho-organic decay eventually sets in when enough neurons have been lost.

Geriatric specialists estimate that 15 percent of people sixty-five to seventy-five years old and 25 percent of those seventy-five and older are suffering from senile dementia, one of the forms of psycho-organic (PSO) decay. Thus, senility or dementia is in no way the same as aging, for if you can prevent PSO decay you will avoid senile dementia, but will continue to age. Senility or dementia is the term applied to destructive changes in the functioning cells of the brain. It is a brain disease and a mental disease. While there are senile physical changes as well, they are not always present in the brain of the senile person.[5]

DMSO aminoacid therapy and DMSO in combination with vasoactive substances have been proven beneficial in the treatment of senility or dementia and other forms of psycho-organic decay. Gustavo Munizaga, M.D., Professor of Neurology at Chile University, conducted an experiment in July 1970 using these two types of DMSO compounds. Merinex and the vasoactive DMSO, called "Ipran," which is also not approved by the FDA for use in the United States, were given to 104 elderly people suffering from PSO decay. These people were divided into five groups, according to their dominant pathology:

1. PSO decay caused by cerebral vascular arteriosclerosis.
2. PSO decay caused by senility.
3. PSO decay after a stroke.
4. PSO decay as a consequence of a head injury.
5. PSO decay due to a degenerative disease such as Parkinsonism, hyperthyroidism, epilepsy, and others.

The patients with mental decay in the last stage of advanced age treated by Dr. Munizaga received Merinex and Ipran, both orally and by injection. As a general rule, treatment began with intramuscular injections, alternating Merinex one day and Ipran the next, or administering one ampoule of each simultaneously, mixed in the syringe, until a cycle of twenty injections was completed. On the days when the patients received no injections, they took two capsules of Merinex and one capsule of Ipran.

The DMSO aminoacid therapy and DMSO combined with vasoactive substances were of remarkable efficacy in the recovery of patients with PSO decay, the neurologist reported. He established that the therapeutic response was quicker when both medicines were administered simultaneously by injection and by mouth. Munizaga said, "The DMSO aminoacid therapy is undoubtedly valuable in the treatment of numerous organic cerebral diseases. At the same time, thanks to the improved cerebral blood irrigation achieved by DMSO used in combination with vasoactive substances, a highly favorable effect on the psychic and somatic functions of senile dementia patients was achieved."

Another study was performed in Chile on 100 patients of both sexes suffering from cerebrovascular diseases such as infarct, cerebral embolism, hardening of the arteries of the brain, and other conditions. Jorge Grismali, M.D., Chief of the Clinic of the Department and Extraordinary Professor of Neurology, Salvador Hospital, and Luis Varela Barrios, M.D.,

Neurologist in that same department, employed a therapeutic method using Ipran ampoules and capsules. The patients were senile as well as victims of one of the cerebrovascular diseases (CVD). In 70 percent of the cases, CVD was accompanied by high blood pressure, demonstrable in the accessible arteries.

The DMSO therapy was given both orally and intramuscularly. The dose was one intramuscular injection—administered slowly—each day, until twenty ampoules had been given. At the same time, one capsule was dispensed in the morning and another in the afternoon so that the patient could swallow a divided double dose. After the first twenty injections, the ampoules were administered every other day until another total of thirty injections was completed. In this second series, two Ipran capsules were swallowed daily, and no more than two injections were given each week.

Drs. Grismali and Barrios summed up their therapeutic results for the DMSO treatment of CVD with atherosclerosis and high blood pressure in the following manner:

Good	74.35 percent
Fair	21.77 percent
Zero	3.88 percent

The two neurologists reported that "recovery from the general symptoms was positive; there were favorable changes which were reflected in a feeling of well being, the recovery of agility, changes of mood from depressed to gay, improvement of sleeping, and clearer speech. As regards the 'focal' results, accelerated recovery from hemiplegia and hemiparesia was registered. A speedier recovery of speech in cases of defined or indicated aphasia took place."

CHAPTER 11

The DMSO-Cancer Connection

In April, 1974, a fifty-six-year-old Exxon Oil Corporate Executive, Joe B. Floyd, now of Spring, Texas, found himself hemorrhaging from the rectum. Realizing that this was an unhealthy sign, Mr. Floyd consulted with his company's industrial physician, C. Hunter Montgomery, M.D. Dr. Montgomery's physical examination revealed that his patient was suffering from a deadly form of cancer of the colon—adenocarcinoma.

Adenocarcinoma is among the most malignant of cancers. Each year, it kills approximately 9,500 Americans. The cancer occurs in all age groups, but the incidence increases with age. While it usually involves the duodenum portion of the small intestine and sometimes the ileum, producing early obstruction, pain, bleeding, and rapid weight loss, Mr. Floyd's adenocarcinoma had infiltrated the rectosigmoid of the large intestine.

The prediction as to the duration, course, and outcome of the disease depends on the degree of bowel wall involvement and the presence of regional lymph node involvement and distant metastases. Unluckily for Mr. Floyd, his adenocarcinoma had spread to the lymph nodes. They had turned rubbery. It had also metastasized rapidly to the liver. Pressure symptoms developed from the expansion of the lymph nodes in the abdominal cavity so that gastric upset occurred. Weight loss, fever, night sweats, and debilitation were weakening the patient, indicating that his cancer was spreading.

Dr. Montgomery referred Joe Floyd to colon surgeon Wade Harris, M.D., of Houston, who removed thirteen inches of the patient's large colon and the lymph nodes in his peritoneum where the cancer had spread. Dr. Harris advised Mr. Floyd to take chemotherapy, for it was certain that in a matter of only a few months, the adenocarcinoma would occur somewhere else. The surgeon also mentioned that his own wife had the identical condition. Mrs. Harris suffered with adenocarcinoma and was then taking chemotherapy at the M.D. Anderson Cancer Institute, a giant hospital complex in Houston.

Dr. Harris had wanted Mr. Floyd to go through the same chemotherapy program as Mrs. Harris, but the man agonized over this decision and finally refused. He went home after his colon surgery on a Saturday morning. He had viewed a television documentary two years before, presented by newsman Ron Stone of KHOU-TV Houston, depicting cancer cures by another Houston physician, E.J. Tucker, M.D. (now deceased). Mr. Floyd was keen to investigate this alternative treatment.

"Then the next Monday morning my wife and I called on Dr. Tucker and after a lot of hard persuasion, he agreed to give me his treatment on an experimental basis," explained Mr. Floyd. "A dying man can make a pretty good argument to keep on living. Within six weeks, Dr. Harris's wife was dead from taking chemotherapy. But I was back at work in downtown Houston at the Exxon Building and taking treatments every other day at the doctor's office. I had no nausea or any of the symptoms usually accompanying chemotherapy. After approximately eighteen months, my CEA tests were far below normal and Dr. Tucker dismissed me as cured. I was to come by for a checkup every thirty days. Now we make a check every three or four months and my CEA is always below normal." CEA stands for carcinogenic embyronic antigen, a blood test for cancer cell activity in a person with a malignancy. Mr. Floyd's CEA has dropped from a high of eighteen to zero (normal) today.

When we last spoke together, on May 16, 1989, J.B. Floyd at seventy-one was retired from Exxon and was the wealthy owner of twelve Texas oil wells. He received gratification as a retailer in his small health food store, bringing good nutrition to his tiny Texas town. Being a health food entrepeneur was his hobby and source of complete satisfaction; being alive and well was the answer to his prayers, which he attributed to the research of Dr. E.J. Tucker.

Mr. Floyd received his treatment as a result of a discovery made by Tucker in 1966, which until now has been ignored by the cancer medical establishment. M.D. Anderson Hospital, among the largest cancer therapeutic research centers in the world, situated just down the street from Tucker's office, doesn't even experiment with this treatment because half of its components include DMSO as part of the therapeutic compound.

The decision to ignore Tucker's compound is mostly based on politics and economics. Administrators of M.D. Anderson Hospital are aware of where the bulk of the hospital's money comes from. It operates on large government grants and some private contributions. The administrators are likely worried that if the medical staff went against the policy of the Food and Drug Administration by using DMSO for an unapproved purpose, the hospital's grants would be in jeopardy.

Indeed, the FDA knows very well about this treatment's success for certain forms of cancer. FDA officials personally met with Tucker and Floyd to study the doctor's DMSO cancer therapy. "[In] the first part of March 1978 a group of doctors from New York City called and wanted Dr. Tucker to come and bring his medicine and show them how to use it," said J.B. Floyd. "Dr. Tucker called me and asked if I would accompany him and tell my story."

Floyd agreed to go anywhere, anytime to bring information about the treatment that saved his life to the medical community. Before leaving for the Houston airport, Tucker received another telephone call from K.C. Pani, M.D., of the Division of Anti-Infective Drug Products, Bureau of Drugs, Food and Drug Administration, Department of Health and Human Services, Rockville, Maryland, to please come by the FDA on the way to New York and bring him up to date. Tucker had numerous records of cures, X-ray films, and slides to show.

Doctor and patient flew to Rockville where Tucker presented his case histories. When they came to Floyd's record, Dr. Pani asked, "How long did this one last, three months?"

Tucker replied, "He is sitting down in the lobby."

Pani said, "I want to see this dead man."

They sought out Mr. Floyd, and he told his story. Then the FDA official, visibly impressed, said he would be in touch with Tucker soon. He also mentioned that he was in contact with Dr. Stanley Jacob of Oregon and that he was monitoring the use of DMSO. About one week later the drug was approved for the treatment of interstitial cystitis. Nothing further was done to follow up its use in cancer, except that Tucker received a request from the FDA for "more research."

Dr. Jacob also is acquainted with Tucker's work. In fact, he telephoned Tucker a few days before the Mike Wallace 60 Minutes show on CBS-TV to check out progress on the cancer treatment. Jacob plays down the DMSO-cancer connection, because he has enough trouble getting the substance recognized for all of its other special uses. He doesn't want to have to fight off the label of "cancer quackery" as well.

DMSO-HEMATOXYLON ACTION ON ANIMALS

By age seventy-eight, Eli Jordon Tucker, Jr., M.D., had done over 1,000 bone fusions for arthritic backs, ankles, and other joints as an orthopedic surgeon practicing for fifty-two years in Houston. Dr. Tucker's true love was medical research, however, and one of his major discoveries was the technique for grafting bone from one animal species to another. The drug company, E.R. Squibb and Sons of Princeton, New Jersey, purchased the patent rights to his discovery and spent half-a-million dollars developing the method about twenty years ago. Dr. Tucker also perfected an oral treatment with vital bone substances for the correction of bone degenerative conditions. For half a century, he was a respected Fellow of the American College of Surgeons, a member of the Orthopedic Board of the International College of Surgeons, an honorary life member of the American Medical Association, and he was one of the few orthopedists in the State of Texas to be presented with the "Award of Merit" by the American Medical Association for his research work on bone.

Dr. Tucker performed his bone grafting experiments with calf bones that he acquired from a nearby slaughterhouse, the Houston Meat Packing Company. While purchasing specimens, he noticed the butchers were accepting for slaughter white-faced cattle that were eaten up with cancer of the face. In many cases, eye cancer spreading down the animal's muzzle was disintegrating the entire face. Even so, the meat inspectors and veterinarians passed these cattle for human consumption provided there was no cancer metastasis to the animal's internal organs.

It occurred to Tucker in 1962 that there might be such a thing as cancer antibodies. Currently scientists are seeking the same thing through studying interferon, the much-publicized antivirus substance. Aside from his research on developing a bone paste for grafting purposes, Dr. Tucker inaugurated an additional project. He did some laboratory work on the blood of cancerous cows, looking for cancer antibodies. His procedure entailed bleeding the animals after they were slaughtered and making gamma globulin from the blood. Then, he injected the gamma globulin into cancer-ridden rats and mice. The substance seemed to retard some of the rodent tumors, specifically the adenocarcinomas and others involving granulomatosis (a condition marked by tumors of the pink tissue that is formed during wound healing) such as lymphosarcoma (lymphoma). It did not affect fibrosarcoma, melanoma, and some other types.

He required a dye for marking the tumors in order to better see any growth alterations. The dye had to stain the tumor sufficiently and at the same time he gave the gamma globulin injection. Tucker was disappointed by most of the dyes he tried. With methylene blue, everything in the tissue field became overly darkened. Picric acid colored all the tissues yellow. The red coloring safranine stain had no effect on the tumor. But hematoxylon turned out to be the perfect dye because it stained the cancer one color, the normal cells another color. It is a multiple-coloring stain.

Hematoxylon is a long-established dye, used by biologists for over 100 years as a pathologic marker for animal cells, particularly because of its affinity for nucleic acids. Hematoxylon's formula, $C_{16}H_{14}O_6$, has two loose hydrogen bonds so that it oxidizes readily to a red substance known as hematein. This property of rapid oxidation is often used as an indicator in chemistry for alkaloid titrations. Thus, hematoxylon is a substance commonly employed by physical scientists.

It is also used in medicine as an astringent for the relief of diarrhea and for the treatment of urinary infections, because the presence of the dye is rapidly excreted in the urine. The human dose recommended in the past has been from 0.6 to 2 grams.

The one drawback for Tucker with adapting hematoxylon for staining tissue was that it is a resin derived from the bark of the logwood tree. The resin is insoluble in ordinary laboratory solvents such as alcohol and ether. The dye has a special nucleus similar to the nucleic acids, the master molecules of life that cannot be duplicated synthetically.

When DMSO came into use around 1963, Tucker found that getting the dye to go into solution was no longer a problem. DMSO's high solvent properties combined with an amazing affinity for hematoxylon, dissolving almost its own weight of the dye, made it an ideal substance for his purposes. Not only that, DMSO did not alter the hematoxylon at all and carried the chemical directly into the tumor. There was good dispersion; only the cancer cells were stained and stood out under the microscope and in gross dissection.

To his amazement, Tucker discovered he could dissolve 25 grams of hematoxylon powder into 62 cc of DMSO liquid, an exceedingly high concentration. In a medical paper published in the January 16, 1968, issue of *International Surgery*, in collaboration with A. Carrizo, M.D., Director of the National Cancer Control and Cancer Center for the Republic of Panama, Panama City, he described how hematoxylon dissolved in DMSO was used in recurrent neoplasms.[1]

Drs. Tucker and Carrizo injected into dogs a solution of 25 grams of hematoxylon dissolved in 75 cc of DMSO as a parenteral intravenous solution with 5 percent dextrose in saline and normal saline to do an acute toxicity study. They observed no abnormalities in the living animals over a month's time, and autopsies showed no changes in the animals' livers, kidneys, gastrointestinal tracts, hearts, bone marrow, lungs, or brains. No dye was present in any of the sectioned tissues. High doses of DMSO without hematoxylon that had been given into the jugular veins of healthy dogs did cause acute respiratory failure, shock, and death in three of four dogs. The combination of the dye and the solvent proved to be much less toxic than DMSO alone. Albino rats could tolerate four times the amount of the combination hematoxylon solution than the DMSO alone.

Experimental animals with both induced and spontaneous tumors were treated with the combination solution. The induced tumors included a methyl cholantranine transplant tumor (fibrosarcoma) and adenocarcinoma of the breast (Walker's tumor) in albino rats. The fibrosarcoma regressed somewhat but not entirely. The adenocarcinoma was not affected by the intravenous injection of hematoxylon and DMSO until a small dose of androgen caused its rapid regression in practically 100 percent of the rats.

Spontaneous tumors in dogs, horses, and cattle were treated with the DMSO-hematoxylon solution. In some cases, Tucker performed the service out of a feeling of pity for the suffering animal. For instance, William Daniel, former Governor of Guam, one of Tucker's friends, phoned and told the doctor: "E.J., I have a cancerous dog on my ranch who is suffering terribly. Could you do anything to help him, or should I have him put to death?"

"I'd love to try," answered Tucker. "I'll send my technician to pick up the dog right away."

The technician brought the animal to Tucker's veterinarian, Dr. Collins, for examination. The vet diagnosed that large-cell lymphosarcoma was permeating the dog's body. "The poor animal is choking to death from the tumors in his throat, and he has large tumors all over his body," said Dr. Collins over the telephone. "I don't think he'll live long enough to be transported to your laboratory."

Tucker said, "Transfuse him, give him some blood fast, and let me have him for treatment."

The physician took the dog, which was barely alive, into the laboratory and injected DMSO-hematoxylon solution intravenously. His technician took over the work and gave the injections daily. Within two weeks, all the tumors had disappeared. It seemed like a miracle to the technician.

Upon Tucker's examination of the dog, he found that all the large-cell lymphosarcoma tumors had completely regressed. The huge masses in the neck and over the whole body of the animal had gone away, and the dog came out of the treatment completely cured.

The dog was thriving at the laboratory when an unlucky accident caused his death. He ate a large quantity of some meat contaminated with Malathion, an insecticide poison. Tucker performed an autopsy, which revealed no active cancer cells in the vestigial remains of the previously large lymphomatous nodules. Many ghost cells—cells that were formerly cancer but weren't any kind of cells anymore—appeared in the microscopic sections. Not a single distinguishable cancer cell remained in the dog.

The Tucker research organization put out word for another lymphosarcomatous dog, which came from a veterinarian hospital. This animal had a small-cell lymphosarcoma. Injections of DMSO-hematoxylon for this dog were less effective than for the first. Its tumors regressed somewhat but not altogether, and the animal died two months after the withdrawal of treatment from a perforated heart brought about by heartworm infestation. Small-cell lymphosarcoma failed to respond to the DMSO-hematoxylon solution as dramatically as had large-cell lymphosarcoma.

A wild horse with osteogenic sarcoma on the right hind leg was treated by Tucker with local applications of the solution. He sprayed on 25 cc of diluted dye and DMSO in 500 cc of normal saline and glucose. The tumor disappeared after treatment continued for approximately a year. The animal lived for at least five more years with no evidence of recurrence locally or by metastasis.

An Arabian stallion with generalized malignant melanomas in and about the anus and under the tail was treated with 10 cc of the solution in 5 percent dextrose in saline twice weekly for three months. The tumors lodged under the skin regressed and then remained static for two more years.

A small squamous-cell carcinoma of the eye in a white-faced cow was treated by local injection of 15 percent DMSO-hematoxylon solution in normal saline and injected directly into the conjunctival sac daily for three months. The squamous-cell tumor completely disappeared and did not recur.

Tucker determined the human dosage of this DMSO-hematoxylon solution by trial and error intravenous injections into 250-gram rats and 25-pound dogs. He lowered the dose seven times and eventually arrived at the correct figure for its parenteral administration to humans. Made from 25 grams of hematoxylon and 75 cc of DMSO combined, 1 cc of the resultant solution is ideal for each 75 pounds of body weight. This material has been administered to people intravenously, intra-arterially, and topically.

ANTI-CANCER SOLUTION TRIALS ON DYING PATIENTS

Tucker told his hospital associates of his findings. Jack Bevil, M.D., of Houston, approached him about trying this new solution for a patient dying from inoperable fibrosarcoma. The woman was critically ill and comatose. Her husband listened to Tucker tell his story of animal cancer treatment and asked the doctor to try to save his wife.

Tucker sat by this woman's bedside and gave the intravenous infusion exceedingly slowly and cautiously, taking six hours the first time. He gave her weeks of treatment, and her tumor began to recede. When it had shrunk to a small enough size, Dr. Bevil took her back to the operating room and removed it. The woman lived on in Houston uneventfully for two more years and then moved to San Antonio where Tucker lost track of her progress.

Tucker performed a series of hematoxylon-DMSO intravenous injections in an extensive, privately financed research project to record the effect of his treatment on different types of cancer. Table 11.1 shows his results.

Analysis of this series of thirty-seven preterminal American cases of malignancy reveals that the treatment with dimethyl sulfoxide and hematoxylon therapy when combined with current anti-cancer agents resulted in condition improvement in 70.5 percent of the patients. These agents included surgery, radiation, and the anti-cancer drugs 5-fluorouracil (5FU), methotrexate, and thiotepa.

Improvement of the patient was gained in only 5.4 percent of those cases treated with the anti-cancer agents alone and no DMSO-hematoxylon solution.

When DMSO-hematoxylon solution was administered alone, condition improvement jumped to 38.1 percent. This was largely a reduction in symptoms with the exception of one case of leiomyosarcoma (case number 1 in the table in which the tumor regressed and was surgically removed).

The most striking results observed by Tucker were in two cases of large-cell lymphosarcoma (number 17 in the table and an uncharted Panamanian patient) and two cases of malignant giant-cell tumor of the bone (numbers 10 and 14 shown in the table). There was complete regression in both of the cases of large-cell lymphosarcoma with no recurrence up to a time well beyond the date of Tucker's published report in June 1968. One of these DMSO-hematoxylon-treated patients died ten years later of a heart attack and the other is still living today. There was also complete regression in one case of malignant giant-cell tumor of approximately one-third of the femur that underwent new bone regeneration.

Tucker did not publish more papers on the subject of hematoxylon combined with DMSO as a treatment for cancer because of continual colleague criticism of his use of a non-approved drug. He was expelled from the staffs of two hospitals for administering this treatment. The expulsions were separate actions that hurt him deeply. Despite his emeritus status among his peers as the grand old gentleman of orthopedic surgery, this did not stop vindictive reactions to his use of DMSO for cancer treatment. Consequently, he provided treatment only very selectively—when the patient was obviously preterminal and in a destitute state. His fees for cancer therapy were ridiculously low, if he charged any fees at all. Tucker didn't want any more publicity about his anti-cancer therapy. My report is given here because I believe it is about time the medical community, especially oncologists, took hold of this treatment and explored it further for the purpose of aiding those one out of three suffering Americans who will eventually come down with cancer, and one out of five who will die from it.

On an ironic note, Dr. Tucker himself came down with a form of cancer that would have responded to his DMSO-hematoxylon treatment, but before he could administer it to himself, he fell into a coma. No one had access to his formula except the author of this book, and I did not know Dr. Tucker's attendants needed it to save his life. Dr. Tucker died only a few months before this book was first published. Its updating and republication may save lives—I hope so!

HOW TO PREPARE AND USE
THE HEMATOXYLON-DMSO SOLUTION

To prepare a solution of hematoxylon dissolved in dimethyl sulfoxide for anti-cancer application, obtain from almost any chemical company 25 grams of powdered hematoxylon HX-0025. Into an 80 cubic centimeter (cc) volume bottle containing the hematoxylon powder, pour DMSO, stirring continuously, until DMSO fills the bottle by three fourths. Stopper the solution and shake by hand or, better, by machine until all powder is completely dissolved. No solid particles should be showing on the bottom of the bottle after it is left standing. Then, fill the bottle with the balance of the DMSO and shake again. The hematoxylon-DMSO solution is now ready for therapeutic use against cancer.

To insure safety during treatment, start by using only .5 cc of the

Table 11.1 *Hematoxylon-DMSO Treatment*
on Different Types of Cancer

Patient Number	Age	Sex	Primary Tumor and Cell Type	Surgery	Other Chemotherapy and Radiation
1.	66	F	Leiomyosarcoma (inoperable) of abdomen	3 unsuccessful attempts at removal. One successful.	None
2.	27	F	Chondroosteosarcoma. Terminal	2/10/65 Biopsy	None
3.	73	M	Adenoca. of prostate and bladder Generalized metastasis. Pre-terminal	None	None
4.	72	F	Squamous-cell ca. of neck with metastasis	Multiple resections of neck.	Max. radiation only.
5.	58	F	Adenoca. of breast with extensive metastasis—Grade 4	Radical mastectomy.	No chemotherapy, Max. X-radiation at operative site.
6.	84	F	Large fungating adenoca. of breast with metastasis to lung	Simple mastectomy.	None
7.	52	F	Squamous-cell ca. of pelvis with large metastases	Pan-hysterectomy.	Max. radiation, 5 F.U. 1800 mg total dosage.
8.	51	M	Squamous-cell ca. of lung with metastasis to neck	None	None—Max. X-radiation to lungs.
9.	86	F	Adenoca. of breast with fungating postop. area	Radical mastectomy.	Max X-radiation to operative site.
10.	60	M	Malignant giant-cell tumor of femur	None Biopsy only.	Total F.U. 8,810 mg.
11.	52	M	Squamous-cell ca. ulcerating of face	None	Max. local X-radiation. Total F.U. 1,120 mg.

Response to Other Therapy Alone	Date of Administration Hematoxylon DMSO Dosage	Total Dosage and Response	Present Status
Removal of necrotizing tumor.	10/23/67 2 cc H-D.M.S.O., IV	50 injections. Tumor regressed and was removed June 1966.	November 1967 Patient still surviving.
None	4/11/65 1½ cc H-D.M.S.O., IV	48 injections. Tumor regressed for 3 months.	Died 12/24/65.
None	11/5/65 2 cc H-D.M.S.O., IV	56 injections. Tumor regressed for 4 months.	Died 5/12/66.
Retardation of local tumor growth	11/12/65 2 cc H-D.M.S.O., IV	60 injections. Tumor regressed for 5 months.	Died 8/66.
None	11/26/65 2 cc H-D.M.S.O., IV	28 injections. Tumor regressed for 3 months.	Died 4/1966.
None	1/5/66 2 cc H-D.M.S.O., IV Local application of 15% H-D.M.S.O.	47 injections. Local applications 7 months. Complete regression of lung metastasis.	Died 8/5/66. Heart disease.
Poor	1/5/66 2 cc H-D.M.S.O., IV	27 injections. Complete regression of metastatic masses.	2/7/66 in complete remission. Died 5/3/66 of drug addiction.
Poor	2/7/66 2 cc H-D.M.S.O., IV	54 injections. Remission for 6 months.	Died 10/66.
Fungating growth at operative site	10/7/66 Local application to fungating area only. 15% H-D.M.S.O.	Daily for 8 months. Complete relief of pain. Lesion regressed. Odor subsided.	Died 6/67. Heart disease.
Poor	10/5/66 2 cc H-D.M.S.O., IV	102 injections. Complete remission. No tumor formation by biopsy or x-ray.	10/9/67 date of complete remission.
Moderate	4/5/67 2 cc H-D.M.S.O., IV Local application of 15% H-D.M.S.O.	72 injections. Local applications daily for 7 months. Complete relief of pain and odor.	11/9/67 tumor continues to regress.

Patient Number	Age	Sex	Primary Tumor and Cell Type	Surgery	Other Chemotherapy and Radiation
12.	50	M	Adenoca. of prostate. Metastasis to verte-brae	Suprapubic cys-totomy.	None
13.	45	M	Squamous-cell ca. of mouth. Preterminal	Radical neck resection and hemimandibulec-tomy.	Total F.U. 1,600 mg.
14.	24	F	Malignant giant cell tumor of upper ⅓ left femur, advanced	None	Max. X-radiation. To-tal F.U. 4,800 mg.
15.	45	F	Mixed tumor of uterus (undifferen-tiated)	None	Total F.U. 400 mg.
16.	44	F	Adenoca. of breast Preterminal	Radical mastectomy. Exploratory laparotomy.	Max. X-radiation. To-tal F.U. 1,600 mg.
17.	63	F	Large-cell lymphosar-coma. Generalized metastasis	Splenectomy.	Total Cytoxan 1,050 mg.
18.	50	F	Squamous-cell ca. of cervix. Preterminal	No surgery.	None
19.	40	F	Squamous-cell ca. of cervix	No surgery.	No radiation. No drug therapy
20.	48	F	Adenoca. of cervix advanced	None	None
21.	50	F	Squamous-cell ca. of cervix. Preterminal	None	None

Response to Other Therapy Alone	Date of Administration Hematoxylon DMSO Dosage	Total Dosage and Response	Present Status
None	2 cc H-D.M.S.O., IV	54 injections. Prostatic tumor regressed.	7/17/67 discharged 11/15/67 still in remission.
Moderate	4/2/67 2 cc H-D.M.S.O., IV	36 injections. Remission.	Dismissed 8/67 11/15/67 still in remission.
Poor	5/2/67 2 cc H-D.M.S.O., IV	72 injections. Tumor regressing rapidly, with bone regeneration.	11/16/67 patient continued to improve.
Poor	3/4/67 2 cc H-D.M.S.O., IV Local application of 15% H-D.M.S.O.	16 injections. Pain, hemorrhage and odor ceased.	Died 4/2/67
Poor	9/14/67 1½ cc H-D.M.S.O., IV	27 injections. Complete regression of abdominal masses.	11/22/67 patient continues to improve.
Fair	8/5/67 2 cc H-D.M.S.O., IV	21 injections. Complete regression.	11/23/67 complete regression.
None	8/5/67 2 cc H-D.M.S.O., IV Local application of 15% H-D.M.S.O.	12 injections. Remission.	11/10/67 progress continues.
Poor	10/24/67 2½ cc H-D.M.S.O., IV Local application daily by vaginal pack 15% H-D.M.S.O.	5 injections. Regression of pain, odor and hemorrhage.	11/9/67 patient continues to improve.
Poor	10/2/67 2 cc H-D.M.S.O., IV Local application by vaginal pack 15% H-D.M.S.O.	12 injections. Patient has relief of odor, pain and bleeding.	10/11/67 patient continues to improve.
None	9/7/67 2 cc H-D.M.S.O., IV	13 injections. Patient free of pain and softening of parametrium.	10/11/67 patient continues to improve.

Patient Number	Age	Sex	Primary Tumor and Cell Type	Surgery	Other Chemotherapy and Radiation
22.	68	M	Squamous-cell ca. of soft palate	None	M.T.X., I.A. Total dose 200 mg.
23.	60	M	Adenoca. of stomach. Inoperable	None	Total F.U. 800 mg.
24.	56	M	Adenoca. of bladder and prostate.	Suprapubic cystos-tomy.	None—M.X.T. Total dose 200 mg. F.U. to-tal 2,800 mg.
25.	22	F	Advanced adenoca. of ovary, with metas-tasis to abdomen.	Exploratory and biopsy only.	No. radiation. Total thio-tepa I.A. 200 mg.
26.	64	F	Squamous-cell ca. of soft palate.	None	None
27.	90	F	Squamous-cell ca. of soft palate.	None	M.T.X., I.A. Total dose 650 mg.
28.	84	F	Squamous-cell ca. of mouth	None	M.T.X., I.A. Total dose 650 mg.
29.	28	F	Chorioepithelioma. Terminal.	None	None
30.	56	F	Bronchogenic ca. with metastasis to left lung	Removal of right lung.	No X-radiation or other cancer drug.
31.	58	M	Ca. of stomach. Pre-terminal	None	None
32.	70	F	Squamous-cell ca. of soft palate	None	None

Response to Other Therapy Alone	Date of Administration Hematoxylon DMSO Dosage	Total Dosage and Response	Present Status
Fair	5/25/67 2 cc H-D.M.S.O., IV	36 injections. Had remission and dismissed from hospital. Had recurrence 1 mo. later.	Released after 24 injections, with another remission & same remission as of 11/10/67.
None	10/9/67 2 cc H-D.M.S.O., IV	24 injections. Patient free of pain and able to eat without pain. No hemorrhage.	11/9/67 continues in state of symptomatic remission.
Moderate	9/19/67 2 cc H-D.M.S.O., IV	22 injections. Patient dismissed from hospital in remission.	10/11/67 progress of patient continues.
Fair	8/15/67 2 cc H-D.M.S.O., IV	23 injections. Palpable tumor reduced 50% of original size and patient free of pain.	10/11/67 progress of patient continues.
Poor	1/26/67	11 injections. Tumor static.	11/15/67 patient free of pain.
Fair	10/21/67 2 cc H-D.M.S.O., IV	11 injections. Tumor static.	11/15/67 patient free of pain.
Fair	9/18/67 2 cc H-D.M.S.O., IV	24 injections. Marked regression of size of tumor.	11/11/67 regression continues.
Poor	10/5/67 2 cc H-D.M.S.O., IV	Immediate response after 12 injections. Gononadotrophin hormone level reduced from 350,000 I.U. to 35,000 I.U.	Died 11/5/67.
Poor	5/23/66 2 cc H-D.M.S.O., IV	59 injections	patient survived 16 months. Died 9/6/67.
None	11/7/66 2 cc H-D.M.S.O., IV	40 injections	Died 4/3/67. Massive hemorrhage.
None	9/7/66 2 cc H-D.M.S.O., IV	36 injections. Patient had remission.	No treatment for 4 months—deserted. Died 4/4/67.

Patient Number	Age	Sex	Primary Tumor and Cell Type	Surgery	Other Chemotherapy and Radiation
33.	40	M	Adenoca. of penis with metastasis	Amputation of penis.	None
34.	42	M	Squamous-cell ca. of penis	Amputation of penis.	None
35.	89	M	Squamous-cell ca. of larynx	Laryngectomy.	None
36.	50	F	Advanced adenoca. of cervix	None	M.T.X., I.A. total dose 650 mg.
37.	66	M	Adenoca. of stomach	None	Total F.U. 1,200 mg.

Ca.	Carcinoma		H.	Hematoxylon
D.M.S.O.	Dimethyl sulfoxide		MTX	Methotrexate
F.U.	Fluorouracil			

solution injected into a 250-milliliter (ml) bottle of 5 percent dextrose water. For diabetic patients, substitute normal saline for the dextrose. Increase the treatment solution concentration by one-tenth daily until the doctor administering the treatment determines that his patient's tolerance level is reached. Beyond tolerance will tend to cause the patient to go into a high fever about 35 minutes after the treatment ends. For this reason, it is advisable for the patient to always carry either Demerol or 50-milligram tablets of Benadryl to counteract the intolerance.

The physician will intravenously administer hematoxylon-DMSO in 5 percent dextrose water. A vein in the arm is usually chosen for the injection, and the drip speed averages approximately 47 drops per minute. If the patient has a low tolerance to the intravenous injection, a Benadryl tablet swallowed 30 to 40 minutes before the IV starts can prevent the onset of fever. Please note that the instructions are supplied for application by a duly licensed physician, as potentially dangerous materials are being used here for the destruction of a possibly deadly disease. These instructions are not to be followed frivolously by anyone unskilled in the medical treatment of oncological conditions. For exam-

Response to Other Therapy Alone	Date of Administration Hematoxylon DMSO Dosage	Total Dosage and Response	Present Status
None	9/7/66 2 cc H-D.M.S.O., IV plus local application	52 injections with daily local applications. Tumor remained static. Dismissed 6/17/67.	11/15/67 exact condition unknown but patient surviving.
None	4/10/67 2 cc H-D.M.S.O., IV	54 injections. Daily local injections. Pain reduced.	11/15/67 tumor is static.
Poor	10/30/67 2 cc H-D.M.S.O., IV	12 injections. Relieved of pain.	10/10/67 patient in state of remission.
Fair	10/5/67 2 cc H-D.M.S.O., IV	14 injections. Relieved of pain.	10/10/67 tumor static.
Poor	10/9/67 2 cc H-D.M.S.O., IV	12 injections. Relieved of pain.	11/10/67 patient in symptomatic remission.

ple, the physician may wish to irrigate the injection site with 2 cc of heparin, a blood-thinning agent, to avoid clotting, if the subclavian vein is chosen for infusion.

The treatment solution may be taken orally. If so, the patient should have no food or drink after midnight. Upon arising in the morning, pour about two ounces of 5 percent dextrose water (saline, if a diabetic) into a small paper cup. Then, using a syringe for precise measurement, put into the cup the same volume of hematoxylon-DMSO solution that would be taken intravenously. Drink the mixture. To allow for absorption of the therapeutic solution, wait at least 30 minutes before eating or drinking anything else. Important notation: In cases of stomach cancer, do not drink this therapeutic mixture, because it will have a direct effect on the tumor. The cancer disappears from the stomach lining, leaving behind a hole similar to a gastric ulcer. Intravenous infusions are therefore more effective for gastrointestinal cancer.

For lung cancer, use the Bennett Respirator Machine and install 2 cc of saline solution and 4 drops of DMSO-hematoxylon solution. Inhale the mixture for about 10 minutes twice a day. Use this inhalation therapy when not receiving an IV. Make sure that intervals of at least two hours occur between treatments.

For bone cancer, take the intravenous infusion, but also swallow at least 2,000 mg of bone meal tablets each day.

For facial cancer, reduce the solution by half with distilled water and apply it to the skin, using a cotton-tip applicator. Paint the skin twice daily. Gradually increase the strength of the applied solution as long as the patient does not show any allergic reaction. The therapeutic solution can also be taken orally for facial cancer.

Other adjunctive drugs that sometimes accompany the application of hematoxylon-DMSO-dextrose solution are cytoxin and F5U, but only for short periods. Sometimes the various medications are alternated, using one one day and the other the next. Both cytoxin and F5U lower the red blood cell count so that it is imperative that a complete blood count be performed once or more a week. Also, do not swallow aspirin when taking cytoxin or F5U. Instead, use a painkiller substitute.

Another once-a-week adjunctive injection is comprised of 1 cc of ACTH Gel, 40 units per 5 cc bottle or vial; .5 cc dexamethasone acetate, 4 mg per 30 cc bottle; and .5 cc triamcinolone acetonide, 40 mg per ml from a 5 ml bottle.

A good cancer test is the one for Carcinoma Embryonic Activity (CEA) performed once a month or more. The normal reading for a non-smoker is 2.5; normal for a smoker is 5.0.

Cancer patients taking the DMSO-hematoxylon-dextrose solution should have kidney function tests of their urine (creatine clearance and BUN) performed biweekly. They should always drink plenty of fluids. If swelling occurs, the physician should prescribe Diuril or some other diuretic.

Taking vitamin supplements, especially vitamins A, C, E, and D, is essential. Carrots should be eaten every day, in particular for the treatment of liver cancer. Absolutely no liquor, wine, or beer should be consumed. And, realize that smoking not only retards healing but may have been a contributing source of causing the condition initially.

The DMSO-hematoxylon-dextrose solution should be administered to the cancer victim daily until a reasonably low CEA test reading is obtained.

CASES OF CANCER CURED WITH
HEMATOXYLON AND DMSO

I mentioned that Dr. Tucker had not published the results of his research and treatment since 1968 because of peer pressure and fear of being removed from medical practice. But this didn't completely deter him from attempting to heal those few who made appeals to him for help. For example, two more patients were successfully treated for large-cell lymphosarcoma. One lived for eight years after treatment and finally died from a heart attack, as had a previous lymphosarcoma case. The other is still alive and well today.

In the latter case, Alva Ruth Wilson of Porter, Texas, then age thirty-eight, learned that she was the victim of disseminated large-cell lymphosarcoma in January 1972. She had sizeable tumors in her lungs, the common iliac arteries, and the lymph nodes around her aorta.

Patients with lymphosarcoma (the kind of cancer that killed the Shah of Iran) experience a malabsorption syndrome, a clinical state resulting from impaired assimilation of nutrients from the small bowel. The victim becomes chronically ill and emaciated, with pale mucous membranes and dry scaly skin that becomes dark in color. Blood pressure drops. Fluid accumulates in the abdominal cavity, which swells disproportionately. Anemia develops, and the cancer cells infiltrate the bone marrow. The patient suffers destruction of normal lymph node architecture and invasion of the node capsules and adjacent fat by characteristic lymphosarcoma cells. Death in a relatively short time is predictable.

Mrs. Wilson had the maximum amount of chemotherapy she could take for one month and then chemotherapy and radiation together for another month. Still, the tumors continued to spread and chemotherapy had to be discontinued because of its awful side effects. One of these was the development of dangerous leukopenia, a condition in which the total number of white blood cells in the patient's circulating blood was far less than normal. She practically lost her immunity to infection. As a life-threatening chemotherapeutic side effect, Mrs. Wilson's white blood count dropped too far below the lower limit of 5,000 per cubic mm.

One year later Tucker began hematoxylon and DMSO injections intravenously for the woman. They were given every other day from January 1973 through January 1974. All evidence of her tumors disappeared, and they have not recurred to the present time. Tucker followed Mrs. Wilson's progress continually; she is perfectly well today with no side effects from the treatment or from the tumor.

In another case, Elroy Guerro of Houston, forty-one years old, had a lymphosarcoma of three years duration. After full treatment with maximum radiation and chemotherapy, the opinion of the radiologist was that the patient had no chance to survive longer than a few more months. He had involvement of the mediastinal lymph nodes.

This patient was treated by intravenous injections of hematoxylon and DMSO, 2.015 g every other day from December 1971 to March 1972. By the end of the injection therapy, the tumor had disappeared and Mr. Guerro quit the treatment. Tucker last heard from him in December 1978 and learned that the man was in excellent condition. There was no evidence of recurrence and no side effects from the medication.

Eventually, when Tucker asked about the patient from his former employer, the Ideal Engineering Company, the personnel office advised him that Guerro had died of a heart attack in April 1980, eight years after he had completed the DMSO treatment for deadly lymphosarcoma.

A third patient was less fortunate. Frank T. Guiddy of Kennedy, New York, age forty-four, was admitted to Memorial Baptist Hospital in Houston in a terminal lymphosarcomatous state. He had an obvious tumor, entirely surrounding his neck, lying just under the skin (see Figure 11.1). Mr. Guiddy had been treated five years previously with maximum radiation and chemotherapy. The traditional cancer treat-

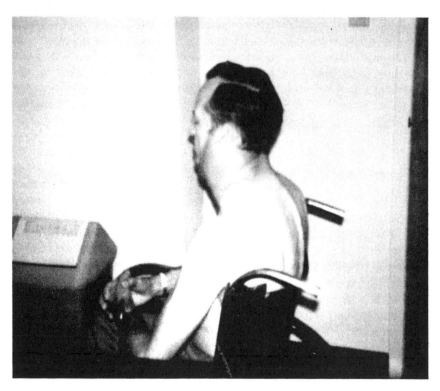

Figure 11.1 Photograph of Frank T. Guiddy, age 44; note large tumor lymphosarcoma of the neck.

ments had brought on severe side effects, mainly absence of white blood cells in the blood stream.

Every day for three weeks, 2.015 g of hematoxylon and DMSO combination solution was injected intravenously into the patient. The tumor in his neck decreased in size from 22.5 inches (in) to 18.75 in (see Figure 11.2), returning Guiddy's neck to normal appearance.

Unfortunately, this man was so riddled with lymphosarcoma, his body was totally assaulted by the process. He died at the hospital September 23, 1980. Autopsy showed that he suffered with cancer in almost every organ of his body. Lymphosarcoma involved the man's cervical lymph nodes, retroperitoneal and abdominal nodes, membranes around his heart, pancreas, left and right lungs, spleen, the entire gastrointestinal tract, kidneys, adrenal glands, and especially his liver, which weighed an immense 3,400 g. He died in bed from liver failure a week after the photograph shown in Figure 11.2 was taken. His liver was a solid mass of dead lymphosarcoma. The DMSO-hematoxylon material had enough anti-tumor quality to destroy the enormous

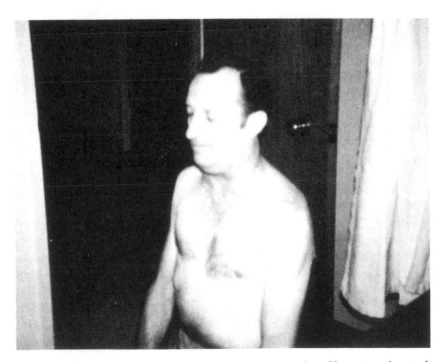

Figure 11.2 Frank T. Guiddy after receiving three weeks of hematoxylon and DMSO treatment. Note the marked decrease in the size of the lymphosarcomatous tumor.

masses of lymphosarcomatous growth permeating the man's body. If Guiddy had had near-normal organs or at least a functioning liver, it's likely he would have survived. But he did not.

MODES OF ADMINISTERING DMSO AND HEMATOXYLON

Cancer of the cervix in the preterminal stage receives the greatest benefit only from local application. The symptoms become less severe. There is very little local regression of the tumor itself in advanced squamous-cell carcinoma of the cervix. However, the patient feels marked relief of pain and a diminution of bleeding and odor, especially when the DMSO-hematoxylon solution follows local radiation treatments.

Vaginal packing with a 15-percent concentration of the Tucker solution has been found to be most effective in controlling hemorrhage and odor from irradiation slough. A small saturated pack is placed against the cervix and left for three hours and then removed.

Topical application has been used in many open lesions of malignancies with encouraging results. A 15-percent solution of hematoxylon and DMSO is made fresh and applied over the sloughing malignancy. Tucker suggested that the doctor should dab the liquid onto the lesion with cotton-tip applicators and, if possible, not cover or dress the area. Often a dressing with the solution causes an irritation of the growth and some increase in its size. No toxicity has been noted by this method's use.

In the administration of the solution intravenously or intra-arterially, the parenteral liquid agent carrying the hematoxylon and DMSO into the blood vessels that Tucker preferred is 5 percent dextrose in saline. This parenteral agent should be started first and when the desired rate of drip is established, then the DMSO-hematoxylon solution is instilled directly into the bottle—not into the tubing. The resultant infusion solution should be a pale yellow to green. In the event the solution turns red, this means hematoxylon has oxidized and should be discarded. A fresh solution must be made up for the infusion.

The intravenous rate of injection should not exceed forty drops per minute. Care must be taken to prevent any of the solution from escaping into the subcutaneous tissue. Otherwise the patient is likely to feel a burning sensation from activation of the underlying nerve endings. Also, such poor technique invariably causes a periphlebitis (inflammation of a vein), which damages the vein for future use. Incidentally, even if the solution has escaped into the underlying tissue, it has never caused a slough (death of tissue).

Too rapid administration results in the patient experiencing shortness of breath and frequent rapid breathing. In the case of large tumor masses, a fever reaction often occurs. Tucker believed that this feverishness is due to rapid absorption of dying tissue. If fever does come on, the treatment should be discontinued and restarted at a later date with a greatly reduced dose of the solution. The antidote for fever is to give aspirin by mouth and to inject Demerol intramuscularly. The Demerol must be given immediately as the intravenous DMSO-hematoxylon solution is unhooked from the patient.

In intra-arterial injections, the same caution should be used as with intravenous infusion. The physician starts the parenteral solution first and establishes a regular amount of instillation before adding the DMSO-hematoxylon into the solution bottle. This method is rarely indicated and should be done with extreme caution.

LABORATORY INVESTIGATION OF DMSO USEFULNESS FOR SKIN CANCER

The effects of dimethyl sulfoxide for the treatment of skin cancer are in some respects similar to those of the skin substances, retinoids. As we know, DMSO has the ability to penetrate cellular membranes and to enhance the penetration of other molecules. Three physicians/biochemists stated in their 1983 published paper, "It may be reasonable to assume that DMSO treatment results in differentiation of cells, possibly through membrane-mediated events. This may be of importance for the study of the carcinogenic process. The release of a certain amount of lysosomal enzymes [natural chemicals that act within and on the organelles called lysosomes] to the extracellular space is a normal function of the cell (Hickman and Neufeld, 1972), and a certain release of the cytoplasmic and lysosomal enzymes to the extracellular space is not necessarily deleterious for the cells (Volden, Haugen, and Skrede, 1980)."

The purpose of the three doctors' investigation was to study the possible effects of DMSO on methylcholanthrene-induced skin cancer. Methylcholanthrene is a toxic agent—a carcinogen—that causes excessive mutagenesis (subdividing) of cells. Since they saw that the uptake of enzymes from the cellular organelles—the lysosomes—took place by cultured cancer cells and involved a cellular membrane receptor process, the effects of the carcinogen, they decided to study HeLa cells and DMSO. HeLa cells are human cancer cells maintained in tissue culture since 1953, originally excised from the cervical carcinoma of a patient named Helen Lane. The cytostatic effect of a medication—that is, the

medication's effect on the status of cells—may be determined by meas-
uring the ademosinetriphosphate (a natural chemical produced within
the cells) of these HeLa cells by means of the laboratory method of
bioluminescence. Bioluminescence is a qualitative analysis of a substance in a compound by visualizing its color in a hot flame. The three
researchers measured the DMSO solvent on the rate of secretion of
lysosomal enzymes and lactate dehydrogenase from the HeLa cells.
Their conclusion was that DMSO has a therapeutic use for skin cancer.[2]

HOW THE ANTI-CANCER DMSO SOLUTION WORKS

Thomas D. Rogers, Ph.D., under the supervision of Vernon Scholes,
M.D., performed experimental work in the cancer research department
at the North Texas State University to determine how Dr. Tucker's
anti-cancer DMSO solution works.

Figure 11.3 shows a controlled lymphosarcoma tumor in a DBA/1J
pure line female mouse. The tumor has not been treated and has been
growing for eleven days between the skin and the muscles of the
abdomen. This lymphosarcoma grows so rapidly, it has no opportunity
to metastisize before destroying the animal.

Figure 11.4 shows another DBA/1J mouse injected intraperitoneally
with the Tucker solution at the same time as the mouse in Figure 11.3. In
this second mouse, the tumor has been present for fourteen days, but it
has hardly grown because the DMSO-hematoxylon solution is destroying
the tumor. Notice that the DMSO-hematoxylon has an affinity only for the
tumor and has flowed nowhere else in the mouse's body. Although the
solution was injected into the abdominal cavity and the tumor lies in the
subcutaneous tissue, the dye substance found its way to the tumor
through the mouse's blood stream.

Figure 11.5 shows an electron microscopy study of the large-cell
lymphosarcoma. The cancer cells are surrounded by ground substance
or interstitial material that looks like ground glass. This is protoplasm
that goes into the cell and feeds the cancer. If the nutritional protoplasm
is eliminated, the cancer cell starves to death.

Figure 11.6 shows that the ground substance around the lymphosarcoma has been destroyed. The cancer cells are separating and dying.
Lymphosarcoma death is taking place because of lack of nutrition. You
can see that the ground glass-like interstitial material is gone because
of the action of the DMSO-hematoxylon combination solution. The host
survives, but the cancer does not.

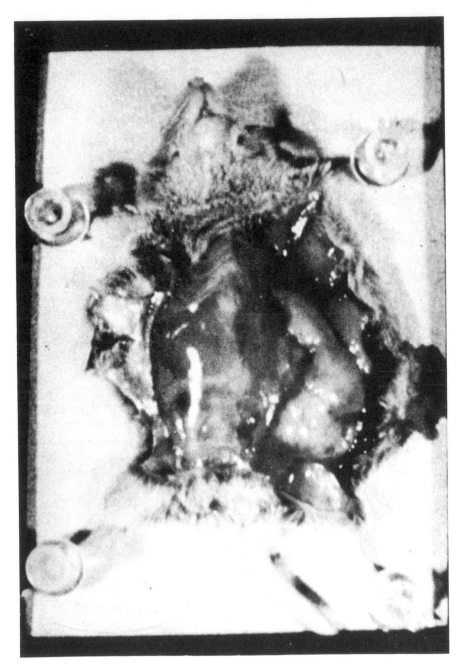

Figure 11.3 An example of a non-treated tumor-bearing mouse with an 11-day tumor.

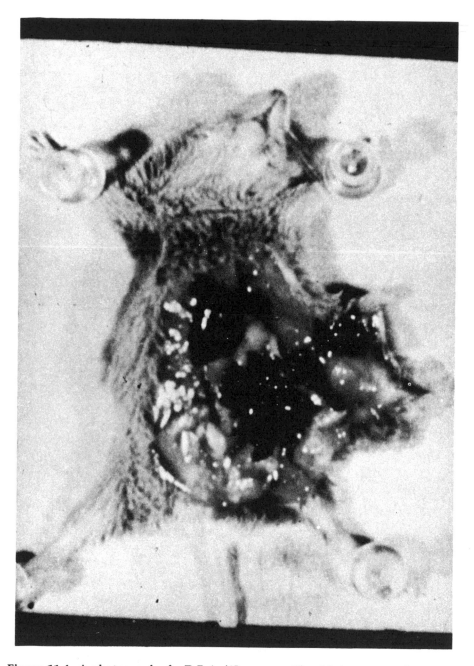

Figure 11.4 A photograph of a D.B.A./1J mouse with a 14-day tumor, showing the affinity of the tumor for the hematoxylon, which is stained, along with the tumor, with no staining of any other tissue.

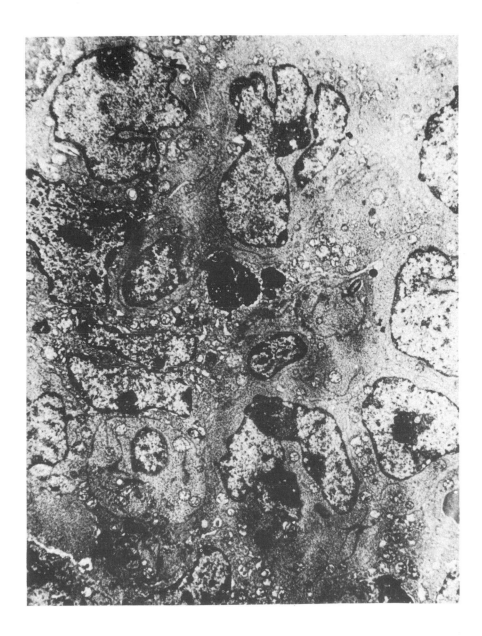

Figure 11.5 An electron micrograph showing a portion of the nucleus and cytoplasm (material outside of a cell nucleus) of the untreated tumor (Figure 11.3). All membrane systems are very distinct and there is an abundant polyribosome aggregate (mass of organelles) distributed in the cytoplasm. X6, 250

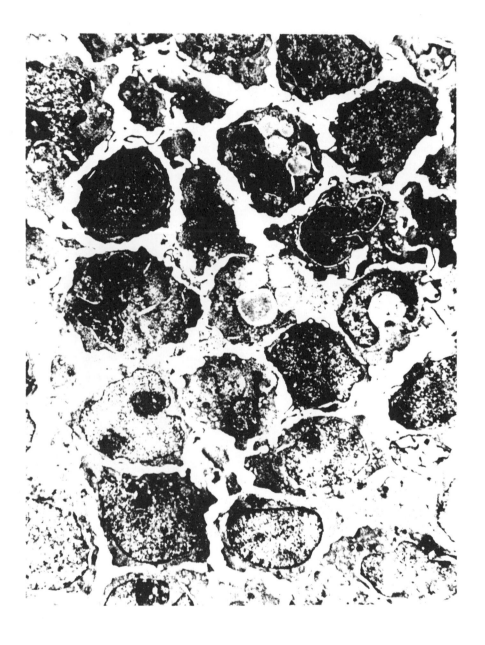

Figure 11.6 An electron micrograph of tumor tissue from the mouse (Figure 11.4). Note the breakdown of tissue structure and separation of cells leading to cell destruction. X6, 250

From the studies of Rogers,[3] we learn that this combination of hematoxylon and DMSO produces a hematein reaction of oxidation with the tumor cells to affect the ground substance, which in turn leads to cancer cell death. The DMSO had no action on the tumor cell itself but remained merely as the remarkable vehicle it is, penetrating the tissues to carry in the hematoxylon. The hematoxylon made the ground substance inactive and therefore starved the cancer cells to death.

Eli Jordon Tucker, Jr., M.D., was a maverick. He bucked the medical establishment to bring a possible cancer cure to the medical consumer. But because he attempted to halt cancer through private research, the physician traditionalists labeled Tucker a "quack." To make matters worse, he used, as part of an anti-cancer compound, a drug that isn't approved by the FDA for any purpose other than treating a urinary bladder condition. In the thinking of traditionalists in medicine, this made the doctor a heretic as well as a quack. But in the hearts and minds of his patients, Tucker was a hero.

Just like Louis Pasteur, who postulated the connection between bacteria and certain diseases, or Ignaz Philipp Semmelweis, who made obstetricians wash their hands, E.J. Tucker braved the wrath of the medical establishment. He was hurt by them, often doubly hurt, especially when his patients were mentally and emotionally assaulted by righteous, self-serving health professionals who use their powers to dispense life or death for their own purposes. Dr. Tucker described such an incident.

A three-year-old boy named Clyde Robert Lindsey of Pasadena, Texas, was brought to Tucker's office by his mother on January 14, 1970. The child had diabetes insipidus, which was being treated by the Texas Children's Hospital of Houston with injections of Pitressin, an anti-diuretic that controlled the excess urination the boy experienced. Worse, he was the victim of a particular type of metastatic endothelioma, also known as Letterer-Siwe disease, which was being treated by the M.D. Anderson Cancer Institute. Multiple cancer lesions had spread through the boy's scalp and over his body. He had draining sinuses from tumors lodged behind the ears on both sides and from inside. These were solid, palpable lumps that you could see and feel. Otolaryngologist George Stout, M.D., at the Houston Eye, Ear, Nose, and Throat Hospital, diagnosed the boy's condition as hopeless. Such a young patient is known not to live over six or seven years.

The mother and son were left destitute by the father, who ran away from his family because his child had come down with cancer. Little Clyde was not getting any better, and Mrs. Lindsey wanted Tucker's treatment for him because she had heard of his particular successful approach. Listening to her pathetic story, the doctor agreed to give the boy care, but only after he explained to the woman that the solution was entirely experimental and might do nothing for her son. He charged nothing for the treatment or for the supplies of solution.

Tucker gave her a small dropper bottle of DMSO-hematoxylon mixture and told her to give the child five drops in distilled water each morning before breakfast while he still had an empty stomach. The doctor also told her to take the medicine to one or both of the hospitals and show the medical personnel taking care of Clyde just what she was having him swallow.

Mrs. Lindsey returned the next day totally distraught. Between heavy sobs and tears, she explained how the Texas Children's Hospital staff became enraged and told her never to come back if she used Tucker's medicine for her son's cancer. This meant that her supply of Pitressin for treating the little boy's water diabetes was completely cut off, since she had no money with which to buy more.

This scene took place within earshot of other patients sitting in Tucker's reception room. They passed the hat and in a couple of minutes raised $75 for the mother to buy her child's diabetic medicine.

Since then, the mother has married a fine and respectable man. She has continued to give Clyde the DMSO-hematoxylon solution all of these years, and today, he is a big, strong young man of twenty-nine who takes his anti-cancer medicine every day. Seeing him again, otolarynogologist George Stout expressed utter amazement that the man was still alive and seemingly so well. Recently I interviewed Clyde and his mother and confirmed the details of this dramatic patient history.

The addition of dimethyl sulfoxide to the intravenous infusion bottles of cancer patients who are undergoing biological (non-drug) therapy has become almost routine today. The pharmaceutical grade of DMSO is broadly adapted by those unconventionally-practicing physicians with open minds and love in their hearts for people who come to them for health assistance. In contrast to so-called orthodox oncologists, the holistic oncologist (and such a physician is rare and should be cherished) does not experiment on his or her patients with toxic ingredients. Side effects are almost nonexistent. Indeed, DMSO is nontoxic altogether, offers little or no side effects, and brings about swift healing qualities for the cancer victim. DMSO—in particular its combination with hematoxylon solution—removes cancer pain and reduces or eliminates free radical pathology that characteristically is present in most cancer patients. Any cancer patient who has received chemotherapy or radiation therapy has, in fact, burdened his or her body with vast amounts of free radicals as manifested by sores at the corners of lips, metallic taste in the mouth, dry mouth, loss of head hair, nausea, and more. Drinking a small quantity of diluted dimethyl sulfoxide will tend to relieve or reduce many of these free radical symptoms and signs.

The 1990s are witnessing a resurgence of interest in dimethyl sulfoxide for the treatment of cancer, especially hard tumor carcinomas and lymphomas. The patient who has not subjected himself to chemotherapy or radiation therapy benefits exceedingly from DMSO intravenous infusions, intramuscular injection, topical applications, and oral solutions. At the start of the third millenium, in the year 2000, DMSO is predicted to be the salvation of cancer patients worldwide. It is medicine's newest therapeutic principle.

A further discussion of DMSO therapy for cancer can be found in the book *Coping With Cancer*, by John L. Sessions, D.O., and Morton Walker, D.P.M., available by mail order from Freelance Communications, 484 High Ridge Road, Stamford, Connecticut 06905-3095, (203) 322-1551.

CHAPTER 12

Infectious Diseases Respond to DMSO

In April 1980, a nutrition and health counselor, Mrs. Vernice Reed of San Francisco, sixty-six years old, contracted a severe infection in her mouth. She sought medical attention from the outpatient department of a general hospital near her home but was turned away with the admonition that her disorder belonged in the province of a dentist.

The next afternoon the woman's dentist told her, "Vernice, you have herpes zoster!"

"Shingles! I don't believe it," she said.

"Well, you've had enough pain, haven't you?"

"Yes!"

"That's what it is, a viral infection," said the dentist. "And I'm sorry, but there's nothing we can do for you, especially when herpes hits the mouth."

Herpes zoster or shingles is a viral nerve infection that produces a painful inflammation of the sections of nerves emerging from the spinal cord. The varicella-zoster virus, the same virus that causes chicken pox, is responsible. Fever and prostration frequently accompany the pain. There are associated chills, gastrointestinal disturbances for three or four days, and a feeling of overall discomfort. On the fourth or fifth day, characteristic crops of tiny, red, acutely sensitive blisters appear on the skin. They mostly erupt on the chest, and spread along one side of the body following the course of the affected nerve. (*Herpes* means "creeping," and *zoster* means "girdle.")

A form of herpes zoster that inflames the nerves leading to the face and eyes, such as the type invading Vernice Reed's mouth, is especially dangerous because it may damage vision.

An ordinary attack of shingles runs its painful course in a few days or weeks and does not leave residual difficulties. One attack will usually confer immunity. In some cases, most frequently in elderly people, there is a persistence of pain called postherpetic neuralgia that may be disabling, and which hangs on long after the blisters of shingles disappear.

Mrs. Reed's dentist was correct in this case. There is no specific therapy for herpes zoster. Sometimes corticosteroids help if given before the symptoms become established; otherwise, the patient just has to wait for the disease to run its course.

Mrs. Reed decided to experiment on her own with DMSO, for she keeps it on hand all the time as a first-aid remedy. She took one teaspoonful of the full strength concentration and combined it with one teaspoonful of distilled water to make a 50 percent swabbing solution for her whole mouth and upper throat. She swabbed and gargled three times through the day and by the evening she had no more pain.

"The next day I did the swabbing again," Mrs. Reed said. "I combined aloe vera with the mixture this time, because aloe vera eases the stinging that accompanies use of DMSO. The following day there were absolutely no more blisters. I didn't need to swab anymore. My mouth has never had any blisters since."

DMSO FOR HERPES ZOSTER: A STUDY
OF FORTY-SIX PATIENTS

Whether you call it shingles or herpes zoster, the disease is a pain for the victim. The condition is especially disconcerting when it appears around the breast area of women and the belt area in men, probably because of constant friction of clothing in those particular places. If it strikes the face or rises in the scalp, the symptoms are a terrible itch and searing pain.

In 1971, Dr. William Campbell Douglass, now of Clayton, Georgia, did a clinical investigation on the local application of DMSO for patients suffering with herpes zoster and had some fine results. Table 12.1 summarizes the study. It illustrates that the sooner DMSO treatment is given for herpes zoster, the better the skin lesion response will be. And it's probably true that when the condition is treated with DMSO early enough in the acute phase, the postherpetic neuralgia syndrome won't occur either.

If you are going to use DMSO to relieve the symptoms of shingles, I suggest you do it under the supervision of a physician following a certain procedure. The material is applied directly to the skin lesions. Put the 75-percent liquid strength onto the sensitive area as often as it is tolerable, realizing that it will sting. If the blisters are too sensitive to accept this high-strength DMSO, dilute it with water to bring down the concentration. Experiment with how much water to add. You may find it comforting to sit in front of a revolving fan to cool the burning feeling from DMSO application on the lesions. Caution: While it is less effective, I recommend only a 50-percent solution be used for treating the face, neck, and scalp.

In his study, Dr. Douglass frequently combined dexamethasone (Decadron) with DMSO. There was no noticeable difference with this drug combination as compared to the DMSO used alone. In Table 12.1, the spinal areas are listed merely as location markers showing the approximate place the herpes zoster was present. Note the unusual cases where good results were acquired even after patient number 24 had the condition for four-and-a-half years and patient number 37 had it for one-and-a-half years.

DMSO has become a specific remedy to overcome the symptoms of herpes zoster, particularly to relieve the pain that follows the course of the involved nerve. Those patients who have itching but no neuralgia do not feel much relief of the itching; in fact it may increase. In general, DMSO applied to herpes zoster with skin eruption appears to shorten the course of the disorder and to prevent postherpetic neuralgia.

AN ENGLISH STUDY OF SHINGLES

Just before the Douglass study took place, a research group in Oxford, England, investigated the use of a combination of the antiviral drug, idoxuridine, and DMSO for treating shingles. Although systemic idoxuridine was tried against this viral nerve disease with equivocal results, the Oxford investigators reasoned that, since the varicella-zoster virus is related to the herpes simplex virus, and since DMSO-idoxuridine has been useful against herpes simplex lesions on the skin and mucous membranes, it was worth a try. The idea was to prevent virus replication, thus ameliorating the disease and, not incidentally, the pain.

The English investigators' trick worked. Continuously applied 40 percent idoxuridine in purified dimethyl sulfoxide clears up the herpes zoster lesions quickly. The continuous administration is achieved with a piece of lint, soaked in the drug, placed over the vesicles, and kept on the skin by a gauze bandage. The lint is resoaked daily.

"The patients were delighted, for the pain disappeared within a median of two days. Healing also appeared to be accelerated," the researchers reported in the *British Medical Journal* of December 26, 1970.[1] Some skin peeling occurred after treatment was ended, but only one subject in this uncontrolled trial had a secondary bacterial infection.

Table 12.1 *DMSO Study on Herpes Zoster (H.Z.)*
and Postherpetic Neuralgia (P.H.N.)

| | William C. Douglass, M.D. | | | | RESULTS | | | |
Patient	Diagnosis	Duration	Location	RX	Good	Fair	Poor	Inconclusive or Unknown
1	Herpes Zoster w/Neuralgia	7 days	T-10	DMSO 90%	X			
2	Post Herpetic Neuralgia	1½ yrs	T-5	DMSO 90%			X	
3	P.H.N.	14 days	T-10	DMSO 90%	X			
4	H.Z. w/Neuralgia	7 days	T-14	DMSO 90% w/Decadron	X			
5	P.H.N.	4 mo.	T-8	DMSO 70%		X		
6	P.H.N.	14 days	T-12	DMSO 90% w/Decadron	X			
7	P.H.N.	3 wks	T-5	DMSO 50% w/Decadron	X			
8	H.Z.	3 days	5th cranial	DMSO 50% w/Decadron	X			
9	H.Z.	7 days	L-5	DMSO 90% w/Decadron		X		
10	H.Z.	4 days	L-5	DMSO 90%	X			
11	H.Z.	5 days	T-5	DMSO 50% w/Decadron	X			
12	H.Z. w/Neuralgia	7 days	T-6	DMSO 9% w/Decadron	X			
13	H.Z. w/Neuralgia	4 days	C-5	DMSO 50% w/Decadron	X			
14	P.H.N.	6 mo.	T-5	DMSO 90% w/Decadron	X			
15	P.H.N.	30 days	T-4	DMSO 90%	X			
16	P.H.N.	5 mo.	5th cranial	DMSO 50% w/Decadron	X			
17	P.H.N.	5 mo.	T-4	DMSO 90% w/Decadron	X			
18	H.Z.	5 days	L-1	DMSO 90% w/Decadron	X			
19	H.Z.	2 days	T-3	DMSO 90% w/Decadron	X			

| | William C. Douglass, M.D. | | | | RESULTS | | | |
Patient	Diagnosis	Duration	Location	RX	Good	Fair	Poor	Inconclusive or Unknown
20	H.Z.	5 days	T-7	DMSO 90%				X
21	P.H.N.	8 wks	T-12	DMSO 70%	X			
22	Neuralgia Post Traumatic	6 mo.	5th cranial	DMSO 70% w/Decadron	X			
23	H.Z.	1 day	L-4	DMSO 90% w/Decadron	X			
24	P.H.N.	4.5 yrs	Left occipital N.	DMSO 70%	X			
25	P.H.N.	3 yrs	T-8	DMSO 90% w/Decadron				X
26	P.H.N. w/Neuralgia	3 wks	T-10	DMSO 70%	X			
27	H.Z. w/Neuralgia	2 wks	T-7	DMSO 70%	X			
28	Neuritis	1 mo.	Dorsum Rt. Foot	DMSO 70%			X	
29	H.Z. w/Neuralgia	1 wk	T-4	DMSO 70%		X		
30	H.Z. w/Neuralgia	2 wks	T-4	DMSO 70%	X			
31	P.H.N.	18 mo.	L-5	DMSO 70%			X	
32	P.H.N.	4 mo.	L-1	DMSO 90% w/Decadron	X			
33	H.Z. w/Neuralgia	2 days	Ulmar N.	DMSO 90% w/Decadron	X			
34	P.H.N.	2 mo.	C-7	DMSO 70%	X			
35	P.H.N.	2 wks	L-1	DMSO 90% w/Decadron	X			
36	H.Z. w/Neuralgia	1 wk	5th cranial	DMSO 50%		X		
37	P.H.N.	1½ yrs	T-7	DMSO 90% w/Decadron	X			

					RESULTS			
William C. Douglass, M.D.								*Inconclusive*
Patient	*Diagnosis*	*Duration*	*Location*	*RX*	*Good*	*Fair*	*Poor*	*or Unknown*
38	H.Z. w/Neuralgia	6 days	T-10	DMSO 70%	X			
39	P.H.N.	10 days	T-5	DMSO 90% w/Decadron	X			
40	H.Z. w/Neuralgia	2 wks	T-5	DMSO 70%	X			
41	P.H.N.	4 mo.	5th cranial	DMSO 50%	X			
42	H.Z. w/Neuralgia	10 days	T-8	DMSO 90% w/Decadron	X			
43	P.H.N.	3 yrs	5th cranial	DMSO 50%	X			
44	H.Z.	1 wk	T-1	DMSO 90%	X			
45	P.H.N.	3½ yrs	T-1	DMSO 90%		X		
46	H.Z.	4 days	T-10	DMSO 90% w/Decadron	X			

The English investigators tried to do a double-blind study by using the 40 percent combination of drugs against DMSO alone, and against salt solution with garlic added. The garlic was supposed to simulate the characteristic odor of DMSO, thus preserving the double-blind feature of the test. I doubt that this can be done, since DMSO has such a distinct odor. Double-blind or not, either the investigating clinician or the subject of the test or both are likely to recognize which solution is the placebo.

This DMSO-idoxuridine treatment worked even better against the simpler virus infection, herpes simplex. By itself, DMSO is only moderately successful against the cold sores (fever blisters) of the simplex virus.

Herpes simplex is a viral skin infection causing clusters of red, fluid-filled blisters on the skin or mucous membranes. The blisters cause burning and itching sensations for from five to ten days, then dry up and form yellowish crusts that fall off easily. Herpes simplex is a latent disease that recurs suddenly within months or sometimes years. It is triggered by exposure to sunlight, emotional upset, intestinal infections, pregnancy, or sexual intercourse. It is, in fact, a venereal-type disease, transferred by personal contact, although it may occur for no apparent reason.

The oral herpes simplex virus type 1 attacks the face, usually near the mouth or on the lips. The genital type, herpes simplex virus type 2, infects the external genital organs; in women it often breaks out in the vagina or on the cervix, and it has been identified as a probable cause of cervical cancer. The type 2 virus is spread by coitus.

Note to doctors treating the herpes venereal disease: Mixing DMSO with vitamin C crystals appears to be quite an effective treatment for herpes labialis or other genital herpes.

In an interview with Orville J. Davis, M.D., formerly in medical practice in San Diego, California, he said he had success with this vitamin C combination for herpes simplex and herpes zoster, too. "What we did was give 60,000 milligrams of vitamin C by intravenous injection, and paint the lesions with the DMSO-vitamin C solution. You have to keep the lesions wet. After two-and-a-half hours of IV, the redness is gone."

One woman, age fifty-eight, that Dr. Davis had treated, got rid of her scalp herpes simplex problems permanently within three days. The lesions on the right side of her head ran from the back of her head, over her scalp, and down to her right eye. She could have had an ophthalmic herpes—highly dangerous to eyesight—if the vitamin C and DMSO did not work so fast.

RESPIRATORY INFECTIONS ELIMINATED WITH DMSO

In Chile, respiratory diseases rate among the principal causes of death for children less than one year old. Doctors in private medical practice there find it necessary to hospitalize babies most often for acute inflammatory obstruction of the lower respiratory tract. For this reason, Chilean pediatricians have been on the lookout for some technique or medication to act with a good, fast therapeutic effect. Three research physicians at the Manuel Arriarn Pediatric Hospital in Chile have found it in DMSO spray. Rodolfo Burdach, M.D., head of the Department of Bronchopulmonary Diseases, Aristides Zuniga, M.D., ear, nose, and throat specialist, and Santiago Rubio, M.D., pediatrician, ran a study using DMSO on babies having respiratory problems.

Generally, the first sign of acute inflammatory obstruction in a baby is the sudden appearance of progressive respiratory difficulties. These difficulties take the form of snoring while awake or sleeping, and repeated coughing. The baby's lung problem is associated with swelling infiltration and fibroid death of the bronchial lining. Great accumulations of mucous secretion develop in the bronchial channels leading into the lungs. This often provokes secondary bacterial infection. The three research physicians labeled the entire syndrome as "bronchiolitis."

Bronchiolitis should not be confused with bronchopneumonia, asthma, whooping cough, interstitial pneumonitis, obstructive laryngitis, or acute obstructive bronchitis. These conditions were treated as well, but bronchiolitis was the three doctors' main area of interest.

As indicated in Table 12.2, they treated a group of thirty babies suffering from bronchiolitis and acute obstructive bronchitis with a DMSO spray containing biguanide hydrochloride, hydrocortisone, n-propylcarbinol, and lidocaine as added ingredients. In Chile, this combination is sold commercially as "Plus-Par." The Plus-Par product is bactericidal and virustatic. It had found use previously for treating wounds, chronic ulcers, recent ulcers, herpes zoster, burns, and fungus infections of the skin. The spray is applied on the affected skin area once or twice a day.

The researchers adapted the spray for respiratory disorders. Their method of application consisted of vaporizing the baby's throat with DMSO spray for a few seconds. The doctors coated the area with approximately 2 ml of the compound in order to uniformly cover the lower part of the larynx to the mouth cavity and the region of the tonsils and palate. One spray application was made twice daily until some therapeutic response was obtained. Then they increased the daily applications from one to four. In ten cases a single application was sufficient; two sprayings were used for nine cases; three sprayings in five cases; and six cases had vaporizing four times. In addition, these cases received antibiotics. The young patients were observed every thirty

Table 12.2 *Distribution of Patients According to Diagnosis*

Diagnosis	Number of Control Cases	Number of DMSO Spray Cases
Bronchiolitis	19	14
Bronchopneumonia	3	7
Atelectasis	1	1
Pneumonitis	5	6
Obstructive bronchiolitis	2	2
Total Patients	30	30

minutes and their physical changes were recorded as to temperature, respiratory frequency, and pulse rate. Results of these clinical trials are recorded in Tables 12.2 and 12.3.

Besides the improvements recorded in Table 12.3, other signs of favorable responses in the babies were: the sticky bronchial secretion, which tends to dry into a troublesome respiratory obstruction, lost its thickness and became more fluid so that the patient could cough it out; and the rapid heartbeat and prolonged exhalation associated with respiratory infections tended to disappear shortly after administering the DMSO spray.

Summarizing, the three doctors wrote, "It may be said that the use of DMSO spray in this clinical experience has been efficacious in the cases of bronchiolitis and obstructive inflammatory bronchial syndromes. The therapeutic response was more rapid and significant in children treated with DMSO spray than in those of the control group, who received medication of antibiotics, corticoids, and stayed in croupettes [humid oxygen chambers]. In view of these favorable changes, the time of permanence in the croupette can be considerably reduced or its use may be dispensed with altogether.

"The advantages of this therapy are its easy application, its rapid action, and the fact that no special instruments or apparatus are required. We therefore believe that this is a therapeutic resource which is particularly indicated in rural and in remote areas, where the physician has no specialized services available and where the treatment can be used on a large scale when the children are threatened by an outbreak of such an epidemic."[2]

THE RELIEF OF TINNITUS

There are two kinds of sounds taken into account in medicine. One is the bruit, a noise that may be heard by the examiner as well as the

Table 12.3 *Variation Mean Percentages in the Immediate Effect With DMSO Spray*

Variations	Percentages
Sensorial and general improvement	80%
Decrease of adenoids	76%
Decrease of intercostal retraction	75%
Change in chest sounds	80%

patient. Then there is a tinnitus, a subjective experience of the patient in which the perception of sound occurs in the absence of acoustic stimulus. It is an annoying experience that may have psychological impact on the victim.

Tinnitus may take the form of a buzzing, ringing, roaring, whistling, or hissing in the ears. Or, it may involve more complex sounds that vary over time. The sounds might come and go or be continuous, and sometimes there's an associated hearing loss.

The condition could be a symptom of nearly all ear disorders, including obstruction of the external auditory canal due to ear wax or foreign bodies, tumors, other degenerative diseases, or as a reaction to some substance that the individual is allergic to. Much of the time, tinnitus comes from an infectious process such as external otitis (ear inflammation), myringitis (inflammation of the tympanic membrane), otitis media (middle ear inflammation), labyrinthitis (inflammation of the internal ear), petrositis (inflammation of the temporal bone and its air cells), syphilis, meningitis, or some other infection.

Until now, there has been no specific medical or surgical therapy for tinnitus. But DMSO used together with vasoactive and anti-inflammatory substances has brought cessation of the sounds to adults of both sexes suffering from this chronic disease.

For fifteen people suffering from chronic tinnitus, DMSO in combination with vasoactive drugs was administered by injection, and DMSO in combination with anti-inflammatory preparations was applied externally. None of the people had responded to any other treatment. Any patient that showed psychotic tendencies or had acoustic trauma or aneurysm was eliminated from the study, because these problems would cause an erratic reading of the results.

A variety of laboratory and physical tests was carried out to determine the modification of tone, intensity, and character of the tinnitus. The treatment consisted of one daily intramuscular injection of "Ipran," a preparation based on DMSO in combination with buphenine and amino acids. The same investigator who was part of the Chilean study, Dr. Aristides Zuniga, performed the second study, in which he took audiometry and tympanic temperature measurements on all patients before and after the treatment.

In addition to the injections, the external ear canal of the particular ear hearing the irritating sound was treated with 2 ml of a medicinal spray containing DMSO and anti-inflammatory drugs described as Plus-Par. The spray applications were made every four days during the entire period of treatment.

Even though all of the patients suffered from chronic tinnitus for more than six months prior to starting the treatment and none had adapted to the noise each heard, in nine out of the fifteen, the subjective discomfort and head noise disappeared completely after one month of treatment. In two others the noise diminished considerably in intensity but did not totally disappear. Four patients retained tinnitus but described it as changed and sporadic, especially when they were exposed to the cold in the morning. Patients who had complained of nausea and positional dizziness from the condition before treatment didn't have these sensations after it. They also lost their persistent insomnia, as well as headache, neurotic anguish, and ear pain.

Dr. Zuniga said, "The disappearance of the tinnitus was permanent and no recurrence of the symptoms was noted on the occasion of the periodic checkups made during the course of one year. The tolerance of the Ipran injections and external Plus-Par applications was satisfactory in all cases. The only undesirable side effects were the garlic odor emanating from the patients undergoing DMSO treatment and on rare occasions a slight tachycardia (rapid heartbeat) and/or feeling of nausea shortly after the intramuscular injection. These temporary side effects can be avoided if the patient remains seated and rests for a short while after each injection."[3]

Since the early use of dimethyl sulfoxide for the protection of biological specimens against freezing damage, this chemical has been put to use in microbiology.[4] A bacteriostatic agent, DMSO retards the growth of bacteria. It is also suspected of being quite a good bactericidal agent, an antiseptic that kills bacteria. It definitely controls fungi, as was shown by its beneficial effect in eliminating athlete's foot, as described in Chapter 8.

One of DMSO's most encouraging characteristics is its ability as an antiviral agent and a transporter of certain antiviral drugs. It carries antiviral compounds directly into the cell where they are most effective against intracellular parasites. This is illustrated by its action against the herpes organisms, described earlier.

The more recently discovered and unexpected DMSO results against animal parasites are really exciting to many clinicians. The drug can be administered for various encysted helminthes (worms). Such hard-to-reach conditions as amebic abscess of the liver, trichinosis of the striated muscles, schistosomiasis, and other problems from animal parasites are now treatable by combining DMSO with antihelmintic compounds. For instance, creeping eruption (cutaneous larva migrans) has lent itself to experimental therapy with DMSO.[5,6]

ADDITIONAL MISCELLANEOUS INFECTIONS
BENEFITTED BY DMSO

In 1984, three Russian physicians reported that dimethyl sulfoxide was incorporated into the program of critical care given to patients suffering from many different types of infections. As an illustration, they utilized the case history of an adolescent adult who overcame his infectious process more swiftly by the addition of DMSO to their medical armamentarium.[7]

Reporting in the June 1984 issue of the *Annals of Rheumatic Diseases*, three American physicians described their use of DMSO in cases of leprosy resulting in complications for the patients' kidneys. Explaining that generalized amyloidosis of the kidneys can be treated only if the underlying disease is eliminated, they investigated the role of dimethyl sulfoxide in leprosy associated with secondary amyloidosis. At first the physicians found that there was no effect on the patients' creatinine clearance or twenty-four-hour proteinuria of the kidneys when a placebo using colchicine was employed. However, when DMSO was added to the therapy, renal function was considerably improved in three patients with moderate kidney failure. But in those with severe renal impairment (a creatinine clearance of less than 10 ml per minute), no particular improvement was observed. The investigators wrote: "These findings point to a beneficial effect of DMSO in human secondary amyloidosis when given at an early stage of renal involvement."[8]

DMSO found use for venereal disease complications in 1989. An unusual localization of lichen amyloidosus (a skin disease) in a patient with IgG k benign monoclonal gammopathy (a non-malignant immune disease) was reported. After topical treatment with dimethyl sulfoxide the skin lesions improved, but histological examination still showed amyloid deposits.[9]

The Russians stated in a 1988 published paper that they are routinely instilling DMSO into surgical wounds to speed their healing and to provide general infection control. As a result, their surgical patients are finding great advantages from faster postoperative wound closure.[10]

Boosting of the immunity among patients suffering from osteomyelitis (a bone disease resulting from infection) occurred from the adjunctive use of DMSO, as indicated in another 1986 Russian study. Their bone infections improved markedly from a boosting of lymphocytes to fight off the chronic disease process. The investigators stated in their clinical journal article, "The application of Dimexid and Dekaris [their two brands of DMSO] is shown to give better results in the treatment of patients with chronic osteomyelitis."[11]

Orchitis, an inflammation of the testis that causes pain, redness, and swelling of the scrotum, and may be associated with inflammation of the epididymis (part of the spermatic duct system), usually is caused by infection. It is a condition that affects one or both testes as the infection spreads down the vas deferens. The orchitis may develop in mumps, and mumps orchitis affecting both testes may result in sterility. Treatment of epididymo-orchitis often is by local support and administration of analgesics for pain and antibiotics for infection. However, a Russian urologist, Dr. V.N. Glozman, reported in a November/December 1986 Russian journal of urology that his patients suffering with orchitis and epididymitis benefitted when he added dimethyl sulfoxide to the treatment regimen.[12]

As recently as September 1992, biological physicians reported to the Pharmacological and Biological Therapies panel of the newly created Office for the Study of Unconventional Medical Practices that DMSO has found use for infection with HIV, the virus suspected of causing AIDS (acquired immune deficiency syndrome). This new office of the National Institutes of Health is looking at DMSO and other unconventional medical practices as a means of expanding health care in the United States.

DMSO has opened up a way to control practically all infections. Medical scientists must now experiment with the substance in laboratories and clinics to discover and label its vast storehouse of applications. For this purpose alone, DMSO should be legalized for use nationally.

CHAPTER 13

Misreporting of DMSO for Scleroderma and Interstitial Cystitis

It was nine years before that Jean Puccio of Washington, D.C., had had a diagnosis of scleroderma leveled at her. Supposedly this was a death sentence. But on July 31, 1980, Mrs. Puccio sat smiling at the United States Senate Subcommittee on Health and Scientific Research and told the four presiding senators her story. DMSO was responsible for the woman's being free of pain at last and able to work twelve- or thirteen-hour days as a hair stylist.

"I had been going for about a year and a half to the military doctors, and they did not know what my problem was," explained Mrs. Puccio. "When I finally got to Walter Reed Hospital, I stayed a week and they did muscle biopsies and nerve blocks. I was examined by thirty doctors and several civilian consultants. They told me that I had scleroderma, which I had never heard of."

Scleroderma, also known as progressive systemic sclerosis (PSS), is a potentially fatal disorder of the connective tissues, a chronic rheumatic disease of unknown cause. It is characterized by fibrotic degeneration and blood vessel abnormalities in the skin, joints, and internal organs (especially the esophagus, intestinal tract, lung, heart, and kidney).

Advanced diffuse scleroderma is unmistakable, but the disease also exists in a form in which there is only limited skin change, often confined to the fingers and face. This variant is generally known as the CREST syndrome, which stands for Calcinosis (lime salts deposited in body tissues, hardening them), Raynaud's phenomenon (spasms of tiny arteries), Esophageal dysfunction (blockage of the food tube), Sclerodactyl (hardening of the skin on the fingers and toes), and Telangiectasia (swelling of the small blood vessels). The CREST syndrome may take many years to develop distinctive and fateful internal manifestations. Thus, the disease may occur in a mild form compatible with long life, or it may cause early death due to heart failure, kidney disease, lung complications, or intestinal malabsorption with extreme weight loss and weakness. PSS is more common in women and comparatively rare in children.

Learning that she had this serious form of collagen vascular disease, Mrs. Puccio said to the doctors, "Okay; fine. What are we going to do about it?"

One of the physicians answered, "Unfortunately, there is nothing we can do about it."

She wondered, "No medication?"

He said, "No. The best you can hope for is a wheelchair, and within a short time, you will probably die."

"I went from doctor to doctor to doctor," Mrs. Puccio told the Senate Subcommittee. "I finally found Dr. Jacob through a lady in Pennsylvania. I called him and went to Portland. Dr. Jacob examined me, and he verified the diagnosis. At that time, I was becoming Oriental-looking; my skin was being pulled back. I was having difficulty breathing and walking and eating. He put me on topical DMSO, but it burned my skin, since scleroderma has a tendency to make your skin tissue thin."

Senator Edward Kennedy, Subcommittee Chairman, asked about the woman's troubles with opening her mouth and her problem with eating, which she had told him of before the beginning of the hearing.

"Because it constricts your tissue, it thickens the tissue, and it makes your skin so tight you cannot move. It was difficult for me to drive; it was difficult for me to turn the ignition in my car or turn my body. It was just very difficult. . . . I have a letter here from my dentist. He could not do any dental work on me for a while. Now, I can open my mouth like anybody else does. . . . I went to Dr. Jacob, and he gave me the medication, which I brought back to Virginia. I painted it topically, but it burned my skin. I called him back, and he said, 'Let us try taking it orally,' so I started taking it orally. Within about six months my condition reversed almost immediately. . . . I can do anything anybody else can now. Unfortunately, I have to be on that drug for the rest of my life."

Mrs. Puccio also paints on a form of DMSO called 87-2, which was developed by Robert Herschler (see Chapter 5). This is mixed with different chemical complexes, including urea. It is almost odor-free. She paints it on her skin at night, and by morning the odor is gone. She is extremely conscious of the odor. When she drinks it, she said, she does not go out. "I drink it on Saturday, and I am not out of the house until Monday evening, because I am conscious of it."

Her eyes were examined every year for the seven years she used DMSO. "I have not had problems with my eyes," said Mrs. Puccio. Her statement about experiencing no eye problems is significant, as we shall see.

On April 9, 1980, writing to United States Representative Claude Pepper who had chaired the House Select Committee on Aging to investigate "DMSO: New Hope for Arthritis?" Lillie Forister of Artesia, New Mexico, told of her particular form of arthritis—scleroderma. Mrs. Forister wrote:

> I was twenty-five years old with a five-year-old daughter when I was told I have scleroderma and that there is no cure and very little help for it. About the first thirteen years, it wasn't too bad. I had ulcers on my fingertips. I only had pain while the ulcers were healing, and being cold during the winter months.
>
> But the last six years have been something else. In 1974, I had an amputation of my first toe. And then in 1979, I lost two more. I am enclosing some pictures so you can get an idea of what has happened to me.
>
> The last five years, during the winter months, the only way to get by is to live on pain pills and then it doesn't do the job, just takes the edge off. You lose weight and walk the floor at night, because you can't sleep for the pain. The pain is with you day after day 'til you don't think you can take it any more.
>
> Then the first part of 1979, I started having chest pains and trouble with my lungs. I couldn't even clean up one room without sitting down and resting. I've always been able to take care of myself. And it's very hard for me to have to accept help from others. Another thing about this disease, if you can't get health insurance or [even] if they will [give you insurance], it's so high you can't afford it.
>
> That's the bad side of scleroderma. Now for the good part, the only ray of hope I've had in nineteen years. I went to Portland, Oregon, to see Dr. Jacob last July. He started me on a treatment with DMSO. After the first week, I felt better than I had in nineteen years. I could button my own clothes, reach behind my head. The pain was almost nothing. Four months later I no longer had chest pains.
>
> I have just come through one more winter and it's the best winter I've had in six years. I had a few bad points where the

pain was pretty rough, but they didn't last long. Now when I get ulcers I use DMSO and it clears them up. Also, I didn't have any more amputations. I feel that now I might have a chance to see my children grown and to be able to enjoy my grandchildren.

Please help us, we need you to help us fight for a better, pain-free life.

THE NEW TREATMENT FOR SCLERODERMA

Lillie Forister was begging for help not only for her own problem but also for the approximately 150,000 other Americans suffering from scleroderma. While the disease itself may not immediately kill them, death in adults follows severe and progressive muscle weakness, difficulty in swallowing, malnutrition, and failure of the respiratory system with superimposed lung infection, such as pneumonia. And as they linger, discomfort in general and pain in particular pervade their lives.

The victims of scleroderma experience gradual thickening of the skin of the fingers, aching in most joints, upset of the gut, extreme fatigue, and muscle wasting. The facial features turn masklike. The skin becomes taut, shiny, and inflexible on the fingertips, which develop ulcers. The sclerodermatous patient gets calcification on bony eminences, friction rubs over the knees and tendon sheaths, and the formation of large bursae. Contractures of the fingers, wrists, and elbows resulting from skin hardening prevent fine movements, sometimes even gross movements, such as Jean Puccio's inability to drive her car.

Internally, there is gastric acidity due to an incompetent functioning of the lower food tube sphincter. Poor absorption from the small intestine occurs from an overgrowth of anaerobic bacteria. Large pockets or sacs develop in the large intestine and biliary cirrhosis develops. The lungs don't work right and defective gas diffusion results. Heart failure can hit any time and tends to be chronic and to respond poorly to medication. Kidney disease is a major cause of death in PSS, usually signaled by sudden high blood pressure that drugs won't bring down.

And for all these symptoms of scleroderma there is no specific treatment. No drug has proved valuable—nothing was even somewhat effective—until DMSO.

"There is no doubt in my mind, the drug relieves certain types of pain. It is not a curative agent and all the reports we have read about 'miraculous and outstanding' should be completely disregarded. There is nothing miraculous about this compound at all, but it does relieve pain in a temporary manner. It is not a cure. None of our anti-rheumative drugs are curative. DMSO applied topically is indeed a safe, therapeutic agent to use," said Arthur L. Scherbel, M.D., founder of the Department of Rheumatic Disease at the Cleveland Clinic Foundation in Cleveland, Ohio, and formerly the department's senior consultant.

In his practice, Dr. Scherbel dealt with patients who have very serious diseases that are challenges to any form of therapy. He is expert in the pathology of PSS. There are no good, highly effective therapeutic agents for the rheumatic connective tissue diseases of which scleroderma is one. No drug exists today that is completely effective and without toxicity for providing the victims with relief, and certainly there's no cure.

Dr. Scherbel began using DMSO twenty years ago and found that it blocked pain for sufferers of scleroderma. This pain relief comes about because the solvent blocks conduction in the small nerve fibers—C&A delta, the fibers important in the recognition of pain. If 75 percent DMSO is used directly on the nerve fibers (in laboratory experiments) and not removed, within two days all nerve conduction will cease. If 100 percent DMSO is put on these nerves, the conduction block will occur more rapidly and usually will not be reversible. The conclusion is that the smaller peripheral nerve fibers, when preferentially blocked by DMSO, become diminished in their central response to a stimulus that ordinarily would cause pain.[1]

The healing of ulcers occurs, as well, and this is more difficult to explain. Marvin F. Engel, M.D., of Brunswick, Georgia, delivered a paper before the Section on Dermatology of the Southern Medical Association, at its sixty-fourth annual meeting in Dallas, Texas, November 18, 1970, where he described how the skin's blood vessels look after DMSO use in scleroderma. Dr. Engel said, "One sees dilatation of vessels in the upper dermis and perhaps the increase in blood flow plays a role. DMSO is known to protect cells and tissue from freezing, thawing, necrotic cutaneous changes, inflammatory and hemorrhagic processes."[2] This protection may be related to cellular physiological enlargement.

In a two-year study of twenty sclerodermatous patients, Dr. Engel found beneficial results using DMSO as the exclusive treatment. He said, "They had increased mobility, rapid relief of pain and healing of persistent ulcers, arrest of the spread of cutaneous disease, regrowth of hair, and return of sensation and sweating. There was absolutely no sign of arrest of systemic disease, as shown by the death of three patients while on therapy and two in the immediate posttreatment period, despite evidence of improvement of the cutaneous manifestations of their disorder."

Dr. Engel also noted that "the maximal activity of DMSO, after it is swallowed, is in the organs and the parts of organs primarily involved in the pathologic changes of progressive systemic sclerosis. . . . DMSO might halt or reverse the process of systemic sclerosis."

As it relates to the following section, what Dr. Engel added is quite significant: "No evidence of ocular damage was found by funduscopic or slit lamp examination in any of our patients."

ALLEGED MISREPORTING OF THE SCHERBEL STUDIES

Dr. Scherbel did similar, more extensive studies on patients having scleroderma, and he performed them under the FDA supervisory investigational new drug (IND) application number 10-778. This means the investigator and the sponsoring pharmaceutical company, Research Industries Corporation, were liable to FDA regulations. Violations of them would be a federal crime.

A statement by Jere E. Goyan, Ph.D., former Commissioner of the FDA, made before the Senate Subcommittee on Health and Scientific Research, included the following information:

"We are requiring that eye examinations be conducted as part of any study involving chronic administration of DMSO in order to obtain additional data to determine whether the drug causes ocular toxicity. The labeling for the approved human drug product suggests that patients should receive thorough eye evaluations, including slit lamp examinations, prior to and periodically during treatment. . . . We have issued inspection assignments to audit the data of the scleroderma studies. In all of these investigations our staff is being asked to pay particular attention to whether or not these studies included eye examinations."

Dr. Scherbel did his IND 10-778 studies on eleven patients with severe progressive systemic sclerosis, using DMSO by oral administration. He had them undergo eye examinations before, during, and after DMSO treatment, in accordance with FDA rules, for this IND. The patients received a total daily dose of DMSO ranging from 21 grams to 84 grams in four divided doses diluted in concentrated juice and crushed ice. The duration of the treatment ranged from 1 month to 22 months with a mean average of 9.4 months. Its results were reported to Henry Moyle, President of the Research Industries Corporation, Salt

Lake City, Utah. In his letter, dated May 4, 1977, Dr. Scherbel advised Mr. Moyle that "in four of eleven patients reported at this time, nuclear sclerosis or progressive myopia have appeared during the study."

This report of lens changes with the development of nearsightedness was alarming news. It might have caused cessation of the investigation if the FDA had been aware of the reported eye changes in these patients. Agency officials say that no one at the FDA knew about them until the information was uncovered, almost by accident, nearly three years later.

Michael J. Hensley, M.D., of the Division of Scientific Investigations, Bureau of Drugs, FDA, told Senator Kennedy how this came about: "It was not officially reported, as far as we can tell. We picked up on this during a routine inspection of Dr. Scherbel. . . . On April 22, 1980, I was standing there with an inspection report in my hand of an oral DMSO study—a study of the use of DMSO orally in scleroderma—a study wherein patients had been given doses very nearly approaching the animal studies that had showed ocular toxicity, and it appeared from the material that we had discovered during this very first, initial tipoff inspection that the eye changes that were being reported in these patients were identical to those seen in the animal studies back in the 1960s. . . . It turns out that the initial report of the oral scleroderma patients had been noted by Dr. Scherbel to Research Industries on May 4, 1977. . . . It appeared that Research Industries had reported to them a possible adverse effect in 1977, and yet had never reported it to the agency because, in our files, we found none of these reports."

From the testimony, Senator Kennedy learned that two inspections of the firm uncovered correspondence that indicated the Scherbel report was received. A letter from Moyle was sent in reply to Dr. Scherbel's report indicating that Dr. Jacob verbally informed K.C. Pani, M.D., an officer of the Division of Anti-Infective Drug Products of the Bureau of Drugs, FDA, of this finding. Another letter dated May 17, 1977, from Moyle to Scherbel implied that the Scherbel report may have been provided to Dr. Pani. At least it said that "Dr. Jacob and I showed him your letter of May 4, 1977, and Dr. Pani suggested lowering the DMSO dosage for these patients affected with eye changes."

Dr. Pani was interviewed, and denied he had ever been told any of this. He said he was given no letter for the FDA files. Dr. Hensley said, "We therefore had the possibility of a violation of the Federal Food, Drug, and Cosmetic Act, and also, perhaps, of title 18, section 1001—the making of false reports to the Government."

Compounding this alleged misreporting, on September 7, 1978,

Moyle wrote Merle L. Gibson, M.D., Director, Division of Anti-Infective Drug Products, Bureau of Drugs, a summarized progress report of IND 10-778 saying: "Our investigations under this IND are still ongoing but to date our investigators have reported no abnormalities relating to toxicity of the drug, nor have they reported any ocular abnormalities. All updated patient reports throughout the year have previously been forwarded to the FDA under separate cover."

Commissioner Goyan considered this alleged misreporting extremely serious in view of the fact that it was the eye toxicity that the FDA was most concerned about. Under the IND regulations that govern this human experimental work, it is mandatory that the sponsor shall promptly investigate and report to the FDA and to all investigators any findings associated with the use of the drug that may suggest significant hazards, contraindications, side effects, and precautions pertinent to the safety of DMSO. Eye changes in the scleroderma patients clearly fall within this definition.

It is possible that lens changes are a complication of the disease, but there is nothing reported in the medical literature indicating that eye symptoms are present in scleroderma.

From the correspondence found three years later in the Research Industries corporate files, it appears that Scherbel's letter is the first DMSO report of human eye toxicity ever, and that the pharmaceutical company had furnished the report to Dr. Pani at the FDA. Commissioner Goyan said that if Pani had possessed this information and not provided it to the FDA, it would be grounds for his dismissal from the agency.

It looked like the FDA had a real health problem with DMSO—specifically, eye toxicity in humans. Also, the agency learned that the odor-free DMSO, 87-2, and another DMSO derivative called Satori, had no IND and no animal testing, but were being distributed in interstate commerce and being used by the general public. We saw at the start of this chapter that Jean Puccio almost daily paints on 87-2, which she acquired from Dr. Jacob. Use of this unapproved drug is illegal. Dispensing it is a violation of the Federal Food, Drug, and Cosmetic Act.

Dr. Hensley brought all this information to the Inspector General of the United States. "The Office of Inspector General went to the United States attorney in Baltimore, because it is the judicial district, and briefed them on what they knew of it," said Dr. Hensley. "They interviewed a great many people during that week [May 12, 1980] and had some very definite impressions as to what they ought to do."

The incident with which we opened Chapter 2, where FDA officials holding a Federal warrant entered Dr. Jacob's office on November 10, 1980, looking for documents on eye toxicity, is a direct outgrowth of this discovery and its eventual public disclosure in the Congressional Record. In fact, one of the investigators visiting Dr. Jacob's office was Dr. Alan B. Lisook, who is Dr. Hensley's supervisor at the Division of Scientific Investigations, Bureau of Drugs, FDA. Lisook flew to Portland, Oregon, from Washington, D.C., to grab what reports on eye toxicity he could out of Jacob's files. You'll recall that Lisook wasn't allowed access to the files.

Meantime, the Inspector General, in consultation with the Baltimore United States attorney, investigated possible malfeasance on the part of some employees of the agency. "The allegations have to do with the question of whether the sponsor and the investigators were investigated promptly enough and in a proper fashion," explained Nancy L. Buc, Chief Counsel of the FDA, "and also may have to do with questions that pertain to the sponsor and to the investigators."

Dr. Pani, the medical officer with the primary responsibility for DMSO, who was assigned to the drug in 1968, was transferred from the DMSO project. And then he was forced to retire from the FDA under threat of outright dismissal. The policy management staff at the FDA conducted an investigation of Dr. Pani and his relationship with the sponsors, the clinical researchers, and the physician-monitor. This physician-monitor was responsible for making sure the protocols of investigations were being followed, the product being employed was pure, and the records being kept were accurate. The FDA staff's findings have not been made public, but I have found out that the physician-monitor was Stanley Jacob. Dr. Pani and Dr. Jacob were indicted by the Justice Department on criminal charges rising from the FDA investigations.

A BUSINESSMAN PROTECTS HIS INVESTMENT

Henry Moyle and Louis Haynie created Research Industries Corporation (RIC) in 1968 out of an amalgamation of a land development firm and the Deseret Drug Company. Early in the 1970s they expanded by purchasing three DMSO clinics in Juarez, Tecate, and Nogales, Mexico, where patients were treated under the direction of Mexican doctors. Not quite satisfied that DMSO was safe, the businessmen called in Dr. Jacob to tour the clinics and coach them on suggested changes in their therapeutic procedures.

After persuading Americans, for a time, to cross the border for DMSO treatment, the partners decided to manufacture, market, and legitimize DMSO in the United States. First they had to work with the FDA in trying to get approval of the drug. This became Moyle's almost full-time responsibility. Dr. Jacob became associated with the company and put Moyle in touch with Dr. K.C. Pani for discussions about INDs for DMSO.

The two indications that seemed most promising for INDs were scleroderma and interstitial cystitis. American physicians treating these conditions with DMSO were Dr. Scherbel and Bruce H. Stewart, M.D., respectively, both of the Cleveland Clinic Foundation. Later, Dr. Stewart brought in Sheridan Shirley, M.D., of the University of Alabama, and these two doctors administered DMSO to patients suffering from interstitial cystitis. Their patient experimentation was done under an IND initiated in 1974.

RIC acquired a wholly owned subsidiary known as Terra Pharmaceuticals, Buena Park, California, to manufacture DMSO. It had once been owned by Nutri-Lite, a subsidiary of the Amway Corporation. Twenty to thirty workers now manufacture DMSO at the Terra Pharmaceuticals plant.

Data submitted by Dr. Shirley was a fifty-one-patient study; the data submitted by Dr. Stewart was a fifteen-patient study. The research had gone on for more than a year. Research Industries Corporation was the sponsor who submitted the clinical trial reports to the FDA. The Shirley and Stewart studies sent along for approval of DMSO in the treatment of interstitial cystitis were accepted, and the drug came into legal use for this condition. About a year later, RIC was inspected by the FDA to see what kind of monitoring the company was doing at the time. Then the FDA checked with the two clinical investigators, randomly chosen, to see how the monitoring that had been conducted actually stood up.

Their visit to Dr. Shirley's research facilities was disturbing to the FDA inspectors. Although the researcher had been given ten days' notice, he had difficulty producing the background information and other raw data that would support the safety claims he had made. This led to another inspection the FDA labeled "for cause." The "for cause" inspection was designed to compare case report forms—fifteen were chosen at random—to the patient records. The inspectors wanted to learn if the underlying data that had previously been missing were still missing. Dr. Hensley said, "The intent was also to pursue beyond that; to go, in fact, to the laboratories that had allegedly done that data and, if necessary, to the patients."

The FDA uncovered virtually every possible deficiency in the Shirley studies, according to Dr. Hensley. For example, there were no records of informed consent by the patients. There was no institutional review board approval where it was appropriate and necessary. The University of Alabama seemed not to have been consulted at all about this patient experimentation under its jurisdiction.

More important from the FDA's viewpoint were problems with the safety and efficacy data, which tended to invalidate all prior approval of DMSO for the treatment of interstitial cystitis. In the safety data, the eye examinations that were supposed to have been done before the study began and every three months during its course and after its completion, appeared not to have been done at all. The laboratory work, a battery of patient tests to be accomplished before the study, then on a monthly basis during its course and after its conclusion, could not be verified because the underlying records were not to be found.

The FDA inspectors diligently pursued these failings and were unable to confirm that the testing had been performed. They interviewed patients and learned that neither the laboratory work nor the eye examinations had taken place. The reports of such laboratory and eye tests were allegedly false, even though the case report forms held in house by the FDA showed that all of this work had been done and that the results were normal.

Hensley told Senator Kennedy that the efficacy data were also disturbing. The agency had received two sets of case reports from RIC on Shirley's study—one near the end of 1975. It showed generally good to excellent results with treating interstitial cystitis. The second arrived in early 1976 on a resubmission of the NDA, which showed some of these patients deteriorating.

When the FDA did its "for cause" inspection, the review of Shirley's records looked a good deal worse; people treated had more than just minor deterioration. The patients, although they might initially have had a very good response, generally did seriously deteriorate and often required other medication or bladder surgery.

The Division of Scientific Investigations then declared that the Shirley data simply could not be used. It was unsatisfactory, to say the least, said Dr. Goyan. Dr. Shirley came under FDA investigation; as a consequence his certification as an FDA inspector was rescinded.

The FDA also turned its attention to the study done by Dr. Stewart and, after completing its review, a decision was made as to whether or not a hearing would be held and further action taken. Furthermore, at least three other interstitial cystitis studies came into question. With-drawing approval of interstitial cystitis as the only legal human use of DMSO was considered. A general pattern of disinclination on the part of the investigating physicians to do the drug safety work—the eye examinations and the laboratory tests—seemed to be developing.

Dr. Scherbel explained the reasons for not burdening patients, institu-tions, and researchers with this drug safety work. He told the House Select Committee on Aging: "For those patients who could indeed profit from the use of a very simple drug, we cannot use it unless we carry out a very strict protocol. If I wanted to give this drug to a patient today, I must obtain sophisticated eye examinations every six months. This patient must have blood studies every three months. If this patient lives 150 miles from Cleveland, he or she must come back at a determined time and the studies must be carried out according to FDA regulations.

"Long ago we realized that toxicity was not a problem but we do not dare to give this drug without carrying out a battery of very sophisti-cated laboratory studies. Who pays for this?" asked Dr. Scherbel. "The patient might not have funds to pay. Will the Cleveland Clinic? They will if I ask them to, but it is not fair to the Cleveland Clinic to do this because it is the FDA request.

"If we obtain funds from a pharmaceutical firm and eventually they sense this drug is not going to be approved, where do the funds come from to continue treatment for this group of patients?"

These are valid questions; they require answers if drug safety is to be assured.

Unfortunately, Dr. Hensley disclosed another reason for the FDA's disinclination to accept DMSO studies strictly on the face value of researchers' opinions. The investigating doctors tended to overlook, maybe not see, or perhaps deliberately ignore possible adverse effects. For example, Dr. Hensley described difficulties with accepting addi-tions to the Stewart study. He said, "The original NDA was twice submitted to the agency; the last time in 1976, and finally it was approved in 1978. In September 1979, another package of data was submitted to the agency by Research Industries. This package con-tained not fifteen patients of Dr. Stewart, but forty."

"We have looked at that data, and it is apparent that a good many of those patient reports had been available prior to the NDA submission and were contemporary with Dr. Stewart's other patients," said Dr. Hensley. "It appeared, therefore, that a selective submission of data had been made to the original NDA."

Thus, the researcher chose certain patients to represent his clinical trials and sent them for submission by RIC to the FDA. Or, RIC did the selecting from the whole group of fifty-five patients and sent along just fifteen.

What of the newly introduced batch of forty people who used DMSO and whose cases weren't revealed until three years later? Dr. Hensley said, "Many of the patients—in fact, I guess the majority of those that are truly interstitial cystitis—had either fair or poor responses to the treatment."

So there have been definite questions raised about both of the studies that were the basis for the NDA approval of DMSO employment against interstitial cystitis. No wonder the FDA has been so stubborn about giving approval for DMSO medical usage in general.

Following the Kennedy hearings, the FDA appointed a DMSO "Steering Committee." This committee brought in a new group of investigators—pharmacological, toxicological, chemical, and medical professionals—who had nothing to do with the initial approval of DMSO for interstitial cystitis. These new investigators were paid for their work by the FDA. They reviewed the entire matter, and their conclusion was that Drs. Shirley and Stewart were quite sloppy in recording their data. Because of this they were disqualified as investigators for the FDA thereafter.

However, the FDA, even after this thorough review of the entire matter, allowed the approval of DMSO for use against interstitial cystitis to stand. They found that the two physicians had been careless rather than dishonest in their reporting.

Such carelessness in medical research is simply an expression of human error, particularly in relation to the employees one depends upon. As interstitial cystitis is a rare disease and difficult to find, the FDA physician-investigators in Cleveland or Birmingham, Alabama, had patients come in for checkups from all over the country. (The FDA requires a minimum of fifty patients from two investigators to approve a drug for prescription use in a specific condition.) On the approval sheets, the FDA had listed various parameters for the investigators to follow and fill in. Certain employed research associates—frequently college students—filled in the answers to questions that they asked the participating patients.

One of the questions on the approval forms concerned ophthalmology. The research associates (dental students) would ask the patients, "Have you had your eyes checked?"

The patients most often said, "Yes!"

The next question was, "Have you had any problems with your eyes?"

The patients replied, "No!"

The research associates then wrote on the approval forms: "Ophthalmology negative."

These patients had been examined by ophthalmologists in areas far distant from the research facilities in Cleveland or Birmingham. The physician-investigators did not have those eye examination records as part of the patients' files. Thus, upon "for cause" evaluation of the records, the FDA declared the investigators' record response for vision unsubstantiated. Later, despite being disqualified as FDA investigators, Drs. Shirley and Stewart were able to show that these ophthalmologic examinations were, in fact, carried out. And as the FDA found that the interstitial cystitis protocol was correct, DMSO remains an approved medication for treatment of this bladder problem.

Senator Kennedy emphasized that there were a series of collective failures among the several people involved with this NDA procedure. The FDA found failures by the investigators doing the clinical work, the sponsor supplying the drug, the physician-monitor checking methods, and the FDA medical officer acting as liaison for the NDA. There was a failure to write up accurate case histories, a failure to keep adequate records of drug accountability, a failure to obtain institutional review committee approval, and a failure to maintain documentation of informed patient consent. In questioning the patients, the FDA believed that most of the required eye and laboratory examinations possibly were never performed at all and they found the lack of records just sloppy reporting. In some of the cases report forms were, in fact, altered between the first and second FDA inspections so that FDA officials remain suspicious. They still think that there was insufficient reporting or alleged misreporting of toxicological ophthalmic effects in the patients.

Looking at just one of the people who failed in all this, Kennedy wondered whose responsibility at RIC it was to detect the various DMSO problems that apparently went undetected right through the NDA approval process. "Senator, I believe that the ultimate responsibility, certainly, lies with me," said Henry Moyle. "I signed the documents that went into the FDA."

Here we see a businessman who had protected his investment. Kennedy asked Moyle, "What would be the impact on Research Industries if, as a result of these problems, the FDA determined that it could no longer maintain the approval of DMSO for treatment?"

"Well, Senator, we are a small company," answered Moyle. "We believed when we started with this application that it would not take nearly this long, and we have stretched it out. On our marketing, we are not yet breaking even. So, we would have real problems. I suppose we would have to dispose of our subsidiary, Terra; that would be too expensive an operation to be able to continue with. If we did that, we would no longer have a lab approved for good manufacturing practices, and it took us three or four years to get that approval at the FDA. So that would be an impossible burden; I do not know what we would do."

CLEARING UP POTENTIAL CONFLICTS OF INTEREST FOR DR. JACOB

Surgeon Stanley Jacob has treated tens of thousands of patients at his modest office at the University of Oregon Health Sciences Center. He now sees more than 200 people a week, some with the most serious health problems such as spinal cord injuries, Down's syndrome, stroke, spondylitis, burns, cancer, scleroderma, herpes zoster, and worse. Dr. Jacob has become known nationwide and overseas for the excellence of his work in making known the new and varied uses for DMSO. The weight of his discovery of the medical properties of dimethyl sulfoxide is enough to plant him firmly in the medical history books. He is an admirable scientist.

Still, with all these patients coming to his office door and the reputation he has established, Dr. Jacob's annual salary was only about $45,000 ten years ago. With raises in steady increments, his salary probably doubled by 1992. The University of Oregon doesn't pay its research physicians on a par with industry, whose physicians average around the $200,000 a year level. Moreover, Dr. Jacob's current salary is probably 25 percent of what he could earn as a surgeon in solo or group private practice.

Why, then, does he do it? And why has he continued taking DMSO himself since 1963? Dr. Jacob says "not for any medical problem but because if any side effects are going to develop, it's better that they raise their ugly head in my body than anyone else's."

His dedication and sacrifice are undeniable. For almost twenty years Stanley Jacob has been struggling with the FDA and the scientific community to get dimethyl sulfoxide approved for national distribution and generally accepted for medical use. The father of five children ranging in age from fourteen to thirty-nine years, Dr. Jacob believes that the failure of his three marriages may be attributed to his total involvement with the legalization of this pharmaceutical solvent. He says it is his "obsession."

The doctor expects to devote the rest of his working life proving the worthiness of DMSO in the pharmacopeia of every physician for a vast array of health problems. Retirement is not for him. "I might spend a little more time with family," Jacob says, "but my research interests wouldn't change. I couldn't begin to scratch the surface of DMSO's uses in the years remaining to me."

All this sounds highly idealistic; he is a magnanimous individual, the image of a truly good man. And this really may be the case—unless you gain access to certain other facts that don't generally get broadcast.

During Senator Kennedy's devastating cross-examination of Research Industries Corporation President Moyle, the Senator learned that Jacob was the physician-monitor for those series of studies on DMSO for scleroderma and interstitial cystitis, mentioned earlier. Errors in accuracy related to the clinical trials may be Jacob's responsibility rather than Moyle's, as Dr. Jacob was obligated to inspect the trials in progress and check the records being kept.

While the royalties Jacob receives on the patents for DMSO medical uses are still relatively small, as DMSO's popularity in medicine increases, the royalties could become huge. At present he turns over royalty money to the University of Oregon Health Sciences Center for the Department of Surgery and for DMSO research, but at any time Jacob could retain the money for himself. It is not held in trust or transferred to a charitable foundation on behalf of the medical center.

When Jacob was a paid director of Research Industries, he was able to purchase 50,000 shares of stock in the company at $6.50 a share. Today the corporation is a publicly traded stock issued on NASDAQ, the over-the-counter market of the National Association of Securities Dealers. Its 2,050,000 shares traded at a high in 1980–81 of $15.50 a share. Plus, the doctor had the option to purchase an additional 50,000 shares at $6.50 and another 50,000 shares at $9.50, over the next four years. In 1982 the high price per share was $12.50. If he had executed his options at the stock's high 1982 price, the accrued value of all these shares would have come to $1,875,000, for which Jacob paid $1,125,000—a clear gain of $750,000.

Finally, when he ended his function as a physician-monitor for the DMSO investigations, Jacob became, for a time, a consultant to the company at a salary of $24,000 a year, which supplemented his University of Oregon salary.

It seemed not to bode well for Jacob's financial future if the investment made by Research Industries Corporation in DMSO research, manufacturing, marketing, and distribution proved invalid. The physician appeared to have too much invested in RIC for him to let this happen so that an objective observer might see potential conflicts of interest here for Stanley Jacob. Consequently, at the semi-annual scientific conference held in Las Vegas, Nevada, November 19, 20, 21, 1982, by the American College of Advancement in Medicine, I interviewed Dr. Jacob on exactly these potential points of conflict. The following is what Stanley Jacob said:

"When I first went to work for Research Industries Corporation in 1973 they offered to give me a quarter of a million shares of the company's stock. I refused it. At that time the stock sold for fifty cents a share. I turned the stock down because I never wanted anyone to accuse me of vested interests before DMSO was approved by the FDA.

"After DMSO won approval, however, I did take a stock option and executed it for 50,000 shares by borrowing money with other directors (I was myself a director of Research Industries Corporation) cosigning the loan note. I also held an option to acquire another 100,000 shares, but the stock price had risen markedly to $6.50 a share. I borrowed $325,000 to purchase the 50,000 shares.

"My idea of taking the stock at that point was to donate any profits I made to DMSO research. Unfortunately, it got into that time of 20 percent prime rate so that the legal expenses and interest expenses reduced the profit return sharply. I received less than $9.00 per share at the sale of my block of stock when I made the sale two years later. My resultant loss on the entire transaction was $2,000.

"Before the Kennedy hearings, in June 1980, I completely disassociated myself from Research Industries Corporation—dropped my directorship, sold the stock, and gave up all rights to any other of the stock options. The particulars of my disassociations were not in the hearings because I actually made the financial transition with the stock the same month as the Kennedy hearings, in July 1980. That's because there was a legal two-year holding period for the stock. I had acquired the 50,000 shares in July 1978."

RESOLVING THE SCANDAL OF DMSO

What was the outcome of these various revelations? Of consequences connected with irregular practices among DMSO researchers and other principals involved, attorney Buc said, "There are a series of actions that will have to be considered. Any of the clinical investigators who have violated our regulations will have to be considered for potential disqualification as clinical investigators. That is a process that is begun by the Bureau of Drugs. The clinical investigators are entitled to a hearing, and it ultimately reaches the Commissioner."

The FDA did judge whether Dr. Shirley and Dr. Stewart should be eliminated as qualified FDA clinical investigators. They were eliminated.

"In addition, to the extent that the information that the Inspector General or any of us turn up results in allegations of criminal activity," continued Ms. Buc, "I know that we will be considering criminal prosecution as well, for the investigators, if there are allegations of criminality there, and, if it comes to that, the people at the agency as well."

The FDA had already interrogated and discharged Dr. Pani, and the Justice Department brought criminal charges against him. Dr. Pani pleaded guilty to a single misdemeanor count of improperly receiving payments. The Indian-born researcher openly accepted loans of $38,500 from Dr. Jacob to assist in paying for cancer treatments for his wife and also for donations to an Indian religious leader. Dr. Pani's wife subsequently died from cancer.

The supervisor of Dr. Jacob's work at the University of Oregon Health Sciences Center, and a friend of his for many years, William W. Krippaehne, M.D., described the DMSO champion as a compassionate humanitarian who has given large sums of money to friends and strangers alike without question. Dr. Krippaehne said that his friend has treated patients from all over the country, often without charge, has given money to people in need, including members of the university staff, without requiring repayment, and has put extra money back into university research programs. "If he didn't do charity work," Dr. Krippaehne said, "his net income would be significantly into six figures." He also said that Dr. Jacob, an associate professor of surgery and author of over 100 medical journal articles, was a "catastrophe" when it came to business matters.

Dr. Krippaehne made these statements on the witness stand, as the Justice Department also brought criminal charges against Dr. Jacob for three counts of improper payments to an FDA official and one count of conspiracy. The trial for the surgeon and the FDA official took place in May 1982 but ended in a mistrial. The government bureaucrats continued their attack and pursued Dr. Jacob in a second trial after Dr. Pani pleaded guilty to misdemeanor.

Dr. Jacob welcomed the initial trial, stating that it would give him a chance to vindicate the use of DMSO. At the second trial not only was he acquitted of all the charges, but the Justice Department actually dropped the charges on the fifth day of the trial, held October 29, 1982. Dr. Jacob was cleared completely and received a semblance of an apology from the government. The grand jury indictment was totally dismissed.

In our interview, Dr. Jacob explained what happened: "Dr. K.C. Pani is a friend of mine. His wife was my patient. I got to know him well. He had horrendous medical bills. I loaned him money by personal check which Dr. Pani returned by personal check. And this exchange of checks was the basis of the indictment for conspiracy and giving an illegal gratuity to a government official.

"I learned a lot from this experience. For instance, I was under the erroneous impression that a Grand Jury of the United States hands down an indictment only after it has sifted through all the evidence and has weighed it carefully. That isn't true at all. Most of the time the United States Grand Jury merely does what the United States attorney tells them to do. This is what happened in my case. The result is that the United States taxpayer has invested one to two million dollars in investigating this case, sending inspectors and investigators across the country several times, preparing for the trial, conducting the trial, and finally dropping the charges to vindicate me and DMSO. Still, the prosecutors seemed to be aboveboard. I developed respect for both United States attorneys. I had the feeling that they were going through the motions of prosecution but that they almost wish they hadn't gotten involved in the case. Their hearts weren't in it.

"The judge had strong feelings that the case should be dismissed and he relayed his feelings to the Justice Department. So, my attorneys and the prosecutors worked out an arrangement where we mutually read statements in open court that said in essence, 'I understand where people could interpret that our exchange of checks was a conflict of interest, and I'm sorry such an interpretation was made.' The federal attorneys in turn stated, 'We are dropping all charges against Dr. Jacob, and we wish to take this opportunity to commend him for his good services to the community.'"

Additionally, Dr. Jacob admitted that it had been "wrong" and "inappropriate" for him to make payments to an FDA scientist even though the payments in no way involved a conspiracy to clear DMSO and win its approval for other uses. The government, furthermore, excused its own action by saying that its sole purpose was to simply "ensure that the integrity of the regulatory process is upheld." In effect, Assistant United States Attorney Richard E. Dunne III said that the Justice Department wasn't after Dr. Jacob as a profiteer because of his early financial connection with Research Industries Corporation, the producer of Rimso-50, but the case was pursued because DMSO could be considered the Laetrile (an anti-cancer drug) of the eighties.

DMSO is a drug that hundreds of thousands of people are using, and for which there is a great public pressure to make legal nationally. There is also tremendous congressional pressure to approve DMSO for general use. But the bureaucratic record thus far is enormously distressing. There is a failure on the part of the FDA to properly handle DMSO. The agency has undergone internal conflict as a result, and the Inspector General is investigating that situation. DMSO has had inefficient and ineffective overall review. Problems that have been discovered were not expeditiously corrected, and it took the FDA an overly long time to make those discoveries. Perhaps the FDA has perpetuated the greatest failure of all those committed, because it is supposed to be the regulator beyond reproach guiding the others to do what is good and true.

The result is, as Senator Kennedy points out, that a travesty has been made on the drug regulatory process and serious questions have arisen in the minds of thousands of physicians and possibly millions of potential patients who need and want to use DMSO. It may alleviate their suffering from a variety of ailments, but the drug is being denied to them because of uncertainty as to its safety and efficacy. The FDA itself has been a blot on the drug regulatory record.

Senator Kennedy assured the public that this entire matter of alleged misreporting, misstatements, and alterations of data was going to be evaluated for criminal content by the United States Department of Justice. And it has been. Overall, charges have not been brought or they've been dropped without definitive conclusions.

Doctors and patients continue to use DMSO in spite of the cloud concerning its safety. In over fifteen years of use, I have not heard of one patient complaining of vision problems, and some of these patients have been using DMSO regularly for ten, twelve, and even fifteen years without complaint. Even if nuclear sclerosis, or progressive myopia, does occur in some people, it is hardly of clinical significance in that patients are unaware of changes and do not complain of visual impairment. All of the studies done up to now show that lens changes seen in experimental animals are reversible simply by discontinuing the medication.

A study by Dr. Jack de la Torre, reported in the *Journal of Toxicology and Environmental Health* 7:49–57, 1981, states: "Daily funduscopic examination during the testing period failed to reveal any abnormalities in any of the monkeys tested. . . . a double-blind slit lamp examination of the lens was performed the day before saline or DMSO administration and then again 10 and 120 days after saline or DMSO. No changes in refraction or translucency of the lens and no other abnormalities were noted in any animal before, during, or eighteen weeks after any drug administration."

There is no therapeutically effective agent on the market that does not have the potential of causing some untoward side effect. Although penicillin, phenylbutazone, clofibrate, and even aspirin can cause death in some patients, no one has suggested that these drugs be taken away from the people. "Adverse eye findings" have been reported with *all* of the arthritis drugs such as Anaprox, Naprosyn, and Motrin (as per their package inserts). Yet, no one has suggested that these minimally effective agents (about the same as aspirin) be taken off the market because of these adverse eye findings.

Even if the Scherbel findings are verified, DMSO will still be one of the safest and most important agents when it's made available. If a person is dying from a stroke or severe burn, it is unlikely that he or his loved ones will worry about clinically insignificant lens changes.

Because of the question of eye changes, and in spite of many studies showing that eye pathology does not occur, most physicians recommend, but do not insist on, a slit-lamp eye examination every six months for patients using DMSO on a continual basis.

I can only hope that this scientific and bureaucratic bungling doesn't set DMSO therapeutics back another twenty years. It seems that the American people are entitled to a better performance from everyone involved—the FDA, the medical researchers, and the private business sector. In the interest of the patients who are suffering and are full of anguish, we must have a quick, accurate, and definitive approval of DMSO for general medical use, as it is, indeed, the new healing power.

INVESTIGATIVE REPORTS CONFIRMING DMSO'S VALUE FOR SCLERODERMA

In 1986, the German journal *Dermatologische Monatsschrift* published a scientific article that verified the value of dimethyl sulfoxide in the treatment of scleroderma. The solvent was combined with dexamethasone, a corticosteroid, and administered as a local treatment that worked well.[3]

In 1983, the Dimexide brand of DMSO was applied to Russian patients for counteracting their scleroderma. Good therapeutic results were reported as circumscribed drug therapy.[4]

Again in 1983, skin manifestations in the form of scleroderma were improved by the patients receiving DMSO. The solvent is known to exert a palliative, therapeutic effect on healing of cutaneous ulcers (ulcers on the skin) in systemic sclerosis (scleroderma). In this study, which was described to the New York Academy of Sciences, the therapeutic response was variable and, therefore, the concentration of DMSO, as well as frequency and duration of treatments, were individualized to obtain maximum healing effect with a minimum of adverse reactions. There was no evidence of ocular (eye) toxicity or other serious toxicity manifestations in this group of patients. They had been treated with topical DMSO for one year or longer. Delayed improvement was observed in the untreated extremity in the majority of patients studied. In no instance did improvement in the untreated extremities exceed improvement in the other, treated limb. It is believed by the investigators that this resulted from a systemic, carryover effect of DMSO rather than spontaneous improvement in the disease course. "DMSO is a worthwhile, supplemental, therapeutic agent providing the limitations of therapy are understood," said the investigator, Dr. A.L. Scherbel.[5]

A prospective, randomized, double-blind trial was carried out in 1985 that compared topical therapy with 0.85 percent normal saline (salt solution as a placebo), 2 percent DMSO, and 70 percent DMSO for treatment of digital ulcers in 84 patients with systemic sclerosis. There were no statistically significant differences among the three treatment groups in the improvement in the total number of open ulcers, total surface area of open ulcers, average surface area per open ulcer, number of infected ulcers, number of inflamed ulcers, or patient pain assessment. While some patients improved during the study, improvement could not be attributed to a specific treatment. Over one-quarter of the patients treated with 70 percent DMSO were withdrawn from the study because of their undergoing significant skin toxicity.[6]

INVESTIGATIVE REPORTS CONFIRMING DMSO'S VALUE FOR INTERSTITIAL CYSTITIS

Interstitial cystitis is not an infectious disease, but it shows clinical manifestations of bladder inflammation and irritation. The condition may be related to the collagen diseases, may be an autoimmune disease or an allergic manifestation, or be secondary to an infectious agent not identified. At any rate, it's apparent that medical science does not know its cause and thus has no viable treatment for interstitial cystitis except the administration of dimethyl sulfoxide.

Histologically, the bladder wall in interstitial cystitis shows a unifocal or multifocal—single-site or multi-site—inflammatory infiltration with ulceration of the bladder's mucosa (lining). Scarring develops, which ultimately results in contraction of the smooth muscle, diminished urinary capacity, and symptoms of frequent, painful urination and hematuria (blood in the urine). Typically, middle-aged women are affected.

To evaluate the effectiveness of dimethyl sulfoxide in the treatment of patients with biopsies suggestive of interstitial cystitis, thirty-three patients underwent a controlled crossover trial in 1988. The results were reported in the *Journal of Urology*. Patients were allocated randomly to receive 50 percent DMSO or salt solution (saline) as placebo. The medication was administered intravesically every two weeks for two sessions of four treatments each. Response was assessed urodynamically (by checking urine) and symptomatically (by observing symptoms). Thirty women and three men having an average age of 48 years and an average duration of symptoms of 5.5 years were entered into the study. No significant side effects to DMSO were noticed by the investigators. When assessed subjectively by the patients, 53 percent of them felt markedly improved compared to 18 percent on the placebo who felt improved. Of the dimethyl sulfoxide group, 93 percent had objective improvement versus 35 percent of the placebo group. Thus, DMSO proved to be superior to placebo in the objective and subjective improvement of patients with interstitial cystitis.[7]

REPORTS SHOWING DMSO'S VALUE FOR OTHER URINARY SYSTEM PROBLEMS

Bladder diseases in general respond well to instillation of DMSO into the urinary tract. For instance, as indicated in a 1985 published paper, complex irritative bladder syndrome responded well to the solvent.[8]

Intravesical instillation of DMSO was used in the treatment of patients with intractable urinary frequency due to chronic prostatitis, chronic cystitis, tuberculous contracted bladder, and interstitial cystitis. A 1985 report from Japan indicated that before the application of dimethyl sulfoxide, all four patients were examined carefully to rule out cases of acute infectious diseases of the urinary tract, active urinary tuberculosis, neurogenic bladder (nerve pain of the bladder), and carcinoma in situ of the bladder (cancer within the bladder). Three of the four patients achieved an excellent response both subjectively and objectively. In the United States, intravesical instillation of DMSO had already been established as the specific method in the treatment of interstitial cystitis and no side effects have been reported so far. Therefore, the Japanese physicians used intravesical instillation of DMSO with success and recommend its application for various forms of intractable urinary frequency.[9]

Urethral syndrome in women is an annoying condition that is not uncommon, but a 1987 report from Poland indicates that it does respond well to DMSO instillation. The chronic urination disorder is relieved by intravesical administration of the solvent solution.[10]

A case of bladder amyloidosis was treated successfully in February 1986, report Japanese researchers, with DMSO bladder instillations. A diagnosis was made by a biopsy of the bladder epithelium (cells lining the inside of the bladder). Amyloid fibrils were confirmed in the biopsy specimen with polarization and electron microscopy. The patient was treated with trans-urethral resection (a surgery) plus DMSO. From these bladder instillations the residual lesion disappeared within four months. DMSO bladder instillations were given twelve times without side effects. Thus DMSO bladder instillation with surgical resection is designated as an excellent therapy for bladder amyloidosis.[11]

Epilogue

"Pain is only four letters, but it means different things to different people," said Ray Peppi of Stamford, Connecticut. Mr. Peppi suffers from excruciating pain caused by undergoing three back operations for relieving spinal arthritis.

"You can't understand great pain unless you have it—unless you can't remember a day in your life when you didn't have it. It makes you want to jump off a roof. It drives you crazy," Peppi explained.

In desperation, because drugs prescribed by his doctors failed to alleviate his pain, four years ago the man acquired DMSO from a nonmedical source. The solvent is not authorized in Connecticut for use on back problems. State residents whose pain is so severe that they are willing to try anything are using the crude industrial grade. DMSO did what other remedies couldn't, said Peppi. It got rid of his pain.

The Public Health Committee of the General Assembly for the State of Connecticut considered legislation that would legalize DMSO for use in Connecticut but rejected it eventually. Texas has passed such legislation, as have Florida, Nevada, Washington, Oregon, Montana, Oklahoma, and Louisiana.

Because of political pressure exerted by interested state assembly members and by members of the United States Congress, the Food and Drug Administration has been prevented from simply ignoring the drug. FDA officials promised the House Select Committee on Aging that they would take another look at it. Dr. J. Richard Crout told committee members that clinical trials of DMSO, which have been around for twenty years, and are still being carried out, haven't been precise enough to merit the drug's general use.

Yet, when the medication proves, in fact, to be as effective and safe as the evidence may show, the American people will certainly be justified in wondering why they have had to wait so many years to use it. Some FDA critics argue that if the Salk vaccine or penicillin were developed today, it would take the same length of time for them to become available to the people. How many would have died in the interim? What numbers are suffering needlessly or dying now because DMSO is unavailable on the legal, open market? This is another of those big questions underlying the whole DMSO controversy.

Government bureaucracy is known for waste and inefficiency in almost all areas of activity. In agriculture, housing, welfare, and other areas it has not solved the problems for which government programs were initially instituted. Often it has compounded them. With DMSO the problem is even more serious. Pain, health, life, and death are involved. To leave an inefficient and ineffective bureaucracy in charge of approving a pain-relieving, life-sustaining drug like DMSO will cost the victims of injury and illness far more than tax dollars.

I believe the medical consumer deserves to have the medicines he or she needs as soon as they have proved to be safe and effective. I ask that the FDA fulfill its mandate to protect Americans from foods and drugs that are unsafe and to facilitate the speedy availability of new foods and drugs that are found to be both safe and worthwhile. DMSO is one of these. DMSO is one of nature's healers—among the safest and most efficacious ever uncovered. We are entitled to it. We must have it generally available.

The life and health of our people lie in the balance. The story I have told highlights the obstacles DMSO has met in getting FDA approval. More than that, I have shown that pain relief is available, pathology reversal is possible, and good health restoration is probable if only DMSO is not denied to us. The crime of denial is senseless. How do we get DMSO to all the people? If there is no medical answer, there may be a political one.

With the former Reagan administration's concern about the regulatory impact on the return on research and development investments, ways were found to lessen the FDA ban. The election of Ronald Reagan as our President meant significant personnel changes for regulators, including the Food and Drug Administration's Bureau of Drugs. FDA Commissioner Jere Goyan, a political appointee during the Carter administration, finally lost his post. Reagan's advisors had searched for highly qualified scientists who understood the problems with regulations. But they wanted regulators who were people-conscious first, then regulation-conscious. They didn't find them. Neither did George

Bush. Instead, David Kessler, M.D., J.D., has turned out to be the most restrictive enforcer of Gestapo-like rules coming out of the FDA. Kessler would remove every American's ability to choose what should be done for or to his or her body. The FDA, by expanding its mandate and reinterpreting the Nutrition Labeling and Education Act of 1990 for its own purposes, is approaching dictatorial powers. I hope his successor will take immediate and decisive steps to reverse this trend. I want my book to move the regulatory process. DMSO, nature's healer, is a new therapeutic treatment for the people. They deserve to have access to it.

APPENDIX I

The Mechanisms of Action of DMSO, Miscellaneous Conditions That Respond Well to DMSO Administration, and Arthritis Treatment Details for Physicians

DMSO lessens platelet adhesiveness, platelet aggregation, and, thus, clot formation. Because of its prostaglandin activity, DMSO is a potent vasodilator. Prostaglandins—long chain hydrocarboxylic acids—are affected in a unique way by dimethyl sulfoxide. The "good prostaglandin," prostaglandin E, which is a powerful vasodilator, is stimulated by DMSO. The "bad prostaglandins," prostaglandin E_2 and prostaglandin F_2 alpha, which are strong vasoconstrictors, are depressed by DMSO. Prostaglandin E_2 and prostaglandin F_2 alpha not only cause vasoconstriction but lysosomal destruction. Lysosomes are cellular "toilets" and their destruction leads to release of the cytotoxic enzyme beta-glucoronidase. This enzyme not only destroys its own cell, but surrounding cells as well, leading to further beta-glucoronidase release, and further destruction.

Prostaglandin E_1, like aspirin and indomethacin, stabilizes lysosomes and probably blocks the release of vasoconstrictive prostaglandins from brain tissue and platelets.

Because of the body's "negative" or destructive responses to injury, including toxic prostaglandin release, beta-glucoronidase destruction of cells, noradrenaline stimulation, reduction of mitochondrial oxidative phosphorylation, release of calcium ions, and other actions, *DMSO may be the initial treatment of choice in all acute destructive bodily processes.* These would include any serious injury to any body part or organ, septicemia, stroke, myocardial infarction, near drowning, heat stroke, etc.

As an example of the fantastically protective effect of DMSO against trauma, consider the work of Dr. Ramon Linn, an Associate Professor of Neurosurgery. As I mentioned in the text, Dr. Linn prepared cultures of glial cells and DMSO, which he subjected to sonic vibrations. The cells were remarkably protected from injury and beta-glucoronidase release.

The other many modes of action of DMSO, such as sensory nerve inhibition, diuretic action, membrane penetrability, free radical neutralization, intracellular water substitution, macrophage stimulation, antigen neutralization, and interferon production, are all discussed in the text.

THE INTRAVENOUS THERAPY TECHNIQUE
USED BY MOST DOCTORS

For intravenous therapy, other than acute stroke, the dose is 1 g DMSO per kg body weight given daily for five to ten days with a rest on the weekend after the first five treatments. A half dose is given the first day to observe the patient's response. An indefinite number of two-week blocks of treatment can be given as long as there is a week's rest in between.

In one type of clinic setup there are two large rooms with rows of reclining chairs for the intravenous (IV) patients. No television is provided, as the patients are encouraged to read nutritional literature and to converse with each other. Also, television sounds disturb those who prefer to sleep during the easy intravenous infusion.

On the first day, blood is drawn for chemistries, CBC, and arthritis profile. Hair analysis, computerized diet analysis, and basal temperature tests are done on all patients no matter what their disease or complaint. The legal consent form must be signed prior to treatment.

The DMSO is mixed in 500 ml of any appropriate isotonic fluid. Physicians usually use D5W. Some clinics use Ringer's Lactate or 0.45 saline in 2.5 percent glucose. For reasons explained later in this section, some doctors add 15 g of ascorbic acid, 100 mg of pyridoxine, 1,000 mg magnesium chloride, 2,000 mcg cobalamin, and 200 mg vitamin B complex. This is infused over a three- to four-hour period.

Occasionally nausea will develop. Phenergan suppositories, 50 mg, usually will take care of it. A good breakfast must be eaten before the treatment to help alleviate the nausea. Infusion nurses also make snacks available to the patients during treatment.

Patients may be advised to apply DMSO to affected areas at home. A 50-percent solution is suggested for the neck and face. Before it was banned by the FDA, the product 75 percent DEMSO was applied to any other affected parts of the body; now Domoso is recommended. Application is two to four times a day depending on skin sensitivity. Oral treatment is continued by the patient at home (one teaspoonful in juice twice a day) along with topical application after the IV program is terminated.

CLINICAL STUDIES SHOWING RESPONSE TO DMSO IN AMYLOIDOSIS

Amyloidosis is the accumulation in the tissues of the fibrillar glycoprotein amyloid in amounts sufficient to impair normal function. As stated a few times in the body of this text, amyloid is a glycoprotein, resembling starch, that is deposited in the internal organs. The cause of amyloid production and its deposition is unknown. A defect in cellular immunity to a specific antigen is suspected. Amyloid is a homogeneous, highly refractile substance with an affinity for Congo red dye, both in prepared tissues and *in vivo*. It is made up primarily of a well-defined fibril, distinct from other extracellular structural proteins, which occurs in two forms.

Chemical analyses of the various forms of amyloid causes classification of the substance as *primary* when there is no associated disease, and *secondary* when it's associated with chronic diseases, either the infectious form such as tuberculosis, osteomyelitis, leprosy, and bronchiectasis, or the inflammatory form such as rheumatoid arthritis and granulomatous ileitis. Amyloid is also found in association with multiple myeloma, Hodgkin's disease, and other tumors. It may accompany aging and may appear in familial forms unassociated with other disease. Increasing numbers of familial amyloid syndromes with distinctive types of neuropathy, nephropathy, and cardiopathy have been described in the medical literature. DMSO has found successful use by clinicians for the treatment of familial amyloidosis.

A report delivered by a half-dozen Japanese medical scientists to the New York Academy of Sciences in 1983 indicated that DMSO was therapeutically administered to patients with familial amyloidosis of the adult onset type. In about half of the treated people there was some clinical improvement. Urinary proteins were analyzed biochemically and immunochemically before and after administration of the dimethyl sulfoxide in seven patients. Increased excretion of various proteins of different molecular weights in the patients' urine was observed by the Japanese investigators, depending on cases and examined organs. The *in vitro* effects of DMSO on amyloid proteins were examined. DMSO-degraded amyloid proteins showed void-volume materials and lower molecular weight components on a special urine test (the Sephadex G column elution profiles and the guanidine-degraded amyloid protein profile). While DMSO is the least potent in dissolving amyloid fibrils among the various denaturing or reducing agents, prealbumin-related proteins (proteins that are the source of albumin) were found from the testing. This proved that scleroderma improves somewhat from oral ingestion of diluted dimethyl sulfoxide.[1]

In another case of familial amyloidosis—only of the polyneuropathic type (related to a disease of multiple nerves)—two case histories were presented in this 1984 paper from Italy. DMSO produced a positive response for those patients having peripheral nerve disease.[2]

Other patients with the primary type of amyloidosis and the kind associated with multiple myeloma usually have the immunoglobulin light-chain form of amyloid fibrils. Patients with secondary amyloidosis have demonstrated the presence of the unique AA protein that consists of non-immunoglobulin.

In primary amyloidosis, the heart, lung, skin, tongue, thyroid gland, and intestinal tract may be involved. Peculiar localized amyloid "tumors" may be found in the involved patient's respiratory tract or other sites. Parenchymal organs of the liver, spleen, and kidney and the vascular system are frequently involved, as well.

Secondary amyloidosis tends to show up in the spleen, liver, kidney, adrenal glands, and lymph nodes. However, no organ system is spared, and vascular involvement may be widespread. The liver and spleen are often enlarged, firm, and rubbery. The kidneys are usually enlarged. Sections of the spleen show large translucent, waxy areas, where the normal malpighian bodies (normally present inclusion cells) are replaced by pale amyloid, producing the "sago" spleen.

Amyloid associated with certain tumors such as multiple myeloma and skin diseases such as lichen planus may be widespread and may show unique sites of involvement. Amyloid may have a strictly local occurrence in association with some malignancies such as medullary carcinoma of the thyroid gland.

In a 1985 clinical paper, the result of topical treatment by dimethyl sulfoxide in a patient with lichen amyloidosis was reported. DMSO improved the patient's itching within five days of therapy. Remarkable flattening of the papules usually present in this condition was obtained within two weeks. The clinical result was confirmed by histological examination, which revealed partial disappearance of amyloid deposits.[3]

Characteristic standard symptoms or signs of amyloidosis are lacking. Manifestations are nonspecific and usually originate in the organ or system affected. Often they are obscured by the underlying disease, which may be fatal before secondary amyloidosis is suspected. The kidney's nephrotic syndrome (series of signs and symptoms present in a diseased kidney) is the most striking manifestation. In the early stages only slight proteinuria may be noted; later the distinctive symptom complex develops with massive swelling of the legs, trunk, and genitalia due to retention of fluid, hypoproteinuria, and massive proteinuria. The urine sediment often contains red blood cells. All kinds of strange changes in the body take place with amyloidosis. For instance, it caused a sudden whitening and loss of hair, as described in an August 1987 Japanese case report. Yet, as shown below, for this amyloidosis patient, treatment with dimethyl sulfoxide solved his difficulty.

Here, a sixty-seven-year-old Japanese man presented himself with rapid progression of whitening and loss of his head hair within two months. It was suspicioned by the attending medical specialists that he suffered with hypothyroidism. He had been told that he had enlargement of the heart, a condition suspected of being present for three years. Thyroid function for the man was within normal limits, however. A prostate biopsy was performed on him because of his obvious prostatic hypertrophy and mild elevation of serum acid phosphatase. Then, amyloid accumulation was observed by the pathologist in the biopsy specimen. Subsequent skin biopsies revealed the same result.

The patient's scalp hair and beard grew and turned to a black color gradually, several months after DMSO treatment was administered to him. The researchers came to the firm conclusion that some manifestations of amyloidosis such as show up in skin, scalp, and hair pathology do respond well to DMSO treatment.[4]

Amyloid disease of the liver produces an enlargement of this organ, but rarely jaundice. Liver function tests usually are normal although an elevated alkaline phosphatase may be observed. Occasionally, portal hypertension may occur with varicose veins of the esophagus, and fluid in the abdomen. Massive liver enlargement with a weight of 7 kg has been reported. Skin lesions as indicated by the case of hair whitening and hair loss described previously may be waxy or translucent; purpura may result from amyloidosis of small skin blood vessels. Cardiac involvement is common and may manifest itself as intractable heart failure or show up as any of the common heart arrhythmias. Atrial standstill has been found in several kinships.

Gastrointestinal amyloid may cause bleeding and malabsorption in the bowel. A firm, symmetric, nontender goiter resembling Hashimoto's or Riedel's struma may result from amyloidosis of the thyroid gland. Amyloid athropathy may mimic rheumatoid arthritis in some cases of multiple myeloma. Peripheral neuropathy is seen in a few cases of primary or myeloma-associated amyloid. It is common in some familial amyloidosis.

With all these amyloid-associated pathologies, DMSO demonstrates a positive therapeutic benefit. It affects systemic amyloidosis efficaciously.

In August 1986, three Japanese clinicians reported to the American medical community on the positive response of systemic amyloidosis to dimethyl sulfoxide. It was a case report of systemic amyloid pathology as a manifestation in the skin. This sixty-five-year-old woman with systemic amyloidosis was given DMSO orally for four years without her having experienced any side effects. Her cutaneous lesions improved markedly after the treatment, and she still survived in satisfactory condition at the time of the article's publication.[5]

Secondary amyloidosis should be suspected by the doctor when the condition of his or her patient with a chronic suppurative (pus-producing) disease progressively deteriorates and the common manifestations of amyloidosis, such as spleen and liver enlargement and/or albumin in the urine appear. Biopsy of rectal mucosa is the best screening test. Other useful sites for biopsy are gingiva, skin, nerve, kidney, and liver. All tissue sections should be stained with Congo red dye and observed with the polarizing microscope for green birefringence (color shadings).

A 1982 report in the *Annals of Rheumatic Diseases* told of continuous oral DMSO treatment of 7 to 15 g per day that was given to three patients with amyloidosis of familial Mediterranean fever (FMF), three patients with idiopathic amyloidosis—amyloidosis having no known cause—and seven patients with secondary amyloidosis. The medically recognized kidney syndrome and various degrees of renal insufficiency were the major clinical manifestation in all cases. Renal function was used as the main parameter for evaluation of the DMSO therapy. DMSO treatment administered for seven to sixteen months produced no effect in the FMF patients and in the patients with idiopathic amyloidosis; they all ran the predictable clinical course of their disease and either died of cardiac failure or have been maintained on chronic hemodialysis. In the seven patients with secondary amyloidosis, an unequivocal improvement of the renal function was observed following from three to six months of DMSO treatment.

The improvement of kidney function was shown by a 30 to 100 percent rise of creatinine clearance and a decline in the amount of protein in the urine (proteinuria). This new equilibrium had been maintained for the patients as long as DMSO was administered. No serious side effects of DMSO were encountered; mild nausea and an unpleasant breath odor were the patients' main concern. The four medical researchers concluded that a therapeutic trial with oral DMSO definitely is warranted in all patients with secondary amyloidosis. "This treatment is unpleasant," they write, "but bears no exceptional risks. It may significantly prolong life, though its effect on amyloid deposits themselves is doubtful."[6]

In secondary amyloidosis, prognosis depends on successful treatment of the underlying disease. All forms of amyloid renal involvement carry a poor prognosis, but with supportive therapy such as the instillation of dimethyl sulfoxide, patients may remain healthy. Amyloidosis associated with multiple myeloma has the poorest prognosis, early death within one to two years being common. However, localized amyloid tumors may be removed without recurrence. Myocardial amyloidosis may cause death from arrhythmias or intractable cardiac failure. Prognosis in the familial amyloidoses varies with each kinship.

An early report of the use of DMSO therapy for amyloid deposits and amyloidosis casts doubt on its value. Writing in the September 1981 issue of *Veterinary Research Communications*, the three clinicians state: "Data from the literature on DMSO therapy for amyloidosis in laboratory animals and man are reviewed and found to be inconclusive. In hamsters with casein-induced amyloidosis, as well as in dogs with spontaneous amyloidosis, therapeutic experiments with DMSO were performed. In these investigations no effect of DMSO on amyloid and amyloidosis was found."[7]

Finally, a urologist, Dr. S. Yachiku, writing in the March 1986 issue of the *Journal of Urology*, reported on a case of primary localized amyloidosis of the bladder that responded well to instillation with dimethyl sulfoxide. Dr. Yachiku first successfully performed a transurethral resection and then did intravesical instillation with DMSO. He concluded that the patient's swift recovery from the primary localized amyloidosis was directly due to DMSO.[8]

CLINICAL STUDIES SHOWING RESPONSE TO DMSO IN DISSOLVING GALLSTONES

A 1988 report by French clinicians confirmed that DMSO is useful for the dissolving of cholesterol gallstones. It is known that methyl tert-butyl ether, which is a powerful cholesterol monohydrate solvent, does not completely dissolve mixed cholesterol gallstones when directly infused into the biliary tree (the stream of bile into the gallbladder). In the current paper, the clinicians compared the effect of various solvents containing different proportions of methyl tert-butyl ether and dimethyl sulfoxide in anhydrous and aqueous systems on the *in vitro* solubilization of human cholesterol stones.

The dissolution rates of cholesterol obtained in the presence of methyl tert-butyl was markedly decreased when 10 parts were added to 100 parts of water. In contrast, the addition of 30 parts of DMSO per 100 parts of water (a 30-percent solution) to the methyl tert-butyl ether-water system enhanced the stone-solvent contact, improved the cholesterol dissolution rates, and left less gallstone debris.

Better yet, a subsequent dissolution with an alkaline (pH = 8.8) aqueous dimethyl sulfoxide–ethylene diamine tetraacetic acid (DMSO-EDTA) solution strongly reduced the noncholesterol residues.

In vivo, nearly complete dissolution of human cholesterol stones implanted in the gallbladders of rabbits were obtained within eight hours when methyl tert-butyl ether–DMSO (in a proportion of 70 to 30 parts) solvent was infused at a rate of 0.6 ml/h/kg. With methyl tert-butyl ether, only 84 parts per 100 of the original stone weight was dissolved.

As for side effects, the infusion of these solvents leads to morphological changes in the gallbladder wall with some focal ulcerations. These alterations can be almost completely recovered after two weeks. No histologic evidence of liver, duodenal, or kidney damage was found.

The four clinicians write: "We conclude that the mixture methyl tert-butyl ether/dimethyl sulfoxide (70/30) constitutes a good solvent for mixed cholesterol stones. Compared with pure methyl tert-butyl ether, the mixed system allows for a more rapid and a more complete dissolution of gallstones."[9]

The above report was a semi-verifier of an earlier Japanese paper that indicated DMSO is a chelator and dissolver of calcium stones in the gallbladder. In 1983, hepatobiliary surgeons (surgeons who operate on the liver and gallbladder) described how they must face the difficult task of treating patients with intrahepatic gallstones (gallstones derived from the liver) in spite of considerable progress in operative methods or mechanical techniques. It was tough for them to remove intrahepatic gallstones completely, and under such circumstances, the development of a solubilizer that could dissolve the intrahepatic bilirubinate calcium stones proved to be a tremendous boon for the patients. The surgeons accomplished this step by injecting DMSO through a postoperative catheter or PTCD catheter. Up to that time a chelating agent, so-called hexametaphosphate (HMP) had been used for removing the calcium from calcium bilirubinate. But this chelating agent, in itself, could not dissolve the bilirubin.

Then the three Japanese surgeons found a direct solubilizer for bilirubin, dimethyl sulfoxide, which they knew to be a bi-polar, non-protonic solvent, and used it as an accelerator for bilirubin determination. After purifying the DMSO to 99.98 percent, they examined its toxicity by oral administration, intravenous administration, and infusion into biliary tracts of animals. No toxicity or side effects were detected on biochemical and pathological examinations. Next they used their solution on humans in the amount of 90 percent DMSO together with 5 percent HMP and achieved a satisfactory effect by attaining the solubilizing of their patients' bilirubinate calcium stones.[10]

CLINICAL STUDIES SHOWING RESPONSE TO DMSO IN MISCELLANEOUS CONDITIONS

Successful treatment of lupus erythematosus, a chronic inflammatory disease of connective tissue, affecting the skin and various internal organs, including the bladder, was carried out using dimethyl sulfoxide. Typically, lupus exhibits a red scaly rash on the face, affecting the nose and cheeks; arthritis; and progressive damage to the kidneys. Often the heart, lungs, and brain are also affected by progressive attacks of inflammation followed by the formation of scar tissue (fibrosis). In a milder form of the disease only the skin is affected.

Lupus erythematosus is regarded as an autoimmune disease and can be diagnosed by the presence of abnormal antibodies in the blood stream, most easily detected by a test that reveals characteristic white blood cells (LE cells). In 1984, four physicians joined together in reporting on two female patients who were victims of systemic lupus erythematosus with pathologically confirmed lupus interstitial cystitis. Their urinary bladders were highly symptomatic. Treatment with prednisone had been tried but without success. Then the two patients responded very well to instillations of DMSO intravesically (into the bladder) and had their conditions disappear.[11]

DMSO works well to alleviate an unhealed wound at the site of a tooth extraction, the well-known "dry socket" that defeats the surgical skills of many dentists. Characterized by intense pain, discharge of pus, and sequestra (residual symptoms, signs, and other ill effects), dry socket is most often associated with a difficult extraction. Dripping DMSO directly into the extraction site tends to prevent this problem from arising.[12]

Lastly, dimethyl sulfoxide has been used to offset inflammations associated with sunburn. Phytophotodermatitis arising in the summer months in temperate climates varies from mild to severe erythematous reactions (inflammation of the skin due to widening or clogging of capillaries near the skin surface) with or without vesicles or bullae (blisters) on the exposed parts of the body. By treating the skin with a membrane labilizing agent (an agent that causes chemical change) such as DMSO and a membrane stabilizing agent such as the steroid desoximethasone, comfort for the patient is achieved.[13]

DMSO ANTI-ARTHRITIS THERAPY

DMSO is not a cure for arthritis. It is one part of a five-part treatment program that consists of:

1. Nutrition
2. Microendocrinology
3. Immunotherapy
4. Food allergy elimination
5. DMSO

Powerful chemical agents such as cortisone, phenoprophins, phenylbutazones, and gold have no place in this arthritis treatment program.

Nutrition writer Adelle Davis, the idol of health food enthusiasts who has been wrongly, in my opinion, sneered at by numerous medical traditionalists, was way ahead of her time. Many of her nutritional suggestions have been confirmed by good scientific research. The ultimate traditionalist in nutrition, the United States Department of Agriculture, has, in fact, adapted much of her wisdom in its "Dietary Goals" for Americans. The National Research Council of the National Academy of Science proved Adelle Davis correct when it issued its 1982 report—two years in the making—on *Diet, Nutrition, and Cancer.* The Council was chaired by Dr. Clifford Grobstein of the University of California, and made up of fourteen highly respected medical scientists.

As we know from high school biology, and were reminded in college and medical school, the anterior pituitary gland is the so-called "master gland." Through the action of ACTH, it directly controls the adrenals.

But something we were not taught, and which is of great clinical significance, is that the highest concentration of certain nutrients is in the adrenals and pituitary gland. The highest concentration of vitamin

E in the body is stored in the pituitary; the highest concentration of vitamin C is held by the adrenals. Also, the pituitary gland needs sufficient protein for efficient function, and the greatest concentration of pantothenic acid lies in the adrenal glands.

Adelle Davis reasoned that if the adrenals were excreting enough natural cortisone, exogenous cortisone would not be needed in the treatment of arthritis. She knew from the work of Dugal (*Endocrinology* 44: 420, 1949) that animals under stress need *seventy times* the normal requirement of vitamin C to protect the adrenals and that people in the "arthritis years" require twice as much vitamin C as the young.

As we can see from my simple little diagram (see Figure A-1), vitamin E deficiency will lead to pituitary insufficiency and, from hyposecretion of ACTH, adrenal insufficiency follows.

Therefore, a *deficiency* of vitamin C, vitamin E, pantothenic acid, and protein, or perhaps certain combinations of these deficiencies, will, over a period of years, lead to arthritis. Because of the high intake of sugar and junk food in this country, subclinical deficiencies of these nutrients (and others) are common.

Vitamin C deficiency is the easiest to measure. Studies of the night nursing personnel of the Emergency Department at Memorial Hospital in Sarasota, Florida, were revealing. These women were under extreme stress (which decreases vitamin C levels) due to the abnormal hours they worked and the nature of the cases they saw—such as gunshot wounds—with the concomitant responsibility. All of the nurses smoked cigarettes, which drastically depresses vitamin C levels. Most of them were on the birth control pill, which depresses vitamin C. They ate large amounts of sugar-filled foods and drank copious amounts of cola drinks, which drive down vitamin C levels. And they took frequent doses of aspirin (C-depressing) for the headaches induced by their usual hypoglycemic swings brought on by the colas and other junk food they ate.

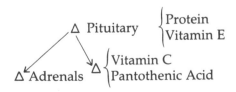

Figure A-1 Diagram showing that adrenal insufficiency follows vitamin E deficiency.

Eighty percent of these young women, who appeared to be in good health, were vitamin C deficient. Over a period of years they have had chronic adrenal exhaustion, and arthritis is likely to follow. Yet, these workers were registered nurses who should have known how to take care of themselves.

I have barely scratched the surface on the importance of nutrition and arthritis. But, contrary to the pronouncements of the Arthritis Foundation, nutritional deficiencies play a major role in the etiology of arthritis, something the writings on orthomolecular nutrition by Adelle Davis and other authors will teach you.

MICROENDOCRINOLOGY

Dr. Melvin Page's extensive work with the calcium-phosphorus ratio, anthropometric measurements, and microendocrinology is a major advance in the treatment of arthritis in particular and degenerative disease in general.

ALLERGY TESTING

For good results in the treatment of arthritis, food allergies must be investigated. The method I like best is cytotoxic testing of the blood. But, unfortunately, cytotoxic labs are available in only a few cities. Sublingual testing or the cumbersome elimination diet technique might possibly be used as a substitute.

For excellent assistance with the various sophisticated allergy tests, including the paper radioimmunosorbent (PRIST) test, the cytotoxic (or leukocytotoxic) test, the radioallergosorbent (RAST) test, the fluoroaller-gosorbent (FAST) test, the autoradiographic (MAST) test, the immunoper-oxidase (IP) test, and the enzyme-linked immunosorbent assay (ELISA) test, you might use the services of several laboratories that I am listing here. Note: of all the tests, the RAST and the ELISA have proven most popular among those physicians specializing in environmental medicine, because these two diagnostic procedures seem to be most accurate. Since this is not a book about food allergy, hypersensitivity, cytolytic reaction, immune complex mediated reaction, delayed hypersensitivity reaction, food intolerance, food idiosyncrasy, food metabolic reaction, toxicity reactions, or anaphylaxis, I won't go into detail describing the various tests. Instead, acquire information from the following laboratories, which are quite accommodating to the health professional:

- Immuno Laboratories, 1620 West Oakland Park Boulevard, Ft. Lauderdale, Florida 33311; toll-free nationally (800) 231-9197, in Florida (305) 486-4500, teleFAX (305) 739-6563.
- Meridian Valley Clinical Laboratory, 24030 132nd Avenue SE, Kent, Washington 98042; toll-free nationally (800) 234-6825, in Washington (206) 631-8922, teleFAX (206) 631-8691. (This is the laboratory with which Jonathan Wright, M.D., was associated and that was raided at gunpoint by agents of the FDA in May 1992.)
- Metametrix Medical Laboratory, 5000 Peachtree Industrial Boulevard, Suite 110, Norcross, Georgia 30071; telephone (404) 446-5483, teleFAX (404) 441-2237.
- Great Smokies Diagnostic Laboratory, 18A Regent Boulevard, Asheville, North Carolina 28806; toll-free nationally (800) 522-4762, in North Carolina (704) 253-0621, teleFAX (704) 253-1127.
- National BioTechnology Laboratory, Inc., 13215 SE 240th Street, Suite C, Kent, Washington 98042; telephone (206) 630-2295, (800) 846-6285.

IMMUNOTHERAPY

Another weapon in our treatment armamentarium is immunotherapy. Bernard A. Bellew, M.D., discovered that patients receiving immunization for influenza and for bacterial infection who had arthritis greatly improved following immunization. Dr. Bellew theorized that rheumatoid arthritis was secondary to chronic infection. With serial injections of flu and bacterial vaccines, he has had impressive results in treating rheumatoid arthritis.

DMSO is, of course, the tool against arthritis that this book favors most. If you have any further questions about the employment of DMSO in arthritis or other treatment modalities, please call or write to William Campbell Douglass, M.D., P.O. Box 888, Clayton, Georgia 30525, telephone (706) 782-7222. He is an expert on this therapy.

For literature and other information on pain relief for chronic joint, ligamentous, and tendon disabilities, send a check or money order for $18 (U.S.) along with a self-addressed, nine-inch by twelve-inch manilla envelope with enough postage for ten ounces of articles to Dr. Morton Walker, Freelance Communications, 484 High Ridge Road, Stamford, Connecticut 06905-3095; telephone (203) 322-1551, teleFAX (203) 322-4656.

FINAL RANDOM COMMENTS

In the treatment of massive stroke, extremely large doses of DMSO are required for a good result. The initial dose is 2 g per kg of body weight. By the usual standards, this is an incredibly large dose of medication, a comment on the lack of toxicity of the drug. What other medication can be safely used even at one tenth of that dose?

One potentially serious side effect can occur at these high dosage levels—hemolysis.

The first IV arthritis patient treated by my medical consultant, Dr. Douglass, had hemolysis with hemoglobinuria at a dosage of one g per kg. This is not a common occurrence but occurs with enough frequency to warrant frequent blood hemoglobin and hematocrit determinations and urine monitoring during the initial phase of treatment.

If hemolysis occurs, treatment should be continued at the same dosage level as long as kidney function remains within normal limits and the hemogram doesn't change significantly. Transfusion will rarely be necessary but packed cells can be given if indicated.

A final word about the legality of DMSO in your state: Most people, including doctors, don't understand the FDA rules and regulations concerning the use of "approved" drugs. Once a drug has been approved by the FDA for any condition, a licensed physician in any state, whether the legislature of that state has passed special legislation or not, has the right to use that drug in any way that he feels will benefit his patient. There are many precedents for this, such as xylocaine in cardiac arrhythmia, propranalol in hypertension and headache, diphenhydramine for sedation, and phentoin for arrhythmias. Another example is the use of the phenopropins for menstrual cramps.

As DMSO has been approved for use in interstitial cystitis by the FDA, *DMSO is also legal in all fifty states for use in stroke, burns, arthritis, and for whatever other purpose the doctor deems appropriate.*

APPENDIX II

Titles of Scientific Papers on DMSO Therapy in the Order They Were Presented at the Dimethyl Sulfoxide Symposium Held Under the Auspices of the New York Academy of Sciences in January 1974

Pharmacologic and Biochemical Considerations of Dimethyl Sulfoxide. Don C. Wood, Ph.D., Medlab Computer Services, Salt Lake City, Utah.

Influence of Non-Ionic Organic Solutes on Various Reactions of Energy Conservation and Utilization. Thomas Conover, Ph.D., Hahnemann Medical College, Philadelphia, Pennsylvania.

Effects of DMSO on Subunit Proteins. Thomas R. Henderson and Rogene F. Henderson, Lovelace Fnd., Albuquerque, New Mexico, and J.L. York, University of Arkansas School of Medicine, Little Rock, Arkansas.

The Effect of Dimethyl Sulfoxide on a Lysosomal Membrane. Donald W. Misch and Margaret S. Misch, Department of Zoology, University of North Carolina, Chapel Hill, North Carolina.

Specific Modifications of the Na+, K+ -ATPase by DMSO. Joseph D. Robinson, State University of New York, Upstate Medical Center, Syracuse, New York.

Toxicology of DMSO and DMSO in Chemical Combinations. Lionel F. Rubin, V.M.D., School of Veterinary Medicine, University of Pennsylvania, Philadelphia, Pennsylvania.

Metabolism and Excretion of DMSO in Calves and Cows After Topical and Parenteral Application of Labelled DMSO. J. Tiewst, E. Scharrer, N. Harre, L. Flogel, and W. Jochle.

The Effect of Dimethylsulfoxide and Dimethylformide on Tumor Cells in Vitro. Ellen Borenfreund and Aaron Bendich, Memorial Sloan-Kettering Cancer Center, New York, New York.

Effect of DMSO on the Hepatic Disposition of Chemical Carcinogens. W.G.

Levine, Department of Pharmacology, Albert Einstein College of Medicine, Bronx, New York.

Potentiation of Anti-Neoplastic Compounds by Oral DMSO in Tumor-Bearing Rats. Joel Warren, Ph.D., Miriam R. Sacksteder, B.S., Harriet Jarosz, B.S., Bruce Wasserman, B.S., and Peter E. Andreotti, Leo Goodwin Institute for Cancer Research, Nova University, Fort Lauderdale, Florida.

Effect of DMSO on Skin Carcinogenesis. F. Stenback and H. Garcia, Eppley Institute, Omaha, Nebraska.

Report on the Use of DMSO on the Treatment of Extensive Superficial Wounds in Dogs and Horses. S.W.J. Seager, M.A., M.V.B., M.R.C.V.S., Department of Surgery, University of Oregon Medical School, Portland, Oregon.

Anti-Inflammatory and Anti-Thrombotic Effects of Topically Applied Dimethyl Sulfoxide (DMSO). Peter Gorog, Ph.D., Egypt Pharmacochemical Works and Irene B. Kovacs, M.D., Otto Korvin Hospital, Budapest, Hungary.

Fate and Metabolism of DMSO in 30 Agricultural Crops. Bernard C. Smale, Ph.D., Neil J. Lasater, and Bruce T. Hunter, Crown Zellerbach Central Research, Camas, Washington.

Accumulation and Persistence of Sulfur 35 in Peach Foliage and Fruit Sprayed With Radiolabeled Dimethyl Sulfoxide. Harry L. Kell, Ph.D., United States Department of Agriculture, Agricultural Research Service, Northeastern Region, Agricultural Research Center–West, Beltsville, Maryland.

Use of DMSO to Control Aflatoxin Production. George A. Bean and George W. Rambo, Division of Agriculture and Life Sciences, University of Maryland, College Park, Maryland.

Current Concepts Concerning Radioprotective and Cryoprotective Properties of Dimethyl Sulphoxide in Cellular Systems. M.J. Ashwood-Smith, Department of Biological Sciences, University of Victoria, Victoria, British Columbia, Canada.

The Effect of Dimethyl Sulfoxide on Forelimb Regeneration of the Adult Newt. Gerald G. Slattery, Ph.D., College of Osteopathic Medicine and Surgery, Des Moines, Iowa, and Anthony J. Schmidt, Ph.D., University of Illinois, Medical Center, Chicago, Illinois.

In Vitro and In Vivo Effects of Dimethylsulfoxide on Streptomycin Sensitive and Resistant Escherichia Coli. W.E. Feldman, J.D. Punch, and P.C. Holden, Richmond, Virginia.

Tolerance of In Vitro Neuritic Development to DMSO. Fred Jerrold Roisen, Ph.D., College of Medicine and Dentistry of New Jersey, Rutgers Medical School, Piscataway, New Jersey.

DMSO: A Tool in Sperm Motility Control Studies. Leonard Nelson, Ph.D., Medical College of Ohio, Toledo, Ohio.

Interferon Production in the White Mouse by Dimethyl Sulfoxide (DMSO). Michael Kunze, M.D., Institute of Hygiene, University of Vienna, Austria.

Effect of Dimethyl Sulfoxide and Hydrogen Peroxide on Tissue Gas Tensions. Beart Myers, M.D., and William Donovan. Surgical Research Laboratory, Veterans' Administration Hospital, and Louisiana State University School of Medicine, New Orleans, Louisiana.

Effect of DMSO on the Hypothalamic-Pituitary Adrenal Axis of the Rat. J.P. Allen, M.D., Brooks Air Force Base, and C.F. Allen, Southwest Foundation for Clinical Research, San Antonio, Texas.

Effects of DMSO and a Corticosteroid on Normal and Infected Anal Sacs of Dogs. J.G. Kilian, Syntex Research, Palo Alto, California.

The Effect of Dimethylsulfoxide (DMSO) on Cholinergic Transmission in Aplysia Ganglion Cells. Makoto Sato, M.D., Ph.D., and Masashi Sawada, Ph.D., Neuroscience Laboratory, Division of Neurosurgery, University of Oregon Medical School, Portland, Oregon.

Protective Effect of Dimethyl Sulfoxide on Brain Cells Against Sonic Stress. Ramon Lim and S. Mullan, University of Chicago, Chicago, Illinois.

DMSO in CNS Trauma. J.C. de la Torre, H.M. Kawanaga, C.M. Johnson, D.W. Goode, K. Kajihara, and S. Mullan, University of Chicago, Chicago, Illinois.

Experimental Design of Clinical Trials Testing the Efficacy of 90% DMSO Solution in Diseases of the Musculoskeletal System in the Dog. E.G. Averkin, Syntex Research, Palo Alto, California, and T. O'Brian, D.V.M., Tauton, Massachusetts.

Introduction Study for a New Topical Medication With DMSO in Dermatology. Dr. Lazaro Schatman, Alvear and Israelita Hospitals and Railway Polyclinic Services, Buenos Aires, Argentina.

Experimental and Clinical Evaluation With Topical DMSO in Vascular Disorders of the Extremities. A. Kappert, M.D., University of Bern, Switzerland.

DMSO Therapy in Chronic Skin Ulcers. Rene Miranda, M.D., University of Chile.

DMSO Therapy as Toxicity Reducing Agent and Potentiator of Cyclophosphamide in the Treatment of Different Types of Cancer. Jorge Cornejo, M.D., Military Hospital, Santiago, Chile.

Clinical Experience With DMSO as a Solvent for Antiviral Agents. B.E. Juel-Jensen, H.A., D.M., University of Oxford, England.

DMSO Therapy in Severe Mental Retardation in Mongoloid Children. M. Aspillaga, M.D., M. Sanchez, M.D., G. Morizon, M.D., and Lucila Capdeville, M.D., Santiago, Chile.

DMSO Therapy Applied to Non-Mongoloid Children Oligophrenia. Dra. Ana Giller and Dra. Maria E.M. de Bernadou, Buenos Aires, Argentina.

Oral DMSO in Mental Retardation: A Preliminary Controlled Study. J.M. Gabourie, J.W. Becker, B.D. Bateman.

DMSO Therapy in Brochiolitis, Tinnitus, and Diminished Hearing. Aristides Zuniga, M.D., Manuel Arriaran Children's Hospital, Santiago, Chile.

Evaluation of DMSO Therapy in Chronic Respiratory Insufficiency of Broncho-Pulmonary Origin. Renato Eulufi, M.D., University of Chile.

DMSO in Retinal Disease. Robert V. Hill, M.D., University of Oregon Medical School, Portland, Oregon.

DMSO Therapy in the Treatment of Secondary Sterility (Inflammatory Tubal Obstruction). Hugo Venegas, M.D., Naval Hospital, Valparaiso, Chile.

APPENDIX III

Directory of Physicians Worldwide Who Can Provide Information on DMSO Treatment

The physicians recorded here who can provide information on DMSO treatment follow the protocol of the American College of Advancement in Medicine. The listing is based on the membership directory of the American College of Advancement in Medicine (ACAM). Please be aware that the use of DMSO is not approved or disapproved by ACAM. The listing of ACAM members is provided here because these are open-minded, progressive, knowledgeable, skilled, and trustworthy physicians who know more about the applications and effects of DMSO than any other health professionals in the world. Oftentimes many of them instill DMSO as part of their chelation therapy for patients.

A key giving information about each physician is provided before the list. For an updated directory or the most current listing of ACAM doctors in a particular geographic region, contact the American College of Advancement in Medicine, 23121 Verdugo Drive, Suite 204, Laguna Hills, California 92653; (714) 585-7666 within California or (800) 532-3688 outside California.

Members of the American College of Advancement in Medicine include diplomates (indicated by **DIPL**), diplomate candidates (indicated by **D/C**), and licensed physicians who may administer DMSO therapy (indicated by **P**).

A **diplomate** of the American College of Advancement in Medicine is an individual who:

1. Is a graduate of an approved school of medicine (D.O. or M.D., or foreign equivalent);
2. Is currently licensed to practice in the state or territory where he/she conducts practice;
3. Has been recommended (by letter) by two ACAM diplomates;
4. Has successfully completed the written examination of ACAM;
5. Shows evidence of being responsible for the administration of therapeutic programs approved by ACAM;

6. Has satisfied the requirements for preceptor training as outlined in the protocol of preceptorship;

7. Has successfully completed the oral examination of the American Board of Chelation Therapy (ABCT);

8. Submits ten acceptable questions and answers with references for use in future written exams.

A **diplomate candidate** of the American College of Advancement in Medicine is an individual who:

1. Is a graduate of an approved school of medicine (D.O. or M.D., or foreign equivalent);

2. Is currently licensed to practice in the state or territory where he/she conducts practice;

3. Has been recommended (by letter) by two diplomates;

4. Has successfully completed the written examination of the American Board of Chelation Therapy, and is in the process of completing the remaining requirements for ABCT.

To get in touch with the American College of Advancement in Medicine, contact one of the following:

ACAM HEADQUARTERS ADMINISTRATIVE STAFF

Edward A. Shaw, Ph.D.
Executive Director

Sally Bonebrake
Administrative Services Coordinator

Grace Claus
Membership Services Coordinator

Nancy Morgan
Books and Literature Coordinator

HEADQUARTERS ADDRESS

American College of Advancement in Medicine
Suite 204
23121 Verdugo Drive
Laguna Hills, CA 92653
(714) 583-7666
(800) 532-3688

Please note that this directory of physicians who use alternative healing methods may not be republished, reprinted, sold, or duplicated in whole or in part in any form or by any means for any commercial purpose or for the compilation of mailing lists without the prior written permission of this book's author or the American College of Advancement in Medicine.

Key to Worldwide American College of Advancement in Medicine Physician's List

PROFESSIONAL LEVEL CODES

DIPL Diplomate
D/C   Dilomate candidate
P   Licensed physician who follows the program now
      put forth by the American College of Advancement
      in Medicine.

SPECIALTY CODES

A	Allergy	IM	Internal Medicine
AC	Acupuncture	LM	Legal Medicine
AN	Anesthesiology	MM	Metabolic Medicine
AR	Arthritis	NT	Nutrition
AU	Auriculotherapy	OBS	Obstetrics
BA	Bariatrics	OME	Orthomolecular Medicine
CD	Cardiovascular	OPH	Ophthalmology
CS	Chest Disease	OSM	Osteopathic Manipulation
CT	Chelation Therapy	P	Psychiatry
DD	Degenerative Disease	PD	Pediatrics
DIA	Diabetes	PH	Public Health
EM	Environmental Medicine	PM	Preventive Medicine
END	Endocrinology	PMR	Physical Medicine & Rehabilitation
FP	Family Practice		
GE	Gastroenterology	PO	Psychiatry Orthomolecular
GER	Geriatrics	PUD	Pulmonary Diseases
GP	General Practice	R	Radiology
GYN	Gynecology	RHI	Rhinology
HGL	Hypoglycemia	RHU	Rheumatology
HO	Hyperbaric Oxygen	S	Surgery
HOM	Homeopathy	WR	Weight Reduction
HYP	Hypnosis	YS	Yeast Syndrome

American College of Advancement in Medicine (ACAM) Physicians—United States

ALABAMA

Birmingham

P. Gus J. Prosch Jr., M.D. **(P)**
759 Valley Street
Birmingham, AL 35226
(205) 823-6180
A,AR,CT,GP,NT,OME

ALASKA

Anchorage

Sandra Denton, M.D. **(DIPL)**
Suite 200
4115 Lake Otis Parkway
Anchorage, AK 99506
(907) 563-6200
FAX (907) 561-4933
Emergencies, EM

F. Russell Manuel, M.D. **(P)**
Suite 304
4200 Lake Otis Boulevard
Anchorage, AK 99506
(907) 562-7070
CT,GP,PM

Robert Rowen, M.D. **(DIPL)**
Suite 300
615 East 82nd Avenue
Anchorage, AK 99518
(907) 344-7775
AC,CT,FP,HYP,NT,PM

Soldotna

Paul G. Isaak, M.D.
Box 219

Soldotna, AK 99669
(907) 262-9341
(Retired)

Wasilla

Robert E. Martin, M.D. **(P)**
PO Box 870710
Wasilla, AK 99687
(907) 376-5284
AU,CT,FP,GP,OS,PM

ARIZONA

Glendale

Lloyd D. Armold, D.O. **(DIPL)**
Suite 2
4901 West Bell Road
Glendale, AZ 85306
(602) 939-8916
AR,CT,GP,MM,OSM,PM

Mesa

William W. Halcomb, D.O. **(P)**
Suite 109
4323 East Broadway
Mesa, AZ 85206
(602) 832-3014
A,CT,GP,HO,OSM,PM

Parker

S.W. Meyer, D.O. **(D/C)**
332 River Front Drive
PO Box 1870
Parker, AZ 85344
(602) 669-8911
CD,CT,DD,FP,OS,RHU

Phoenix

Terry S. Friedmann, M.D. **(DIPL)**
Suite 381
2701 East Camelback Road
Phoenix, AZ 85016
(602) 381-0800
A,CT,FP,HGL,HYP,NT

Stanley R. Olsztyn, M.D. **(P)**
Whitton Place
Suite 210
3610 North 44th Street
Phoenix, AZ 85018
(602) 954-0811
A,CT,DD,PM

Prescott

Gordon H. Josephs, D.O. **(P)**
315 West Goodwin Street
Prescott, AZ 86303
(602) 778-6169
CT,GP,NT,PM,S

Scottsdale

Gordon H. Josephs, D.O. **(P)**
7315 East Evans
Scottsdale, AZ 85250
(602) 996-9232
CT,GP,NT,PM,S

Tempe

Garry Gordon, M.D. **(DIPL)**
5535 South Compass
Tempe, AZ 85283
(602) 838-2079
CT,NT,PM

ARKANSAS

Hot Springs

William Wright, M.D. **(P)**
Suite 211
1 Mercy Drive
Hot Springs, AR 71913
(501) 624-3312
A,CT,GP,IM

Leslie

Melissa Tallaferro, M.D. **(DIPL)**
Cherry Street
PO Box 400
Leslie, AR 72645
(501) 447-2599
FAX (501) 447-2917
AC,CT,DD,IM,NT,PM,RHU

Little Rock

Norbert J. Becquet, M.D. **(DIPL)**
115 West Sixth Street
Little Rock, AR 72201
(501) 375-4419
CT,OPH,PM,RHU

John L. Gustavus, M.D. **(D/C)**
4721 East Broadway
North Little Rock, AR 72117
(501) 758-9350

Springdale

Doty Murphy III, M.D. **(P)**
812 Dorman
Springdale, AR 72764
(501) 756-3251
CD,CT

CALIFORNIA

Albany

Rose B. Gordon, M.D. **(DIPL)**
405 Kaine Avenue
Albany, CA 94706
(510) 526-3232
FAX (510) 526-3217
BA,CT,NT,PM

Bakersfield

Ralph G. Selbly, M.D. **(D/C)**
1311 Columbus Street
Bakersfield, CA 93305
(805) 873-1000
CT,GP,NT,PM

Campbell
Carol A. Shamlin, M.D. **(D/C)**
Suite 11A
621 East Campbell
Campbell, CA 95006
(408) 378-7970
A,CT,GP,MM,OME,PM

Chico
Eva Jalkotzy, M.D. **(P)**
Suite E
156 Eaton Road
Chico, CA 95926
(916) 893-3080
CT,FP,GP,NT,PM

Concord
John P. Toth, M.D. **(D/C)**
Suite 10
2299 Bacon Street
Concord, CA 94520
(510) 682-5660
A,FP,GP

Corte Madera
Michael Rosenbaum, M.D. **(P)**
Suite B-130
45 San Clemente Drive
Corte Madera, CA 94925
(415) 927-9450
FAX (415) 927-3759
A,HGL,MM,NT,P,YS

Covina
James Privitera, M.D. **(D/C)**
105 North Grandview Avenue
Covina, CA 91723
(818) 966-1618
A,MM,NT

Daly City
Charles K. Dahlgren, M.D. **(P)**
Suite 604
1800 Sullivan Avenue
Daly City, CA 94015

(415) 756-2900
A,NT,RHI,S

El Cajon
William J. Saccoman, M.D. **(P)**
Suite 103
505 North Mollison Avenue
El Cajon, CA 92021
(619) 440-3838
CT,NT,PM

Encino
A.Leonard Klepp, M.D. **(DIPL)**
Suite 725
16311 Ventura Boulevard
Encino, CA 91436
(818) 961-5511
FAX (818) 907-1468
CT,FP,HGL,NT,PM

Fresno
David J. Edwards, M.D. **(P)**
360 South Clovis Avenue
Fresno, CA 93727
(209) 251-5066
CT,GYN,PM

Grand Terrace
Bruce Halstead, M.D. **(P)**
22807 Barton Road
Grand Terrace, CA 92324
(No Referrals)

Hollywood
James J. Julian, M.D. **(P)**
1654 Cahuenga Boulevard
Hollywood, CA 90026
(213) 467-5555
AR,BA,CT,NT,PM

Joan Priestley, M.D. **(P)**
Suite 603
7080 Hollywood Boulevard
Hollywood, CA 90028
(213) 957-4217
A,EM,FP,NT

Huntington Beach

Joan M. Resk, D.O. **(D/C)**
Suite 203
18821 Delaware Street
Huntington Beach, CA 92648
(714) 842-5591
FAX (714) 843-9580
CD,CT,DD,NT,OSM,PM

Kentfield

Carolyn Albrecht, M.D.
10 Wolfe Grade
Kentfield, CA
(Retired)

La Jolla

Pierre Steiner, M.D.
1550 Via Corona
La Jolla, CA 92037
(No Referrals)

Lake Forest

David A. Steenblock, D.O. **(DIPL)**
Suite 500
22706 Aspen
Lake Forest, CA 92630
(714) 770-9616
FAX (714) 770-9775
CD,CT,DIA,IM

Laytonville

Eugene D. Finkle, M.D. **(P)**
PO Box 309
Laytonville, CA 95454
(707) 984-6151
FAX (707) 984-6151
CT,GP,GYN,MM,NT,PM

Long Beach

H. Richard Casdorph, M.D., Ph.D.,
  F.A.C.A.M. **(DIPL)**
Suite 201
1703 Termino Avenue
Long Beach, CA 90804
(310) 597-8716

FAX (310) 597-4616
CD,CS,CT,DIA,IM,NT

Los Altos

Robert F. Cathcart III, M.D. **(P)**
Suite 4
127 Second Street
Los Altos, CA 94022
(415) 949-2822
A,AR,CT,DD,OME,PM

Claude Marquette, M.D. **(P)**
Suite 110
5050 El Camino Real
Los Altos, CA 94022
(415) 964-6700
A,BA,CT,NT,PM

Los Angeles

Laszlo Belenyessy, M.D. **(P)**
Suite D
12732 Washington Boulevard
Los Angeles, CA 90066
(213) 822-4614
A,AC,BA,CT,GP,NT

M. Jahangiri, M.D. **(P)**
2156 South Santa Fe
Los Angeles, CA 90058
(213) 587-3218
A,AC,CT,FP,GP

Monterey

Lon B. Work, M.D. **(P)**
Suite D
841 Foam Street
Monterey, CA 93940
(408) 655-0215
CT,DD,GYN,HGL,NT,RHU

Newport Beach

Julian Whitaker, M.D. **(D/C)**
Suite 100
4321 Birch Street
Newport Beach, CA 92660

(714) 851-1550
FAX (714) 851-9970
CD,CT,DD,DIA,NT,PM

North Hollywood

David C. Freeman, M.D. **(P)**
Suite 103
11311 Camarillo Street
North Hollywood, CA 91602
(818) 985-1103
CD,CT,END,HGL,NT,PM

Oceanside

A. Hal Thatcher, M.D.
2552 Cornwall Street
Oceanside, CA 92054
(Retired)

Oxnard

Mohamed Moharram, M.D. **(P)**
Suite B
300 West 5th Street
Oxnard, CA 93030
(805) 483-2355
CS,CT,DD,DIA,GP,PM

Palm Desert

David H. Tang, M.D. **(D/C)**
Suite 6
74133 El Paseo
Palm Desert, CA 92260
(619) 341-2113
FAX (619) 341-2724
AC,CT,IM,MM,NT,PM

Palm Springs

Sean Degnan, M.D. **(D/C)**
Suite 200
2825 Tahquitz McCallum
Palm Springs, CA 92262
(619) 320-4292
AC,CT,NT,PM

Porterville

John B. Park, M.D. **(D/C)**
131 East Mill Avenue

Porterville, CA 93527
(209) 781-6224
AN,BA,FP,GP,PM,S

Rancho Mirage

Charles Farinella, M.D. **(P)**
Suite 106A
69-730 Highway 111
Rancho Mirage, CA 92270
(619) 324-0734
CT,GP,PM

Redding

Bessie J. Tillman, M.D. **(D/C)**
2054 Market Street
Redding, CA 96001
(916) 246-3022
A,CT,DD,NT,PM,YS

Reseda

Ilona Abraham, M.D. **(P)**
19231 Victoria Boulevard
Reseda, CA 91335
(818) 345-8721
A,AC,CD,CT,P

Sacramento

J.E. Dugas, M.D.
Suite 206
3400 Cottage Way
Sacramento, CA 95825
(Retired)

Michael Kwiker, D.O. **(P)**
Suite 3
3301 Alta Arden
Sacramento, CA 95825
(916) 489-4400
A,CT,DIA,NT

San Clemente

William Doell, D.O. **(DIPL)**
971 Calle Negocio
San Clemente, CA 92672
(No Referrals)

San Diego

Lawrence Taylor, M.D. **(P)**
Suite 402
3330 Third Avenue
San Diego, CA 92103
(619) 296-2952
A,CT,FP,NT,PM,YS

San Francisco

Richard A. Kunin, M.D. **(P)**
2698 Pacific Avenue
San Francisco, CA 94115
(415) 346-2500
CT,DD,HYP,P,PM,PO

Russell A. Lemesh, M.D.
Suite 320
595 Buckingham Way
San Francisco, CA 94132
(415) 731-5907
CD,END,GER,IM,MM,PM

Paul Lynn, M.D. **(DIPL)**
345 West Portal Avenue
San Francisco, CA 94127
(415) 566-1000
A,AR,CT,DD,NT,PM

Gary S. Ross, M.D. **(P)**
Suite 300
500 Sutter
San Francisco, CA 94102
(415) 398-0555
A,AC,CT,DD,FP,NT,PM

San Leandro

Steven H. Gee, M.D. **(DIPL)**
595 Estudillo Street
San Leandro, CA 94577
(510) 483-5881
AC,BA,CT,GP

San Marcos

William C. Kubitschek, D.O. **(DIPL)**
1194 Calle Maria

San Marcos, CA 92069
(619) 744-6991
AC,FP,NT,OSM,PM,PMR

San Rafael

Ross B. Gordon, M.D. **(DIPL)**
4144 Redwood Highway
San Rafael, CA 94903
(415) 499-9377
BA,CT,NT,PM

Santa Ana

Ronald Wempen, M.D. **(D/C)**
Suite 306
3620 South Bristol Street
Santa Ana, CA 92704
(714) 546-4325
A,AC,MM,NT,PO,YS

Santa Barbara

H.J. Hoegerman, M.D. **(DIPL)**
Suite D
101 West Arrellaga
Santa Barbara, CA 93101
(805) 963-1824
A,CD,CT,DIA,FP,GP,RHU

Mohamed Moharram, M.D. **(P)**
Suite B
101 West Arrellaga
Santa Barbara, CA 93101
(805) 965-5229
CS,CT,DD,DIA,GP,PM

Santa Maria

Donald E. Reiner, M.D. **(P)**
1414-D South Miller
Santa Maria, CA 93454
(805) 925-0961
CT,GP,OME,PM,S

Santa Monica

Michael Rosenbaum, M.D. **(P)**
Suite 110
2730 Wilshire Boulevard
Santa Monica, CA 90403

(310) 453-4424
A,HGL,MM,NT,P,YS

Murray Susser, M.D. (DIPL)
Suite 110
2730 Wilshire Boulevard
Santa Monica, CA 90403
(310) 453-4424
FAX (310) 828-0261
A,CT,NT,OME

Santa Rosa

Terri Su, M.D. (D/C)
Suite 3
1038 4th Street
Santa Rosa, CA 95404
(707) 571-7560
AC,AN,CT,FP,NT,PM

Seal Beach

Allen Green, M.D. (P)
Suite 212
909 Electric Avenue
Seal Beach, CA 90740
(310) 493-4526
AC,CT,FP,NT,PM

Sherman Oaks

Rosa M. Ami Belli, M.D.
13481 Cheltenham Drive
Sherman Oaks, CA 91423
(No Referrals)

Smith River

JoAnn Hoffer, M.D. (D/C)
12559 Highway 101 North
(Mini-Mart)
Smith River, CA 95567
(707) 487-3405
CT,NT,PM

James D. Schuler, M.D. (DIPL)
12559 Highway 101 North
(Mini-Mart)
Smith River, CA 95567

(707) 487-3405
A,CT,DIA,PM,S,YS

Stanton

William J. Goldwag, M.D. (P)
7499 Cerritos Avenue
Stanton, CA 90680
(714) 827-5180
CT,NT,PM

Studio City

Charles E. Law, Jr., M.D. (P)
Suite I
3959 Laurel Canyon Boulevard
Studio City, CA 91604
(818) 761-1661
AC,BA,CT,GP,NT,PM

Torrance

Anita Millen, M.D. (P)
Suite 170
1010 Crenshaw Boulevard
Torrance, CA 90501
(310) 320-1132
CT,DD,FP,GYN,NT,PM

Van Nuys

Frank Mosler, M.D. (P)
14426 Gilmore Street
Van Nuys, CA 91401
(818) 785-7425
BA,CT,GP,HGL,NT,PM

Walnut Creek

Alan Shifman Charles, M.D. (P)
1414 Maria Lane
Walnut Creek, CA 94596
(510) 937-3331
AC,CT,DD,FP,OM

Peter H.C. Mutke, M.D. (P)
1808 San Miguel Drive
Walnut Creek, CA 94596
(510) 933-2405
CT,HGL,HYP,NT,PM,YS

COLORADO

Colorado Springs

James R. Fish, M.D. **(DIPL)**
3030 North Hancock
Colorado Springs, CO 80907
(719) 471-2273
CT,HYP,PM

George Juetersonke, D.O. **(D/C)**
Suite 200
5455 North Union
Colorado Springs, CO 80918
(719) 528-1960
A,AC,CT,HGL,NT,OSM,P

Englewood

John H. Altshuler, M.D. **(P)**
Building 10
Greenwood Executive Park
7485 East Peakview Avenue
Englewood, CO 80111
(303) 740-7771
HYP,IM

Grand Junction

William L. Reed, M.D. **(D/C)**
Suite A-4
591 - 25 Road
Grand Junction, CO 81505
(303) 241-3631
A,CT,NT,PM

CONNECTICUT

Torrington

Jerrold N. Finnie, M.D. **(P)**
Suite 204
333 Kennedy Drive
Torrington, CT 06790
(203) 489-8977
A,CT,CS,NT,RHI,YS

DISTRICT OF COLUMBIA

Washington

Paul Beals, M.D. **(P)**
Suite 100
2639 Connecticut Avenue NW
Washington, DC 20037
(202) 332-0370
CT,FP,NT,PM

George H. Mitchell, M.D.
Suite C-100
2639 Connecticut Avenue NW
Washington, DC 20008
(202) 265-4111
A,NT

FLORIDA

Atlantic Beach

Richard Worsham, M.D. **(D/C)**
303 - 1st Street
Atlantic Beach, FL 32233
(No Referrals)

Boca Raton

Leonard Haimes, M.D. **(P)**
Suite 107
7300 North Federal Highway
Boca Raton, FL 33487
(407) 994-3888
A,BA,CT,IM,NT,PM

Narinder Singh Parhar, M.D. **(D/C)**
Suite 220
7840 Glades Road
Boca Raton, FL 33434
(407) 479-3200
A,CT,FP,NT,PM,S,WR

Bradenton

Eteri Melnikov, M.D. **(D/C)**
116 Manatee Avenue East
Bradenton, FL 34208

(813) 748-7943
CD,CT,DIA,GP,PM,YS

Fort Lauderdale

Bruce Dooley, M.D. **(P)**
1493 SE 17th Street
Fort Lauderdale, FL 33316
(305) 527-9355
A,CT,GP,NT,PM,YS

Fort Myers

Gary L. Pynckel, D.O. **(DIPL)**
Suite 115
3940 Metro Parkway
Fort Myers, FL 33916
(813) 278-3377
CT,FP,GP,OSM,PM

Hollywood

Herbert Pardell, D.O. **(DIPL)**
7061 Taft Street
Hollywood, FL 33020
(305) 989-5558
CT,DD,IM,MM,NT,PM

Homosassa

Carlos F. Gonzalez, M.D. **(D/C)**
7991 South Suncoast Boulevard
Homosassa, FL 32646
(904) 382-8282
A,CD,CS,END,PMR,RHU

Jupiter

Neil Ahner, M.D. **(DIPL)**
1080 East Indiantown Road
Jupiter, FL 33477
(407) 744-0077
CT,NT,PM

Lakeland

Harold Robinson, M.D. **(P)**
Suite 27
4406 South Florida Avenue
Lakeland, FL 33803

(813) 646-5088
CT,FP,GP,HGL,NT,PM

Lauderhill

Herbert R. Slavin, M.D. **(D/C)**
Suite 210
7200 West Commercial Boulevard
Lauderhill, FL 33319
(305) 748-4991
CT,DD,DIA,GER,IM,NT

Maitland

Joya Lynn Schoen, M.D. **(D/C)**
Suite 200
341 North Maitland Avenue
Maitland, FL 32751
(407) 644-2729
FAX (407) 644-1205
A,CT,HGL,HOM,OSM

Miami

Joseph G. Godorov, D.O. **(P)**
Suite 307
9055 SW 87th Avenue
Miami, FL 33176
(305) 595-0671
CT,END,FP,HGL,NT,PM

Bernard J. Letourneau, D.O. **(P)**
6475 SW 40th Street
Miami, FL 33155
(305) 666-9933
FP,GP,NT,OS

North Lauderdale

Narinder Singh Parhar, M.D. **(D/C)**
1333 South State Road 7
North Lauderdale, FL 33068
(305) 978-6604
A,CT,FP,NT,PM,S,WR

North Miami Beach

Martin Dayton, D.O. **(DIPL)**
18600 Collins Avenue
North Miami Beach, FL 33160

(305) 931-8484
CT,FP,GER,NT,OSM,PM

Ocala

George Graves, D.O. **(P)**
3501 NE Tenth Street
Ocala, FL 32670
(904) 236-2525 or (904) 732-3633
CT,DD,PM

Orange City

Travis L. Herring, M.D. **(P)**
106 West Fern Drive
Orange City, FL 32763
(904) 775-0525
CT,FP,HOM,IM

Palm Bay

Neil Ahner, M.D. **(DIPL)**
1200 Malabar Road
Palm Bay, FL 32907
(407) 729-8581
CT,NT,PM

Pensacola

Ward Dean, M.D. **(P)**
PO Box 11097
Pensacola, FL 32524
(No Referrals)

Pompano Beach

Dan C. Roehm, M.D. **(P)**
Suite 3450
3400 Park Central Boulevard North
Pompano Beach, FL 33064
(305) 977-3700
FAX (305) 977-0180
CD,CT,IM,MM,NT,OME

Port Canaveral

James Parsons, M.D. **(D/C)**
Suite 110
707 Mullet Drive
Port Canaveral, FL 32920

(407) 784-2102
A,CT,MM,NT,PO,RHU

Sarasota

Thomas McNaughton, M.D. **(D/C)**
1521 Dolphin Street
Sarasota, FL 34236
(813) 365-6273
FAX (813) 365-4269
CT,GP,NT,PM

Joseph Ossorio, M.D. **(P)**
Suite H-5
3900 Clark Road
Sarasota, FL 34277
(813) 921-6338
HYP,P,PM

St. Petersburg

Ray Wunderlich, Jr., M.D. **(DIPL)**
666 - 6th Street South
St. Petersburg, FL 33701
(813) 822-3612
A,BA,CT,DD,HGL,MM,PO

Sunrise

Leon L. Shore, D.O.
10111 West Oakland Park Boulevard
Sunrise, FL 33351
(305) 741-1533
GP,OS

Tampa

Donald J. Carrow, M.D. **(P)**
Suite 206
3902 Henderson Boulevard
Tampa, FL 33629
(813) 832-3220
FAX (813) 282-1132
AR,CD,DIA,HGL,HO

Eugene H. Lee, M.D. **(P)**
Suite A
1804 West Kennedy Boulevard
Tampa, FL 33606

(813) 251-3089
AC,CT,GP,HGL,NT,PM

Venice

Thomas McNaughton, M.D. (D/C)
540 South Nokomis Avenue
Venice, FL 34285
(813) 484-2167
CT,GP,NT,PM

Wauchula

Alfred S. Massam, M.D. (P)
528 West Main Street
Wauchula, FL 33873
(813) 773-6668
CT,FP,PM

Winter Park

James M. Parsons, M.D. (D/C)
Great Western Bank Building
#303 2699 Lee Road
Winter Park, FL 32789
(407) 628-3399
A,CT,MM,NT,PO,RHU

Robert Rogers, M.D. (P)
Suite 204
1865 North Semoran Boulevard
Winter Park, FL 32792
(407) 679-2811
A,CD,CT,NT,PM

GEORGIA

Atlanta

Stephen B. Edelson, M.D. (P)
3833 Roswell Road
Atlanta, GA 30342
(404) 841-0088
A,CT,FP,NT,OME,PM,YS

David Epstein, D.O. (P)
Suite 100
427 Moreland Avenue
Atlanta, GA 30307
(404) 525-7333
BA,CT,GP,NT,OSM,PM

Milton Fried, M.D. (DIPL)
4426 Tilly Mill Road
Atlanta, GA 30360
(404) 451-4857
A,CT,IM,NT,PM,PO

Bernard Mlaver, M.D. (DIPL)
4480 North Shallowford Road
Atlanta, GA 30338
(404) 395-1600
CT,NT,PM

Camilla

Oliver L. Gunter, M.D. (DIPL)
24 North Ellis Street
Camilla, GA 31730
(912) 336-7343
CT,DD,DIA,GP,NT,PU

Decatur

Naima ABD Elghany, M.D. (P)
3455H North Druid Hill Road
Decatur, GA 30033
(404) 639-3385
A,CD,IM,PH,PM,PUD

Warner Robins

Terril J. Schneider, M.D. (P)
Suite 19
205 Dental Drive
Warner Robins, GA 31088
(912) 929-1027
A,CT,FP,NT,PM,PMR

HAWAII

Kailua-Kona

Clifton Arrington, M.D. (P)
PO Box 649
Kealakekua, HI 96750
(808) 322-9400
BA,CT,FP,NT,PM

IDAHO

Coeur d'Alene

Charles T. McGee, M.D. **(P)**
Suite 108
1717 Lincolnway
Coeur d'Alene, ID 83814
(208) 664-1478
A,CT,NT,OME,PM

Nampa

John O. Boxall, M.D. **(P)**
824 - 17th Avenue South
Nampa, ID 83651
(208) 466-3517
AC,CT,GP,HYP

Stephen Thornburgh, D.O. **(P)**
824 - 17th Avenue South
Nampa, ID 83651
(208) 466-3517
AC,CT,HOM,OS

Sandpoint

K. Peter McCallum, M.D. **(DIPL)**
2500 Selle Road
Sandpoint, ID 83864
(208) 263-5456
CT,NT,MM,OME,PM

ILLINOIS

Arlington Heights

Terrill K. Haws, D.O. **(D/C)**
Suite 111
121 South Wilke Road
Arlington Heights, IL 60005
(708) 577-9451
CT,DD,FP,GP,OSM

William J. Mauer, D.O., F.A.C.A.M.
  (DIPL)
3401 North Kennicott Avenue
Arlington Heights, IL 60004
(800) 255-7030

FAX (708) 255-7700
CT,DIA,GP,NT,OSM,PM

Aurora

Thomas Hesselink, M.D. **(D/C)**
Suite 1735
888 South Edgelawn Drive
Aurora, IL 60506
(708) 844-0011
FAX (708) 844-0500
A,Candida,CT,GP,NT,PM

Belvidere

M. Paul Dommers, M.D. **(P)**
554 South Main Street
Belvidere, IL 61008
(815) 544-3112
AR,AU,CT,MM,PM

Chicago

Razvan Rentea, M.D. **(P)**
3354 North Paulina
Chicago, IL 60657
(312) 549-0101
GP,MM,PM

Downers Grove

Guillermo Justiniano, M.D. **(P)**
1430 Parrish Court
Downers Grove, IL 60515
(708) 964-8083
(No Referrals)

Geneva

Richard E. Hrdlicka, M.D. **(D/C)**
Suite 206
302 Randall Road
Geneva, IL 60134
(708) 232-1900
A,BA,FP,NT,PM,YS

Glen Ellyn

Robert S. Waters, M.D. **(DIPL)**
739 Roosevelt Road
Glen Ellyn, IL 60137

(708) 790-8100
CT,OME,PM

Homewood

Frederick Weiss, M.D.
3207 West 184th Street
Homewood, IL 60430
(No Referrals)

Metamora

Stephen K. Elsasser, D.O.,
  F.A.C.A.M. (DIPL)
205 South Engelwood
Metamora, IL 61548
(309) 367-2321
FAX (309) 367-2324
CT,GP,HO,NT,OSM,PM

Moline

Terry W. Love, D.O. (DIPL)
2610 - 41st Street
Moline, IL 61252
(309) 764-2900
CT,NT,PM

Oak Park

Paul J. Dunn, M.D. (D/C)
715 Lake Street
Oak Park, IL 60301
(708) 383-3800
CT,HGL,NT,OSM,PM,YS

Ottawa

Terry W. Love, D.O. (DIPL)
645 West Main
Ottawa, IL 61350
(815) 434-1977
AR,CT,GP,OSM,PM,RHU

Woodstock

John R. Tambone, M.D. (P)
102 East South Street
Woodstock, IL 60098
(815) 338-2345
A,CT,GP,HYP,NT,PM

Zion

Peter Senatore, D.O. (P)
1911 - 27th Street
Zion, IL 60099
(708) 872-8722
CT,FP,GP

INDIANA

Clarksville

George Wolverton, M.D. (DIPL)
647 Eastern Boulevard
Clarksville, IN 47130
(812) 282-4309
CD,CT,FP,GYN,PD,PM

Evansville

Harold T. Sparks, D.O. (D/C)
3001 Washington Avenue
Evansville, IN 47714
(812) 479-8228
A,AC,BA,CT,FP,PM

Highland

Cal Streeter, D.O. (DIPL)
9635 Saric Court
Highland, IN 46322
(219) 924-2410
FAX (219) 924-9079
A,CD,CT,FP,OSM,PM

Indianapolis

David A. Darbro, M.D. (DIPL)
2124 East Hanna Avenue
Indianapolis, IN 46227
(317) 787-7221
A,AR,CT,DD,FP,PM

Mooresville

Norman E. Whitney, D.O. (P)
PO Box 173
Mooresville, IN 46158
(317) 831-3352
AR,CD,DD,DIA,FP,NT

South Bend

David E. Turfler, D.O. **(P)**
336 West Navarre Street
South Bend, IN 46616
(219) 233-3840
A,FP,GP,HGL,OBS,OSM

Valparaiso

Myrna D. Trowbridge, D.O. **(D/C)**
850-C Marsh Street
Valparaiso, IN 46383
(219) 462-3377
AC,AR,CT,GP,NT,OSM

IOWA

Des Moines

Beverly Rosenfeld, D.O. **(P)**
Suite 10
7177 Hickman Road
Des Moines, IA 50322
(515) 276-0061
GP,HGL,NT,OS,PM,YS

Sioux City

Horst G. Blume, M.D. **(P)**
700 Jennings Street
Sioux City, IA 51105
(712) 252-4386
Neurology,S

KANSAS

Andover

Stevens B. Acker, M.D. **(DIPL)**
Suite D
310 West Central
PO Box 483
Andover, KS 67002
(316) 733-4494
CT,DD,FP,MM,PM

Garden City

Terry Hunsberger, D.O. **(P)**
602 North 3rd
PO Box 679
Garden City, KS 67846
(316) 275-7128
BA,CT,FP,NT,OSM,PM

Hays

Roy N. Neil, M.D. **(P)**
105 West 13th
Hays, KS 67601
(913) 628-8341
BA,CD,CT,DD,NT,PM

Kansas City

John Gamble, Jr., D.O. **(D/C)**
1509 Quindaro
Kansas City, KS 66104
(913) 321-1140
DD,DIA,FP,GP,NT,OSM

KENTUCKY

Berea

Edward K. Atkinson, M.D.
PO Box 3148
Berea, KY 40403
(No Referrals)

Bowling Green

John C. Tapp, M.D. **(P)**
414 Old Morgantown Road
Bowling Green, KY 42101
(502) 781-1483
CT,GYN,MM,P,PD,RHU

Louisville

Kirk Morgan, M.D. **(DIPL)**
9105 U.S. Highway 42
Louisville, KY 40059
(502) 228-0156
CD,CT,FP,MM,NT,YS

Nicholasville

Walt Stoll, M.D. **(P)**
6801 Danville Road
Nicholasville, KY 40356

(606) 233-4273
CT,FP,NT,PM

Somerset

Stephen S. Kiteck, M.D. (P)
1301 Pumphouse Road
Somerset, KY 42501
(606) 678-5137
FP,IM,PD,PM

LOUISIANA

Baton Rouge

Steve Kuplesky, M.D.
5618 Bayridge
Baton Rouge, LA 70817
(No Referrals)

Chalmette

Saroj T. Tampira, M.D. (P)
812 East Judge Perez
Chalmette, LA 70043
(504) 277-8991
CD,DD,DIA,IM

Mandeville

Roy M. Montalbano, M.D. (P)
4408 Highway 22
Mandeville, LA 70448
(504) 626-1985
CT,FP,NT,PM

Natchitoches

Phillip Mitchell, M.D. (P)
407 Blenville Street
Natchitoches, LA 71457
(318) 357-1571 or (800) 562-6574
FP

Newellton

Joseph R. Whitaker, M.D. (P)
PO Box 458
Newellton, LA 71357

(318) 467-5131
CT,GP,IM

New Iberia

Adonis J. Domingue, M.D. (D/C)
Suite 600
602 North Lewis
New Iberia, LA 70560
(318) 365-2196
GP

New Orleans

James P. Carter, M.D. (P)
1430 Tulane Avenue
New Orleans, LA 70112
(504) 588-5136
GP,NT,PM

Shreveport

R. Denman Crow, M.D. (P)
Suite 222
1545 Line Avenue
Shreveport, LA 71101
(318) 221-1569
A,FP,GP,GYN,PM,PUD

MAINE

Van Buren

Joseph Cyr, M.D. (P)
62 Main Street
Van Buren, ME 04785
(207) 868-5273
CT,GP,OBS

MARYLAND

Laurel

Paul V. Beals, M.D. (P)
Suite 205
9101 Cherry Lane Park
Laurel, MD 20708
(301) 490-9911
CT,FP,NT,PM

Pikesville

Alan R. Gaby, M.D. **(P)**
31 Walker Avenue
Pikesville, MD 21208
(410) 486-5656
GP,NT,PM,YS

Silver Spring

Harold Goodman, D.O. **(P)**
Suite 405B
8609 Second Avenue
Silver Spring, MD 20910
(301) 881-5229
AC,AU,CT,OS,PMR

MASSACHUSETTS

Barnstable

Michael Janson, M.D., F.A.C.A.M.
  (DIPL)
275 Mill Way
PO Box 732
Barnstable, MA 02630
(508) 362-4343
FAX (617) 661-8651
A,CD,CT,NT,OME,YS

Cambridge

Michael Janson, M.D., F.A.C.A.M.
  (DIPL)
2557 Massachusetts Avenue
Cambridge, MA 02140
(617) 661-6225
FAX (617) 661-8651
A,CD,CT,NT,OME,YS

Hanover

Richard Cohen, M.D. **(DIPL)**
Suite 1
51 Mill Street
Hanover, MA 02339
(617) 829-9281
A,CD,CT,NT,PM,YS

Lowell

Svetlana Kaufman, M.D. **(P)**
Suite 323
24 Merrimack Street
Lowell, MA 01852
(508) 453-5181
A,AC,GER,GP,PM,RHI

Newton

Carol Englender, M.D. **(P)**
1340 Centre Street
Newton, MA 02159
(617) 965-7770
A,EM,FP,NT,PM

West Boylston

N. Thomas La Cava, M.D. **(D/C)**
Suite 107
360 West Boylston Street
West Boylston, MA 01583
(508) 854-1380
NT,PD,PM

Williamstown

Ross S. McConnell, M.D.
732 Main Street
Williamstown, MA 01267
(413) 663-3701
DD,HO,NT,PM

MICHIGAN

Atlanta

Leo Modzinski, D.O., M.D. **(DIPL)**
100 West State Street
Atlanta, MI 49709
(517) 785-4254
FAX (517) 785-2273
BA,CT,FP,GP,NT,OSM

Bay City

Doyle B. Hill, D.O. **(P)**
2520 North Euclid Avenue
Bay City, MI 48706

(517) 686-5200
A,CT,FP,GP,NT,OSM

Farmington Hills

Paul A. Parente, D.O. **(DIPL)**
30275 Thirteen Mile Road
Farmington Hills, MI 48334
(313) 626-9690
BA,CT,GP,PM

Albert J. Scarchill, D.O. **(DIPL)**
30275 Thirteen Mile Road
Farmington Hills, MI 48334
(313) 626-9690
BA,CT,FP,GP,MM,OSM,PM

Flint

William M. Bernard, D.O. **(P)**
1044 Gilbert Street
Flint, MI 48532
(313) 733-3140
A,CT,FP,GER,OSM,PM

Kenneth Ganapini, D.O. **(P)**
1044 Gilbert Street
Flint, MI 48532
(313) 733-3140
FP,GP,OSM,PM,YS

Grand Haven

E. Duane Powers, D.O. **(DIPL)**
PO Box 170
Grand Haven, MI 49417
(Retired)

Grand Rapids

Grant Born, D.O. **(DIPL)**
2687 - 44th Street SE
Grand Rapids, MI 49512
(616) 455-3550
A,CT,FP,GYN,PM,PMR

Linden

Marvin D. Penwell, D.O. **(DIPL)**
319 South Bridge Street
Linden, MI 48451

(313) 735-7809
A,CT,FP,GE,GYN,OSM

Pontiac

Vahagn Agbabian, D.O. **(P)**
Suite 1105
28 North Saginaw Street
Pontiac, MI 48058
(313) 334-2424
CT,DD,DIA,GER,IM,OME

St. Clair Shores

Richard E. Tapert, D.O. **(DIPL)**
23550 Harper
St. Clair Shores, MI 48080
(313) 779-5700
CT,GP,NT,PM

Williamston

Seldon Nelson, D.O. **(P)**
4386 North Meridian Road
Williamston, MI 48895
(517) 349-2458
AR,CT,GP,NT,OSM

MINNESOTA

Minneapolis

Michael Dole, M.D. **(D/C)**
Suite 350
10700 Old County Road 15
Minneapolis, MN 55441
(612) 593-9458
FP,PM,YS

Jean R. Eckerty, M.D. **(DIPL)**
Suite 350
10700 Old County Road 15
Minneapolis, MN 55441
(612) 593-9458
CT,IM,NT,OME,PM

Tyler

Keith J. Carlson, M.D. **(D/C)**
210 Highland Court
Tyler, MN 56178

(507) 247-5921
AC,CT,GP

Wayzata

F.J. Durand, M.D. **(D/C)**
3119 Groveland School Road
Wayzata, MN 55391
(No Referrals)

M.S.C. Durand, M.D.
3119 Groveland School Road
Wayzata, MN 55391
(No Referrals)

MISSISSIPPI

Coldwater

Pravinchandra Patel, M.D. **(P)**
PO Drawer DD
Coldwater, MS 38618
(601) 622-7011
CT,FP

Columbus

James H. Sams, M.D. **(D/C)**
1120 Lehmburg Road
Columbus, MS 39702
(601) 327-8701
AN,CT,GP

Ocean Springs

James H. Waddell, M.D. **(P)**
1520 Government Street
Ocean Springs, MS 39564
(601) 875-5505
AC,AN,AU,CT

Shelby

Robert Hollingsworth, M.D. **(DIPL)**
Drawer 87
901 Forrest Street
Shelby, MS 38774
(601) 398-5106
CT,FP,GYN,OBS,PD,S

MISSOURI

Festus

John T. Schwent, D.O. **(D/C)**
1400 Truman Boulevard
Festus, MO 63028
(314) 937-8688
A,CT,FP,NT,OBS,OSM

Florissant

Tipu Sultan, M.D. **(P)**
11585 West Florissant
Florissant, MO 63033
(314) 921-7100
A,AR,CT,HGL,PM

Independence

Lawrence Dorman, D.O. **(P)**
9120 East 35th Street
Independence, MO 64052
(816) 358-2712
AC,CT,MM,OSM,PM

James E. Swann, D.O. **(DIPL)**
2116 Sterling
Independence, MO 64052
(816) 833-3366
CD,CT,DD,FP,IM,S

Kansas City

Edward W. McDonagh, D.O.,
  F.A.C.A.M. **(DIPL)**
2800-A Kendallwood Parkway
Kansas City, MO 64119
(816) 453-5940
FAX (816) 453-1140
CD,CT,DD,FP,HO,PM

James Rowland, D.O. **(P)**
8133 Wornall Road
Kansas City, MO 64114
(816) 361-4077
AC,CT,DD,GP,HYP,OSM

Charles J. Rudolph, D.O., Ph.D.,
  F.A.C.A.M. **(DIPL)**

2800-A Kendallwood Parkway
Kansas City, MO 64119
(816) 453-5940
FAX (816) 453-1140
CD,CT,DD,FP,HO,PM

Springfield

William C. Sunderwirth, D.O. **(P)**
2828 North National
Springfield, MO 65803
(417) 869-6260
CT,DIA,GP,OSM,PM,S

St. Louis

Harvey Walker, Jr., M.D., Ph.D.,
 F.A.C.A.M. **(DIPL)**
138 North Meramec Avenue
St. Louis, MO 63105
(314) 721-7227
CT,DIA,HGL,IM,NT,PM

Stockton

William C. Sunderwirth, D.O. **(P)**
307 South Street
Stockton, MO 65785
(417) 276-3221
CT,DIA,GP,OSM,PM,S

Sullivan

Ronald H. Scott, D.O. **(P)**
750 Pascal Street
Sullivan, MO 63080
(314) 468-4932
GER,GP,GYN,NT,OSM,PM

Union

Clinton C. Hayes, D.O. **(D/C)**
100 West Main
Union, MO 63084
(314) 583-8911
CT,GP

NEBRASKA

Omaha

Eugene C. Oliveto, M.D. **(P)**
Suite 208
8031 West Center Road
Omaha, NE 68124
(402) 392-0233
CT,HYP,NT,P,PM,PO

Ord

Otis W. Miller, M.D. **(D/C)**
408 South 14th Street
Ord, NE 68862
(308) 728-3251
CT,FP,NT,P,YS

NEVADA

Incline Village

W. Douglas Brodie, M.D. **(D/C)**
848 Tanager
Incline Village, NV 89450
(702) 832-7001
DD,FP,GP,IM,NT,PM

Las Vegas

Ji-Zhou (Joseph) Kang, M.D. **(P)**
5613 South Eastern
Las Vegas, NV 89119
(702) 796-2992
A,AC,GP,IM,NT

Paul McGuff, M.D.
Suite 903
3930 Swenson
Las Vegas, NV 89106
(Retired)

Robert D. Milne, M.D. **(P)**
Suite 446
501 South Rancho
Las Vegas, NV 89106
(702) 385-1999
A,AC,CT,FP,NT,PM

Terry Pfau, D.O. **(P)**
Suite 446
501 South Rancho Drive
Las Vegas, NV 89106
(702) 385-1999
A,AC,CT,OSM

Robert Vance, D.O. **(DIPL)**
Suite F2
801 South Rancho Drive
Las Vegas, NV 89106
(702) 385-7771
A,CT,HO,MM,OSM,PM

Reno

David A. Edwards, M.D. **(P)**
Suite A7
6490 South McCarran Boulevard
Reno, NV 89509
(702) 827-1444
A,AC,CT,DD,PM,YS

Michael L. Gerber, M.D. **(DIPL)**
3670 Grant Drive
Reno, NV 89509
(702) 826-1900
CT,MM,OME

Donald E. Soli, M.D. **(D/C)**
708 North Center Street
Reno, NV 89501
(702) 786-7101
A,AR,CT,HGL,HO,PUD

Yiwen Y. Tang, M.D. **(P)**
380 Brinkby
Reno, NV 89509
(702) 826-9500
A,CD,CT,HGL,HO,PM

NEW JERSEY

Bloomfield

Majid Ali, M.D. **(D/C)**
320 Belleville Avenue
Bloomfield, NJ 07003

Cherry Hill

Allan Magaziner, D.O. **(DIPL)**
1907 Greentree Road
Cherry Hill, NJ 08003
(609) 424-8222
FAX (609) 424-1832
CT,NT,OSM,PM

Denville

Majid Ali, M.D. **(D/C)**
Institute of Preventive Medicine
95 East Main Street
Denville, NJ 07834
(201) 586-4111
FAX (201) 743-1354
A,PM,Pathology

Edison

C.Y. Lee, M.D. **(DIPL)**
952 Amboy Avenue
Edison, NJ 08837
(908) 738-9220
FAX (908) 738-1187
A,AR,AU,CT,DD,OME

Ralph Lev, M.D., M.S., F.A.C.A.M.
 (DIPL)
952 Amboy Avenue
Edison, NJ 08837
(908) 738-9220
FAX (908) 738-1187
CD,CT,S

Richard B. Menashe, D.O. **(D/C)**
15 South Main Street
Edison, NJ 08837
(908) 906-8866
A,CD,CT,HGL,NT,YS

Elizabeth

Gennaro Locurcio, M.D. **(P)**
610 - 3rd Avenue
Elizabeth, NJ 07202
(908) 351-1333
A,AC,AU,CT,FP,HYP

Ortley Beach

Charles Harris, M.D. **(P)**
1 Ortley Plaza
Ortley Beach, NJ 08751
(908) 793-6464
A,BA,CT,DD,FP,GER

Ridgewood

Constance Alfano, M.D. **(P)**
74 Oak Street
Ridgewood, NJ 07450
(201) 444-4622
A(food),Candida,CT

Skillman

Eric Braverman, M.D. **(D/C)**
100-102 Tamarck Circle
Skillman, NJ 08558
(609) 921-1842
A,CT,DD,FP,IM,PM

West Orange

Faina Munits, M.D. **(DIPL)**
51 Pleasant Valley Way
West Orange, NJ 07052
(201) 736-3743
A,CD,DD,DIA,HGL,PM

NEW MEXICO

Albuquerque

Ralph J. Luciani, D.O. **(DIPL)**
Suite G
2301 San Pedro NE
Albuquerque, NM 87110
(505) 888-5995
AC,AU,CT,FP,OSM,PM

Gerald Parker, D.O. **(P)**
Suite D
6208 Montgomery Boulevard NE
Albuquerque, NM 87109
(505) 884-3506
A,AC,AR,CT,GP,HO

John T. Taylor, D.O. **(P)**
Suite D

6208 Montgomery Boulevard NE
Albuquerque, NM 87109
(505) 884-3506
A,AC,AR,CT,GP,HO

Roswell

Annette Stoesser, M.D. **(P)**
112 South Kentucky
Roswell, NM 88201
(505) 623-2444
A,CT,DD,DIA,FP,NT

NEW YORK

Bronx

Richard Izquierdo, M.D. **(P)**
Lower Level
1070 Southern Boulevard
Bronx, NY 10459
(212) 589-4541
A,FP,GP,NT,PD,PM

Brooklyn

Gennaro Locurcio, M.D. **(P)**
2386 Ocean Parkway
Brooklyn, NY 11223
(718) 336-2291
A,AC,AU,CT,FP,HYP

Tsilia Sorina, M.D. **(P)**
2026 Ocean Avenue
Brooklyn, NY 11230
(718) 375-2600
GP,NT,PM

Michael Teplitsky, M.D. **(P)**
415 Oceanview Avenue
Brooklyn, NY 11235
(718) 769-0997
FAX (718) 646-2352
BA,CD,DIA,IM,PM

Pavel Yutsis, M.D. **(D/C)**
1309 West 7th Street
Brooklyn, NY 11204
(718) 259-2122

FAX (718) 259-3933
A,CT,FP,NT,PD,PM,YS

East Meadow

Christopher Calapai, D.O. (D/C)
1900 Hempstead Turnpike
East Meadow, NY 11554
(516) 794-0404
A,CT,FP,NT,OSM,YS

Falconer

Reino Hill, M.D. (P)
230 West Main Street
Falconer, NY 14733
(716) 665-3505
CT,FP,PM

Great Neck

Mary F. Di Rico, M.D. (P)
1 Kingspoint Road
Great Neck, NY 11024
(No Referrals)

Huntington

Serafina Corsello, M.D., F.A.C.A.M.
  (DIPL)
175 East Main Street
Huntington, NY 11743
(516) 271-0222
FAX (516) 271-5992
CT,DD,MM,NT,OME,PM

Lawrence

Mitchell Kurk, M.D. (P)
310 Broadway
Lawrence, NY 11559
(516) 239-5540
CT,FP,GER,NT,OME,PM

Massena

Bob Snider, M.D. (D/C)
HC 61, Box 43D
Massena, NY 13662
(315) 764-7328
A,CT,FP

New York

Robert C. Atkins, M.D. (DIPL)
152 East 55th Street
New York, NY 10022
(212) 758-2110
CT,HGL,OME

Serafina Corsello, M.D., F.A.C.A.M.
  (DIPL)
Suite 1202
200 West 57th Street
New York, NY 10019
(212) 399-0222
CT,DD,MM,NT,OME,PM

Ronald Hoffman, M.D., F.A.C.A.M.
  (DIPL)
40 East 30th Street
New York, NY 10016
(212) 779-1744
FAX (212) 779-0891
A,FP,HGL,NT,PM

Warren M. Levin, M.D. (DIPL)
444 Park Avenue South/30th Street
New York, NY 10016
(212) 696-1900
FAX (212) 213-5872
A,AC,CT,NT,OME,PM

Niagara Falls

Paul Cutler, M.D., F.A.C.A.M. (DIPL)
652 Elmwood Avenue
Niagara Falls, NY 14301
(716) 284-5140
FAX (716) 284-5159
A,CT,NT

Orangeburg

Neil L. Block, M.D. (P)
14 Prei Plaza
Orangeburg, NY 10962
(914) 359-3300
A,CD,FP,IM,NT,PO

Plattsburgh

Driss Hassam, M.D. **(P)**
50 Court Street
Plattsburgh, NY 12901
(518) 561-2023
GE,S

Rhinebeck

Kenneth A. Bock, M.D., F.A.C.A.M.
  (DIPL)
108 Montgomery Street
Rhinebeck, NY 12572
(914) 876-7082
FAX (914) 876-4615
A,CD,CT,FP,NT,PM

Suffern

Michael B. Schachter, M.D.,
  F.A.C.A.M. **(DIPL)**
Suite 202
Two Executive Boulevard
Suffern, NY 10901
(914) 368-4700
FAX (914) 368-4727
A,CT,NT,PO

Watervliet

Rodolfo T. Sy, M.D. **(D/C)**
1845 - 6th Avenue
Watervliet, NY 12189
(518) 273-1325
AC,CT,GP,PMR,WR

Westbury

Savely Yurkovsky, M.D. **(P)**
309 Madison Street
Westbury, NY 11590
(516) 333-2929
A,CD,CS,CT,NT,PM

NORTH CAROLINA

Aberdeen

Keith E. Johnson, M.D. **(P)**
188 Quewhiffle

Aberdeen, NC 28315
(919) 281-5122
DD,GER,GP,NT,PM,PMR

Leicester

John L. Laird, M.D. **(DIPL)**
Route 1, Box 7
Leicester, NC 28748
(704) 683-3101
A,CD,CT,FP,NT,PM

Statesville

John L. Laird, M.D. **(DIPL)**
Plaza 21 North
Statesville, NC 28677
(704) 876-1617 or (800) 445-4762
A,CD,CT,FP,NT,PM

NORTH DAKOTA

Grand Forks

Richard H. Leigh, M.D. **(D/C)**
2314 Library Circle
Grand Forks, ND 58201
(701) 775-5527
CT,GYN,MM,NT

Minot

Brian E. Briggs, M.D. **(D/C)**
718 - 6th Street SW
Minot, ND 58701
(701) 838-6011

OHIO

Akron

Francis J. Waickman, M.D. **(P)**
544 "B" White Pond Drive
Akron, OH 44320
(216) 867-3787
A,Clinical Immunology,EM,YS

Bluffton

L. Terry Chappell, M.D., F.A.C.A.M.
  (DIPL)
122 Thurman Street

Bluffton, OH 45817
(419) 358-4627
FAX (419) 358-1855
AU,CT,FP,HYP,NT,PMR

Canton

Jack E. Slingluff, D.O. **(DIPL)**
5850 Fulton Road NW
Canton, OH 44718
(216) 494-8641
CD,CT,FP,HGL,MM,NT

Cincinnati

Ted Cole, D.O. **(P)**
9678 Cincinnati-Columbus Road
Cincinnati, OH 45241
(513) 779-0300
A,CT,FP,NT,OSM,PD

Cleveland

John M. Baron, D.O. **(DIPL)**
Suite 100
4807 Rockside
Cleveland, OH 44131
(216) 642-0082
CT,NT,PO

James P. Frackelton, M.D.,
   F.A.C.A.M. **(DIPL)**
24700 Center Ridge Road
Cleveland, OH 44145
(216) 835-0104
FAX (216) 871-1404
CT,HO,NT,PM

Derrick Lonsdale, M.D., F.A.C.A.M.
   (DIPL)
24700 Center Ridge Road
Cleveland, OH 44145
(216) 835-0104
FAX (216) 871-1404
NT,PD,PM

Douglas Weeks, M.D. **(D/C)**
24700 Center Ridge Road
Cleveland, OH 44145
(216) 835-0104

FAX (216) 871-1404
AC,CT,HO,NT,PM,PMR

Columbus

Robert R. Hershner, D.O. **(P)**
1571 East Livingston Avenue
Columbus, OH 43255
(614) 253-8733
FP,GP,GYN,IM,P,PD

William D. Mitchell, D.O. **(P)**
3520 Snouffer Road
Columbus, OH 43235
(614) 761-0555
CD,CT,GP,IM,OSM,PM

Dayton

David D. Goldberg, D.O. **(DIPL)**
100 Forest Park Drive
Dayton, OH 45405
(513) 277-1722
CT,GP,OSM,PM

Lancaster

Richard Sielski, M.D. **(P)**
3484 Cincinnati-Zainsville Road
Lancaster, OH 43130
(614) 653-0017
CT,FP,NT,PM

Paulding

Don K. Snyder, M.D. **(P)**
Route 2, Box 1271
Paulding, OH 45879
(419) 399-2045
CT,FP

Youngstown

James Ventresco, Jr., D.O. **(P)**
3848 Tippecanoe Road
Youngstown, OH 44511
(216) 792-2349
CT,FP,NT,OSM,RHU

OKLAHOMA

Jenks

Leon Anderson, D.O. (DIPL)
121 Second Street
Jenks, OK 74037
(918) 299-5039
CT,NT,OSM

Oklahoma City

Charles H. Farr, M.D., Ph.D.,
  F.A.C.A.M. (DIPL)
Suite 107
8524 South Western
Oklahoma City, OK 73139
(405) 632-8868
A,CT,NT,PM

Charles D. Taylor, M.D. (D/C)
3715 North Classen Boulevard
Oklahoma City, OK 73118
(405) 525-7751
GP,GYN,OBS,PM,PMR

OREGON

Ashland

Ronald L. Peters, M.D. (P)
1607 Siskiyou Boulevard
Ashland, OR 97520
(503) 482-7007
A,CT,DD,FP,NT,PM,YS

Eugene

John Gambee, M.D. (P)
Suite 140
66 Club Road
Eugene, OR 97401
(503) 686-2536
A,BA,CT,PM

Grants Pass

James Fitzsimmons, Jr., M.D. (P)
591 Hidden Valley Road
Grants Pass, OR 97527

(503) 474-2166
A,CT

Salem

Terence Howe Young, M.D. (D/C)
1205 Wallace Road NW
Salem, OR 97304
(503) 371-1558
A,CT,GP,OSM,PM

PENNSYLVANIA

Allentown

Robert H. Schmidt, D.O. (P)
Suite 303
1227 Liberty Plaza Building
Allentown, PA 18102
(215) 437-1959
CT,FP,NT,PM

D. Erik Von Kiel, D.O. (D/C)
Suite 200
Liberty Square Medical Center
Allentown, PA 18104
(215) 776-7639
CT,FP,MM,NT,OSM

Bangor

Francis J. Cinelli, D.O. (P)
153 North 11th Street
Bangor, PA 18013
(215) 588-4502
CT,GP,HYP

Bedford

Bill Illingworth, D.O. (P)
120 West John Street
Bedford, PA 15522
(814) 623-8414
AN,CT,GP,NT,Pain Management

Bethlehem

Sally Ann Rex, D.O. (P)
1343 Easton Avenue
Bethlehem, PA 18018

(215) 866-0900
CT,GP,Occupational Medicine,OS,PM

Elizabethtown

Dennis L. Gilbert, D.O. **(D/C)**
50 North Market Street
Elizabethtown, PA 17022
(717) 367-1345
AC,CT,NT,OSM,PM

Fountainville

Harold H. Byer, M.D., Ph.D. **(D/C)**
Suite A-101
5045 Swamp Road
Fountainville, PA 18923
(215) 348-0443
AR,CT,DIA,S

Greensburg

Ralph A. Miranda, M.D. **(DIPL)**
RD #12, Box 106
Greensburg, PA 15601
(412) 838-7632
FAX (412) 836-3655
CT,FP,NT,OME,PM

Hazleton

Arthur L. Koch, D.O. **(DIPL)**
57 West Juniper Street
Hazleton, PA 18201
(717) 455-4747
CT,GP,PM

Indiana

Chandrika Sinha, M.D. **(P)**
1177 South Sixth Street
Indiana, PA 15701
(412) 349-1414
AC,CT,NT,PM,S

Macungle

D. Erik Von Kiel, D.O. **(D/C)**
Suite 101
7386 Alburtis Road
Macungle, PA 18062

(215) 967-5503
CT,FP,MM,NT,OSM

Mertztown

Conrad G. Maulfair, Jr., D.O.,
  F.A.C.A.M. **(DIPL)**
Box 71, Main Street
Mertztown, PA 19539
(215) 682-2104
FAX (215) 682-6693
A,CT,HGL

Mt. Pleasant

Mamduh El-Attrache, M.D. **(P)**
20 East Main Street
Mt. Pleasant, PA 15666
(412) 547-3576
BA,CT,DIA,GER,OBS,PO

Newtown

Robert J. Peterson, D.O.
64 Magnolia Drive
Newtown, PA 18940
(No Referrals)

North Versailles

Mamduh El-Attrache, M.D. **(P)**
215 Crooked Run Road
North Versailles, PA 15137
(412) 673-3900
BA,CT,DIA,GER,OBS,PO

Philadelphia

Frederick Burton, M.D. **(P)**
69 West Schoolhouse Lane
Philadelphia, PA 19144
(215) 844-4660
CT,IM,NT,PM

Jose Castillo, M.D.
228 South 22nd Street
Philadelphia, PA 19103
(215) 567-5845, 46, and 47

Mura Galperin, M.D. **(P)**
824 Hendrix Street
Philadelphia, PA 19116

(215) 677-2337
CT,FP

P. Jayalakshmi, M.D. **(DIPL)**
6366 Sherwood Road
Philadelphia, PA 19151
(215) 473-4226
A,AC,AR,BA,CT,DD,DIA

K.R. Sampathachar, M.D. **(DIPL)**
6366 Sherwood Road
Philadelphia, PA 19151
(215) 473-4226
AC,AN,CT,DD,HYP,NT

Lance Wright, M.D. **(D/C)**
3901 Market Street
Philadelphia, PA 19104
(215) 387-1200
DD,END,HYP,NT,PM,PO

Quakertown

Harold Buttram, M.D. **(DIPL)**
5724 Clymer Road
Quakertown, PA 18951
(215) 536-1890
A,CT,FP,NT

Somerset

Paul Peirsel, M.D. **(P)**
RD 4, Box 257A
Somerset, PA 15541
(814) 443-2521
CT,Critical Care,Emergency Medicine,NT

SOUTH CAROLINA

Columbia

Theodore C. Rozema, M.D. **(DIPL)**
2228 Airport Road
Columbia, SC 29205
(803) 796-1702 or (800) 992-8350
CT,FP,NT,PM

Landrum

Theodore C. Rozema, M.D. **(DIPL)**
1000 East Rutherford Road
Landrum, SC 29356
(803) 457-4141 or (800) 992-8350
FAX (803) 457-4144
CT,FP,NT,PM

TENNESSEE

Jackson

S. Marshall Fram, M.D. **(P)**
135 Weatheridge Drive
Jackson, TN 38305
(Retired)

Morristown

Donald Thompson, M.D. **(P)**
PO Box 2088
Morristown, TN 37816
(615) 581-6367
CT,FP,GER,GP,NT,PM

Nashville

Stephen L. Reisman, M.D. **(D/C)**
417 East Iris Drive
Nashville, TN 37204
(615) 383-9030
CT,GP,HGL,NT,PM,YS

TEXAS

Alamo

Herbert Carr, D.O. **(P)**
PO Box 1179
Alamo, TX 78516
(512) 787-6668
CT,OSM,PM

Abilene

William Irby Fox, M.D. **(P)**
1227 North Mockingbird Lane
Abilene, TX 79603

(915) 672-7863
CT,DIA,GER,GP,PMS,S

Amarillo

Gerald Parker, D.O. **(P)**
4714 South Western
Amarillo, TX 79109
(806) 355-8263
A,AC,AR,CT,GP,HO

John T. Taylor, D.O. **(P)**
4714 South Western
Amarillo, TX 79109
(806) 355-8263
A,AC,AR,CT,GP,HO

Austin

Vladimir Rizov, M.D. **(P)**
8311 Shoal Creek Boulevard
Austin, TX 78758
(512) 451-8149
AR,CT,DD,DIA,GP,IM

Dallas

Brij Myer, M.D. **(D/C)**
Suite 222
4222 Trinity Mills Road
Dallas, TX 75287
(214) 248-2488
CD,DD,MM,PM,PUD

Michael G. Samuels, D.O. **(D/C)**
Suite 230
7616 LBJ Freeway
Dallas, TX 75251
(214) 991-3977
CT,NT,OSM,PM

J. Robert Winslow, D.O. **(P)**
Suite 111
2815 Valley View Lane
Dallas, TX 75234
(214) 243-7711
A,CD,CT,END,PM,R

J. Robert Winslow, D.O. **(P)**
2745 Valwood Parkway
Dallas, TX 75234

(214) 241-4614
A,CD,CT,END,PM,R

El Paso

Edward J. Etti, M.D. **(P)**
3500 North Piedras
PO Box 31397
El Paso, TX 79931
(915) 566-9361
AC,CT,IM,Pathology

Francisco Soto, M.D. **(DIPL)**
Suite 100
424 Executive Center Boulevard
El Paso, TX 79902
(915) 534-0272
CD,CT,DD,HO,PM,S

Houston

Robert Battle, M.D. **(DIPL)**
9910 Long Point
Houston, TX 77055
(713) 932-0552
A,BA,CD,CT,FP,HGL

Jerome L. Borochoff, M.D. **(P)**
Suite 504
8830 Long Point
Houston, TX 77055
(713) 461-7517
CD,CT,FP,HO,PM

Luis E. Guerrero, M.D. **(P)**
Suite 150
2055 South Gessner
Houston, TX 77063
(713) 789-0133
AC,CT,FP,NT,PM,PO

Carlos E. Nossa, M.D. **(P)**
Suite 1007
3800 Tanglewilde
Houston, TX 77063
(No Referrals)

Humble

John P. Trowbridge, M.D.,
  F.A.C.A.M. **(DIPL)**
Suite 205
9616 Memorial Boulevard
Humble, TX 77338
(713) 540-2329
FAX (713) 540-4329
A,CT,MM,NT,PM,YS

Kirbyville

John L. Sessions, D.O. **(DIPL)**
1609 South Margaret
Kirbyville, TX 75956
(409) 423-2166
CT,IM,OSM

La Porte

Ronald M. Davis, M.D. **(P)**
10414 West Main Street
La Porte, TX 77571
(713) 470-2930
CT,GP,PM

Laredo

Ruben Berlanga, M.D.
649-B Dogwood
Laredo, TX 78041
(No Referrals)

Pecos

Ricardo Tan, M.D. **(P)**
423 South Palm
Pecos, TX 79772
(915) 445-9090
AC,AU,CT,FP,NT,PM

Plano

Linda Martin, D.O. **(P)**
Suite C
1524 Independence
Plano, TX 75075
(214) 985-1377
FAX (214) 612-0747
CT,GP,NT,PM

San Antonio

Jim P. Archer, D.O. **(P)**
8434 Fredericksburg Road
San Antonio, TX 78229
(512) 615-8445
A,CT,HO,NT,PM

Ron Stogryn, M.D. **(P)**
Suite 100
7334 Blanco Road
San Antonio, TX 78216
(512) 366-3637
FAX (512) 366-3638
A,CT,MM,NT,PD,YS

Wichita Falls

Thomas R. Humphrey, M.D. **(P)**
2400 Rushing
Wichita Falls, TX 76308
(817) 766-4329
BA,FP,GP,HYP

UTAH

Provo

Dennis Harper, D.O. **(D/C)**
Suite 11E
1675 North Freedom Boulevard
Provo, UT 84604
(801) 373-8500
A,CT,OSM,YS

D. Remington, M.D. **(D/C)**
Suite 11E
1675 North Freedom Boulevard
Provo, UT 84604
(801) 373-8500
A,CT,EM,FP

VIRGINIA

Annandale

Sohini Patei, M.D. **(P)**
Suite 207
7023 Little River Turnpike
Annandale, VA 22003

(703) 941-3606
A,CT,NT,PM

Hinton

Harold Huffman, M.D. **(D/C)**
PO Box 197
Hinton, VA 22831
(703) 867-5242
CT,FP,PM

Midlothian

Peter C. Gent, D.O. **(D/C)**
11900 Hull Street
Midlothian, VA 23112
(804) 744-3551
CT,GP,OSM

Norfolk

Vincent Speckhart, M.D. **(DIPL)**
902 Graydon Avenue
Norfolk, VA 23507
(804) 622-0014
IM,Medical Oncology

Trout Dale

Elmer M. Cranton, M.D., F.A.C.A.M.
  (DIPL)
Ripshin Road, Box 44
Trout Dale, VA 24378
(703) 677-3631
FAX (703) 677-3843
A,CD,CT,FP,HO,NT

WASHINGTON

Bellevue

David Buscher, M.D. **(P)**
Suite 102
1370 - 116th NE
Bellevue, WA 98004-3825
(206) 453-0288
Clinical Ecology/EM,GP,NT

Maurice Stephens, M.D.
5011 133rd Place SE

Bellevue, WA 98006
(No Referrals)

Bellingham

Robert Kimmel, M.D. **(D/C)**
Suite 104
4204 Meridian
Bellingham, WA 98226
(206) 734-3250
AC,CT,DD,FP,NT,PM

Fairchild

James P. De Santis, D.O.
8116 Palm Street
Fairchild AFB, WA 99011
(No Referrals)

Kent

Jonathan Wright, M.D. **(P)**
24030 - 132nd, SE
Kent, WA 98042
(206) 631-8920
A,CT,END,FP,MM,NT

Kirkland

Jonathan Collin, M.D. **(DIPL)**
Suite A-50
12911 120th Avenue NE
PO Box 8099
Kirkland, WA 98034
(206) 820-0547
FAX (206) 385-7703
CT,NT,PM

Port Townsend

Jonathan Collin, M.D. **(DIPL)**
911 Tyler Street
Port Townsend, WA 98368
(206) 385-4555
CT,NT,PM

Seattle

Michael G. Vesselago, M.D. **(P)**
217 North 125th
Seattle, WA 98133

(206) 367-0760
CT,FP,IM,MM,NT,PM

Spokane

Burton B. Hart, D.O. **(P)**
East 12104 Main
Spokane, WA 99206
(509) 927-9922
FAX (509) 927-9922
CT,OSM,PM

Vancouver

Richard P. Huemer, M.D. **(P)**
Building C-303
406 SE 131st Avenue
Vancouver, WA 98684
(206) 253-4445
A,CT,HGL,MM,NT,PM

Yakima

Murray L. Black, D.O. **(P)**
609 South 48th Avenue
Yakima, WA 98906
(509) 966-1780
A,CT,FP,GP,OSM

Yeim

Elmer M. Cranton, M.D., F.A.C.A.M.
  (DIPL)
15246 Leona Drive SE
Yeim, WA 98597
(206) 894-3548
FAX (206) 894-2176
A,CD,CT,FP,HO,NT

WEST VIRGINIA

Beckley

Prudencio Corro, M.D. **(P)**
251 Stanaford Road
Beckley, WV 25801
(304) 252-0775
A,CT,RHI

Michael Kostenko, D.O. **(DIPL)**
114 East Main Street
Beckley, WV 25801
(304) 253-0591
A,AC,CT,FP,OSM,PM

Charleston

Steve M. Zekan, M.D. **(P)**
1208 Kanawha Boulevard East
Charleston, WV 25301
(304) 343-7559
CT,NT,PM,S

WISCONSIN

Green Bay

Eleazar M. Kadile, M.D. **(D/C)**
1538 Bellevue Street
Green Bay, WI 54311
(414) 468-9442
A,CT,P

Lake Geneva

Rathna Alwa, M.D. **(DIPL)**
717 Geneva Street
Lake Geneva, WI 53147
(414) 248-1430
AC,AR,BA,CT,HYP,IM

Milwaukee

William J. Faber, D.O. **(P)**
6529 West Fond du Lac Avenue
Milwaukee, WI 53218
(414) 464-7680
Neuro-Musculoskeletal

Thomas Hesselink, M.D. **(D/C)**
Suite 202
10520 West Blue Mound Road
Milwaukee, WI 53226
(414) 259-1350
A,Candida,CT,GP,NT,PM

Robert R. Stocker, D.O. **(DIPL)**
2505 Mayfair Road

Milwaukee, WI 53226
(Retired)

Jerry N. Yee, D.O. **(D/C)**
2505 North Mayfair Road
Milwaukee, WI 53226
(414) 258-6282
BA,CT,GP,OSM

Wisconsin Dells

Robert S. Waters, M.D. **(DIPL)**
Race and Vine Streets
Box 357
Winsonsin Dells, WI 53965
(608) 254-7178
CT,OME,PM

American College of Advancement in Medicine (ACAM) Physicians—International

AUSTRALIA

Donvale, Victoria
R.B. Allen, M.D. (D/C)
5/90 Mitcham Road
Donvale, Victoria 3111
A,AC,CT,HGL,NT,PM

Gosford, N.S.W.
Heather M. Bassett, M.D. (P)
91 Donnison Street
Gosford, N.S.W. 2250
CD,DD,GYN,NT,OSM,PMR

BELGIUM

Antwerpen
Didier Langouche, M.D. (D/C)
Rubenslei 17
2018 Antwerpen
CT

Ghent
Michel De Meyer, M.D. (D/C)
Nekkersberglaan 11
9000 Ghent
FP,GP,OS,PH

St. Niklaas
A. De Bruyne, M.D. (D/C)
Ankerstraat 152B
2700 St. Niklaas
DD,FP,GER,GP,OBS,PM

BRAZIL

Amazonas
Fernando M. de Souza, M.D. (P)
R. Fortaleza 203
Adrianopolis, Manaus
Amazonas CEP 69050
CT,NT,PM

Curitiba
Oslim Malina, M.D. (P)
Rua Casemiro de Abreu 32
Curitiba, PR
Brazil 82.000
CT,Vascular Surgery

Florianopolis
Jose P. Figueredo, M.D. (P)
PCA Geturio Vargas, 20
Florianopolis, SC
CD,CT,GER,IM,NT,PM

Osorio-RS
Jose Valdai de Souza, M.D. (P)
St. Mal Floriano 1012
s/Iron 1 to 9
Osorio-RS 95520
CD,CT,DD,GER,GP,PM

Pelotas-RS
Antonio C. Fernandes, M.D. (P)
Rua Santa Tecia 470A
Pelotas, RS 96010
CD,CT,GER,GP,IM,PM

Porto Alegre

Moyses Hodara, M.D. **(P)**
Rua Vigario Jose Inacio
368, Sala 102
Porto Alegre-RS
CS,CT,DD,FP,GP,RHU

Carlos J.P. de Sa, M.D. **(P)**
Marcilio Dias-1056
Porto Alegre-RS 90060
CD,CT,DIA,HGL,S

Rio Preto

A.O. Passos Correa, M.D. **(P)**
Ave. Alberto Andalo
3314 Sao Jose do Rio Preto
CEP: 15015
CD,CT,GER,IM,NT,PM

Sao Paulo

Guilherme Deucher, M.D. **(P)**
Rua Borges,
Lagoa 1231/2° Andares
Sao Paulo
CT,PM,S

Fernando L. Flaquer, M.D. **(D/C)**
Rua Prof. Artur Ramos
183y33, Sao Paulo
CS,CT,DD,GER,IM,PM

Sergio Vaisman, M.D. **(P)**
Rua Hilo Torres 123
Sao Paulo, SP 04650
CD,CT,DD,GER,IM,PM

CANADA

BRITISH COLUMBIA

Argenta

Robert Sweeney, M.D. **(D/C)**
General Delivery
Argenta, B.C. V0G 1B0
CT,P

Errington

George Barber, M.D. **(D/C)**
Box 234
Errington, B.C. V0R 1V0
CT,GP

Kelowna

Alex A. Neil, M.D. **(D/C)**
205 Rutland Road
Kelowna, B.C. V1X 3B1
CT,GP,HYP,NT

Vancouver

Kevin R. Nolan, M.D. **(D/C)**
205/2786 West 16th Avenue
Vancouver, B.C. V6K 3C4
A,FP,NT,PM,PO,YS

Saul Pilar, M.D. **(D/C)**
205/2786 West 16th Avenue
Vancouver, B.C. V6K 3C4
A,DD,HYP,NT

Donald W. Stewart, M.D. **(D/C)**
2184 West Broadway, #435
Vancouver, B.C. V6K 2E1
CT,GP

Zigurts Strauts, M.D. **(D/C)**
3077 Granville Street, #201
Vancouver, B.C. V6H 3J9
AC,CT,FP,Thermography,
Manipulative Therapy

Victoria

Deanne Roberts, M.D. **(P)**
1041 Chamberlain Street
Victoria, B.C. V8S 4C1
A,CT,NT,PM

MANITOBA

Winnipeg

Howard N. Reed, M.D. **(P)**
302 Lamont Boulevard

Winnipeg, Manitoba R3P 0G1
(Retired)

ONTARIO

Blythe

Richard W. Street, M.D. (D/C)
Box 100, Gypsy Lane
Blythe, Ont. N0M 1H0
GP,NT,PM

Sarnia

Nazeer Vellani, M.D. (P)
241 Wellington Street
Sarnia, Ont. N7T 1G9
CT,NT,PM

Smiths Falls

Clare Minielly, M.D. (D/C)
33 Williams Street East
Smiths Falls, Ont. K7A 1C3
AN,CT,GP,NT

Willowdale

Paul Cutler, M.D., F.A.C.A.M. (DIPL)
Suite B-4
4841 Yonge Street
Willowdale, Ont. M2N 5X2
A,CT,NT

DENMARK

Aarhus

Kurt Christensen, M.D. (DIPL)
Fredenstorv 8-1
8000 Aarhus C
AC,CT,GP,NT

Bruce P. Kyle, M.D. (P)
Sydtoften 35
8260 Aarhus
CT,GP,NT,OME,PM

Humlebaek

Joergen Rugaard, M.D. (D/C)

23 Kystvej
3050 Humlebaek

Lyngby

Claus Hancke, M.D. (DIPL)
Lyngby Hovedgade 17[1]
DK-2800 Lyngby
CT,FP,GP,NT,OSM,PM

Skodsborg

Bo Mogelvang, M.D. (P)
Strandvejen 123-135
DK-2942 Skodsborg
CT,NT,PM

Niels Ove Pedersen, M.D. (P)
Strandvejen 123-135
DK-2942 Skodsborg
AN,CD,CT,IM,NT,PM

Vejle

Knut T. Flytlie, M.D. (D/C)
Gludsmindevej 39
DK-7100 Vejle
A,AC,AU,GP,OSM,PM

Virum

Pierre Eggers-Lura, M.D. (P)
Furesoevej 141
DK-2830 Virum
AC,CT,NT

DOMINICAN REPUBLIC

Santo Domingo

Antonio Pannocchia, M.D. (P)
Suite 201
Ave. 27 de Febrero
Santo Domingo 6
CT,NT,PM

EGYPT

Cairo

Elham G. Behery, M.D. (P)

94 Sarwat Street, Orman
Cairo
A,DIA,END,HGL,MM,RHU

ENGLAND

Kent

F. Schellander, M.D. **(P)**
8 Chilston Road
Tunbridge Wells
Kent TN4 9LT
CT,GP,HO,MM,NT,PM

West Sussex

Simi Khanna, M.D. **(P)**
34 St. Agnes Road
East Grinstead
West Sussex RH193RP
HOM,NT

FRANCE

Paris

Bruno Crussol, M.D. **(P)**
4 Rue Des Belles Feuilles
75016 Paris
CT,NT,PM,S

Paul Musarella, M.D. **(D/C)**
96 Rue de Miromesnil
75008 Paris
GER,NT,PM,S

GERMANY

Bad Fussing

Karl Heinz Caspers, M.D. **(P)**
Beethovenstrasse 1
D 8397 Bad Fussing
NT,PM

Bad Steben

Helmut Keller, M.D. **(P)**
Am Reuthlein 2

D 8675 Bad Steben
IM,Oncology,PD,S

Rottach-Egern

Claus Martin, M.D. **(P)**
PO Box 244
8183 Rottach-Egern
CT,DD,GER

Werne

Jens-Ruediger Collatz, M.D. **(P)**
Fuerstenhofklinik
Fuerstenhof 2
D 4712 Werne
AC,CT,DD,GER,HO,PM

INDONESIA

Bandung

Benj. Widjajakusuma, M.D. **(P)**
Pasirkaliki 115
Bandung 40172
CD,DIA,GER,IM,NT,PUD

Jakarta

Maimunah Affandi, M.D. **(DIPL)**
Suite 13
Jalan Gandaria 8
Kebayoran-Baru
Jakarta-Selatan
CD,CT,DD,PD

Adjit Singh Gill, M.D. **(P)**
Suite 27A
Jalan Tanah Abang V
Jakarta
CD,CT,PM

Yahya Kisyanto, M.D. **(DIPL)**
71 Diponegoro
Jakarta
CD,CT,DIA,GER,IM,PMR

ITALY

Michele Ballo, M.D. **(P)**
Via Ruggero Settimo, 55
90139 Palermo
CD,CT,GER,IM,PM,PMR

MALAYSIA

Mohamed S.A. Ishak, M.D. **(P)**
40 Jalan Kee Ann,
75100 Melaka
West Malaysia
FP,GP,RHI

MEXICO

Chihuahua

H. Berlanga Reyes, M.D. **(DIPL)**
Antonio de Montes 2118
Col. San Felipe
Chihuahua, Chih. 31240
CT,GER,GP,PM

Guadalajara, Jalisco

Eleazar A. Carrasco, M.D. **(P)**
Chapultepec Norte 140-203
Guadalajara, Jalisco 44600
CT,GP,GYN,OBS,S

F. Navares Merino, M.D. **(DIPL)**
Lopez Mateos Nte. 646, S.H.
Guadalajara, Jalisco 44680
CT,NT,PM

Juarez, Chihuahua

H. Berlanga Reyes, M.D. **(DIPL)**
Insurgentes 2516
Cd. Juarez, Chihuahua 32330
CT,GER,GP,PM

Francisco Soto, M.D. **(D/C)**
16 de Septiembre, 2215
32030 Cd. Juarez
CD,CT,DD,HO,PM,S

Matamoros, Tamp.

Frank Morales, Sr., M.D. **(P)**
1a y Nardos, Cal. Jardin
H. Matamoros, Tamp.
CT,DD,NT,PM

Tijuana

Francisco Rique, M.D. **(P)**
Azucenas 15
Frac. del Prado
Tijuana, B.C.
AC,AR,CT,DD,NT,PM

Rodrigo Rodriguez, M.D. **(D/C)**
Azucenas 15
Frac. del Prado
Tijuana, B.C.
CD,CT,DD,GER,MM,PM

Roberto Tapia, M.D. **(P)**
Azucenas 15
Frac. del Prado
Tijuana, B.C.
CT,DD,END,MM,NT,PM

Torreon, Coahuila

Carlos Lopez Moreno, M.D. **(P)**
Tulipanes 475
Col. Torreon, Jardin
Torreon, Coahuila 27200
CT,NT,PM

NETHERLANDS

Bilthoven

C.J.M. Broekhuyse, M.D. **(D/C)**
Hobbemalaan 11
3723 EP Bilthoven
AC,AU,CT,DD,GP,NT,PM

Etten-Leur

Peter Zeegers, M.D. **(P)**
Beatrixpark 20
4872 BJ Etten-Leur
A,CD,CT,DD,GP

Haarlem

Eduard Schweden, M.D. **(DIPL)**
Kenaupark 22
2011 MT Haarlem
CT,DD,NT,OS,PM

Dirk van Lith, M.D. **(DIPL)**
Kenaupark 22
2011 MT Haarlem
A,DD,CT,GP,HO,NT,PM,S

Leende

Peter van der Schaar, M.D. **(DIPL)**
Renheide 2
5595 XJ Leende
CD,CT,DD,OME,S

Marc Verheyen, M.D. **(DIPL)**
Renheide 2
5595 XJ Leende
CD,CT,DD,OME,S

Loenersloot

A. Verbon, M.D. **(D/C)**
Voorburgstraat 30
NL3634 AW Loenersloot
CT,PUD

Maastricht

Rob van Zandvoort, M.D. **(DIPL)**
Burg. Cortenstraat 26
6226 GV Maastricht
CT

Oudenbosch

E.T. Oei, M.D. **(D/C)**
34 St. Louis Markt
4731 HP Oudenbosch
AC,CT,DIA,END,GER,IM

Rotterdam

Robert T.H.K. Trossel, M.D. **(DIPL)**
Zoutmanstraat 4
3012 EV Rotterdam
A,DD,CT,GP,HO,NT,PM,S

Utrecht

P.J.C. Riethoven, M.D. **(D/C)**
Ramstraat 27-A
3581 HD Utrecht
CT

Velp

J.H. Leenders, M.D. **(D/C)**
344 Arnhemsestraatweg
6881 NK Velp
A,AC,AU,CD,CT,DD,PM

NETHERLANDS ANTILLES

Aruba

Adhemar E. Hart, M.D. **(P)**
Shakespearstraat 13
Oranjestad, Aruba
PD

St. Maarten

Dirk van Lith, M.D. **(DIPL)**
PO Box 3030
Simpsonbay
St. Maarten
A,CT,DD,GP,HO,NT,PM,S

Robert T.H.K. Trossel, M.D. **(DIPL)**
PO Box 3030
Simpsonbay, St. Maarten
A,CT,DD,GP,HO,NT,PM,S,

NEW ZEALAND

Auckland

Maurice B. Archer, D.O. **(P)**
PO Box 2981
Auckland 1
CT,NT,PM

R.H. Bundellu, M.D. **(DIPL)**
173 Tamaki Road
Otara, Auckland
CT,FP,OBS

Christchurch

Robert Blackmore, M.D. **(D/C)**
196 Hills Road
Christchurch 1
AC,CT,FP,GP,NT,OBS

Hamilton

William J. Reeder, M.D. **(D/C)**
PO Box 4187
Hamilton
AC,CT,GP,NT,PM

Masterton

T.J. Baily Gibson, M.D. **(DIPL)**
PO Box 274
Masterton
A,CT,FP,OBS,OME

New Lynn

Raymond Ramirez, M.D. **(P)**
3075 Great North Road
New Lynn, Auckland
AC,AU,CT,GP,OSM,YS

Napier

Tony Edwards, M.D. **(D/C)**
30 Munroe Street
Napier
CT,FP,NT,OBS,PM

Oxford, North Canterbury

Ted Walford, M.D. **(P)**
454 Cameron Road
Tauranga
CT,NT,PM

Tauranga

Michael E. Godfrey, M.D. **(DIPL)**
Willow House
14 Willow Street
Tauranga
CT,OME,PM

PHILIPPINES

Manila

Rosa M. Ami Belli, M.D. **(P)**
Suite 303-501
PDC Building
1440 Taft Avenue
Manila
CT,HGL,NT,P

Leonides Lerma, M.D. **(P)**
#301, Pearl Garden
1700 M. Adriatico Malate
Manila
A,AC,AU,GER,P

Corazon Macawili-Yu, M.D. **(P)**
Suite 303-501
PDC Building
1440 Taft Avenue
Manila
CT,NT,PM

Remedios L. Reynoso, M.D. **(P)**
Suite 303-501
PDC Building
1440 Taft Avenue
Manila
CT,NT,PM

PUERTO RICO

Cidra

Pedro Rivera, M.D. **(P)**
PO Box 1518
Cidra 00639
(Retired)

Santurce

Pedro Zayas, M.D. **(D/C)**
PO Box 14275
B.O. Obrero Station
Santurce
AC,BA,CT,FP,HGL,NT

SPAIN

Malaga
Henning Munksnaes, M.D. **(P)**
Medina Sidonia 192
Urb. Torre Nueva
Mijas Costa / Malaga
CT,DD,GYN,NT,P

SWITZERLAND

Geneva
Robert Tissot, M.D. **(P)**
168 Route de Malagnou
1224 Geneva
AU,NT,OSM,PM,PMR

Montreux
Claude Rossel, M.D., Ph.D. **(P)**
Clinique Bon Port
1820 Montreux
CT,NT,PM

Netstal (Glarus)
Walter Blumer, M.D. **(P)**
8754 Netstal

(Glarus bei Zurich)
CT
(Honorary Life Member)

TAIWAN (R.O.C.)

Taipei
Paul Lin, M.D. **(P)**
5 Lane 85 Sung Chiang Road
Taipei
CT,NT,PM

Yeh-Sung Lin, M.D. **(P)**
154 Sec. 1 Chien Kuo N. Road
Taipei
AN,CD,DD,DIA,END

WEST INDIES

Jamaica
H. Marco Brown, M.D. **(D/C)**
6 Corner Lane
Montego Bay, Jamaica
CT,NT,PM

Notes

Chapter 1
The Painkiller With a Problem

1. Olver, I.N.; J. Aisner; A. Hament; L. Buchanan; J.F. Bishop; and R.S. Kaplan. "A prospective study of topical dimethyl sulfoxide for treating anthracycline extravasation." *Journal of Clinical Oncology* (Nov. 1988); 6(11):1732–1735.
2. Babenko, V.N. "Treatment of patients with generalized periodontitis with a suspension of indomethacin in a dimexide solution." *Stomatologiia* (Mar./Apr. 1987); 66(2):26–28.
3. Goranov, K.; V. Zarankova; M. Velceva; and S. Dermend:zieva. "Clinical results from the treatment of a hemorrhagic form of periodontosis with a complex herb extract and 15 percent DMSO." *Stomatologiia* (Nov./Dec. 1983); 65(6):25–30.

Chapter 2
DMSO's Controversial History

1. "DMSO Documents Sought," *NHF Public Scrutiny.* Vol. XXVII, No. 27, January, 1981, p. 29.

2. Szmant, H. Harry. "Physical properties of dimethyl sulfoxide and its function in biological systems," *Biological Actions of Dimethyl Sulfoxide*, Stanley W. Jacob and Robert Herschler (eds.), New York: Annals of the New York Academy of Sciences, Vol. 243, January 27, 1975, pp. 20–23.
3. Tackett, Michael. "Arthritis victims warned on solvent," *Chicago Tribune*, November 16, 1980, p. 1.
4. Dewitt, Karen. "Drug DMSO studied as unauthorized use rises," *The New York Times*, July 31, 1980, p. A11.
5. Sweeney, Thomas F. "Medicinal uses of marijuana get conflicting reviews," *The Advocate*, January 28, 1981, p.2.
6. "Former Gov. Wallace travels to Oregon for special treatment," *The Advocate*, June 30, 1980, p.3.

Chapter 3
The Therapeutic Principle of DMSO

1. Schlafer, H.L. and W. Schaffernicht. *Angew. Chem*, 72:618, 1960.

2. Ranky, W.O. and D.C. Nelson. *Organic Sulfur Compounds* (N. Kharasch, ed.), Vol. 1, Pergamon, New York, 1961, p. 170.

3. MacGregory, W.S. *Ann. N.Y. Acad. Sci.*, 141:3, 1967.

4. Martin, D.; A. Weise; and H.J. Niclas. *Angew. Chem*, 79:340, 1967.

5. Thomas, R.; C.B. Schoemaker; and K. Eriks. *Acta Cryst.*, 21:12, 1966.

6. Parker, A.J. *Advances in Organic Chemistry, Methods and Results*, (R.A. Raphael, E.C. Taylor, and H. Wynberg, eds.), Vol. 5, Wiley (Interscience), New York, 1965, p. 1.

7. Lindberg, J.J.; J. Kenttamaa; and A. Nissema. *Suomen Kemistilehti*, 34B:98, 1961.

8. Schlafer and Schaffernicht, op. cit.

9. Wiberg, K.B. *Physical Organic Chemistry*, Wiley, New York, 1964, p. 136.

10. Martin, Weise, and Niclas, op. cit.

11. Pruckner, H.; Erdoel; and Kohle, *Acta Shandia Med.*, 16:188, 1963.

12. Lindberg, J.J. *Finska Kemistsamfundets Medd.*, 77:130, 1968.

13. Kauzmann, W. *Advan. Protein Chem.*, 14:1, 1959.

14. Klotz, I.M. *Brookhaven Symp. Biol.*, 13:25, 1961.

15. Tanford, C. *J. Am. Chem. Soc.*, 84:4240, 1962.

16. Typley, J.A. *J. Phys. Chem.*, 68:2002, 1964.

17. Kligman, H.M. *J. Am. Med. Soc.*, 193:11, 1965.

18. Muset, P. Puig, and J. Martin Esteve. *Experientia*, 21:649, 1965.

19. Horita, A., and L.J. Weber. *Life Sci.* (Oxford), 3:1389, 1964.

20. Herskovits, T.T., and M. Laskowski, Jr. *J. Biol. Chem.*, 237: 2481, 1962.

21. Hamaguchi, K. *J. Biochem* (Tokyo), 56:441, 1964.

22. Szmant, H. Harry. "Physical properties of dimethyl sulfoxide and its function in biological systems," *Biological Actions of Dimethyl Sulfoxide*, ed. by Stanley W. Jacob and Robert Herschler. New York: New York Academy of Sciences, 1975, pp. 20–23.

23. Barfeld, H., and T. Atoynatan. "N-acetylcysteine inactivates migration inhibitory factory and delayed hypersensitivity reactions," *Nature New Bio.*, 231:157–159, 1971.

24. Barfeld, H., and T. Atoynatan. "Cytophilic nature of migration inhibitory factor associated with delayed hypersensitivity," *Proc. Soc. Exp. Biol. Med.*, 139:497–501, 1969.

25. Tschope, M., cited in Raettig, H. "The potential of DMSO in experimental immunology," *Dimethylsulfoxyl.*, Internationales Symposium in Wien. G. Laudahn and K. Getrich, eds.:54. Saladruck, Berlin, West Germany, 1966.

26. Jacob, Stanley W. "Dimethyl sulfoxide, its basic pharmacology and usefulness in the therapy of headache," *Headache*, 5:78–81, October 1965.

27. Hucker, H.B. *J. Pharmacol. Exp. Ther.*, 155:309, 1967.

28. Maibach, H.I., and R.J. Feldman. *Ann. N.Y. Acad. Sci.*, 141:423, 1967.

29. Stoughton, R.B. *Arch. Derm.*, 91:657, 1965.

30. Stoughton, R.B. *Toxic. Appl. Pharmacol.*, 7:1, 1965.
31. Brink, J.J., and D.G. Stein. *Science*, 158:1479, 1967.
32. Formanek, and W. Kovak. "Die wirkung von DMSO auf experimentell erzeugte rattenpfotenodeme," *DMSO Symposium*, 1966, Saladruck, Berlin, 1966, p. 18.
33. Gorog, P., and I.B. Kovacs. *Curr. Ther. Resp.*, 10:486, 1968.
34. Weisman, G. *Ann. N.Y. Acad. Sci.*, 141:326, 1967.
35. Ibid.
36. Swanson, B.N. "Medical use of dimethyl sulfoxide (DMSO)," *Reviews in Clinical and Basic Pharmacology* (Jan–June 1985), 5 (1-2):1–33.
37. Walker, Morton. *Chelation Therapy*. Stamford, Conn.: Freelance Communications, 1980.
38. Walker, Morton. *The Chelation Answer*. New York: M. Evans & Co., 1982.

Chapter 4
General Medical Uses for DMSO

1. *Physicians' Desk Reference*, Oradell, N.J.: Medical Economics Company, 1980.
2. "Doctor Claims DMSO Saved 11," *Ocala Star-Banner*, January 11, 1981, p. 10A.
3. Edelson, E. "DMSO," *Daily News*, June 9, 1980, p. 35.
4. Ashwood-Smith, M.H. "The radioactive action of dimethyl sulphoxide and various other sulphoxides," *Intern J. Radiation Biol.* 3:41, 1961.
5. Ashwood-Smith, M.H. "Radioprotective and cyroprotective properties of dimethyl sulfoxide in cellular systems," *Ann. N.Y. Acad. Sci.*, 141:45, 1967.

6. Hagemann, R.F., and J.C. Schaer, "The mechanism of modification of radiation effect by dimethyl sulfoxide," *Experientia*, 27:319, 1971.
7. Grozdov, S.P. "Mechanism of the biological action and radiation-protective effect of DMSO," *Radiobiologiya*, 11:522, 1971.
8. Lappenbusch, W.L. "On the mechanism of radioprotective action of dimethyl sulfoxide," *Radiation Res.*, 46:279, 1971.
9. Bridges, B.A. "The chemical protection of *Pseudomonas* species against ionizing radiation," *Radiation Res.*, 17:801, 1962.
10. Vos, O.; M.C.A. Kaalen; and L. Burdke. "Radiation protection by a number of substances preventing freezing damage. I. Protection of mammalian cells *in vitro*," *Intern J. Radiation Biol.*, 9:33, 1965.
11. Noel, J.F., and E.A. Wright. "*In vitro* radioprotection of mouse tail bones by dimethyl sulphoxide, glycerol and anoxia," *Intern. J. Radiation Biol.*, 18:301, 1970.
12. Dod, J.L., and J. Shewell. "Local protection against x-irradiation by dimethylsulphoxide," *Brit. J. Radio.*, 41:950, 1968.
13. Zharinov, G.M.; S.F. Vershinina; and O.I. Drankova. "Prevention of radiation damage to the bladder and rectum using local application of dimethyl sulfoxide." *Meditsinskaia Radiologiia*, 30(3):16–18, March 1985.
14. Lovelock, J.E., and M.W.H. Bishop. "Prevention of freezing damage to living cells by dimethyl sulphoxide," *Nature*, 183:1394, 1959.

15. De la Torre, J.C.; J. Meredith; and M.G. Netsky. "Cerebral air embolism in the dog," *Arch. Neurol.*, 6:307–316, 1962.

16. De la Torre, J.C.; H.M. Kawanga; D.W. Rowed; C.M. Johnson; K. Kajihara; D. Goode; and S. Mullan. "Dimethyl sulfoxide in central nervous system trauma," *Ann. N.Y. Acad. Sci.*, 243:362–389, 1975.

17. Gabourie, J.; J.W. Becker; B. Bateman; M. Dunn; and S. Jacob. "Oral dimethyl sulfoxide in mental retardation," *Ann. N.Y. Acad. Sci.*, 245:449–459, 1975.

18. Aspillaga, M.J.; G. Morzon; I. Avendano; M. Sanchez; and L. Capdeville. "Dimethyl sulfoxide therapy in severe retardation in mongoloid children," *Ann. N.Y. Acad. Sci.*, 241:423–431, 1975.

19. Engel, M.F. *Ann. N.Y. Acad. Sci.*, 141:638, 1967.

20. Fil'iulia. "Use of dimexide for the local treatment of surface burns," *Klinicheskaia Khirurgiia*, (3):38–40, March 1985.

21. Jacob, S.W. *Current Ther. Res.*, 6:134, 1964.

22. Tsuchiva, T. *Bull. Chem. Soc.*, Japan 57:285, 1962.

23. Gabourie, Becker, Bateman, Dunn, and Jacob, op. cit.

24. Shelest, L.I.; B.M. Brusilovski; B.V. Radionov; and V.S. Kuts. "Prospects of using dimexide with antibiotic therapy." *Problemy Tuberkuleza*, (3):58–63, 1986.

25. Sebert, F.B. *Ann. N.Y. Acad. Sci.*, 243:175, 1967.

26. More, R.C.; J.M. Kabo; F.J. Dorey; R.A. Meals. "The effects of dimethyl sulfoxide on posttraumatic limb swelling and joint stiffness," *Clinical Orthopaedics and Related Research*, 233:304–310, August 1988.

27. Garrido, J.C., and R.E. Lagos. "Dimethyl sulfoxide therapy as toxicity-reducing agent and potentiator of cyclophosphamide in the treatment of different types of cancer," *Ann. N.Y. Acad. Sci.*, 245:412–420, 1975.

28. Friend, C., and W. Scher. "Stimulation by dimethyl sulfoxide of erythroid differentiation and hemoglobin synthesis in murine virus-induced leukemic cells," *Ann. N.Y. Acad. Sci.*, 243:155–163, 1975.

29. Spremulli, E.N., and D.L. Dexter. "Polar solvents: a novel class of antineoplastic agents," *Journal of Clinical Oncology*, 2(3):227–241, March 1984.

30. Ostrow, S.S.; M.E. Klein; N.R. Bachur; M. Colvin; and P.H. Wiernik. "Cyclophosphamide and dimethylsulfoxide in the treatment of squamous carcinoma of the lung. Therapeutic efficacy, toxicity, and pharmacokinetics," *Cancer Chemotherapy & Pharmacology*, 6(2):117–120, 1981.

31. Egorin, M.J.; R.S. Kaplan; M. Salcman; J. Aisner; M. Colvin; P.H. Wiernik; and N.R. Bachur. Cyclophosphamide plasma and cerebrospinal fluid kinetics with and without dimethyl sulfoxide," *Clinical Pharmacology & Therapeutics*, 32(1):122–128, July 1982.

32. Kojima, K.; H. Hasegawa; T. Fujishiro; T. Yanai; S. Murai; N. Funahashi; M. Mizuno; T. Ogawa; and S. Kawashima. "Successful treatments of plasma exchange, hemodialysis, immunosuppressive agents and dimethylsulfox-

ide in a case of myeloma kidney," *Nippon Jinzo Gakkai Shi*, 29(1):115–121, January 1987.

33. Volden, G.; E. Thorud; and O.H. Iversen. "Inhibition of methylcholanthrene-induced skin carcinogenesis in hairless mice by the membrane-labilizing agent DMSO," *British Journal of Dermatology*, 109 Suppl. 25:133–136, July 1983.

34. Jacob, S.W. "Dimethyl sulfoxide, its basic pharmacology and usefulness in therapy of headache," *Headache*, 5:78–81, October 1965.

35. Burton, W.J.; P.W. Gould; M.W. Hursthouse; P.J. Sears; D.A. Larnder; H.C. Stringer; and B.C. Turnbull. "A multicentre trial of Zostrum (5 percent idoxuridine in dimethyl sulphoxide) in herpes zoster," *New Zealand Medical Journal*, 94(696):384–386, November 1981.

36. Sehtman, L. "Dimethyl sulfoxide therapy in various dermatological disorders," *Ann. N.Y. Acad. Sci.*, 245:395–402, 1975.

37. Miranda-Tirado, R. "Dimethyl sulfoxide therapy in chronic skin ulcers," *Ann. N.Y. Acad. Sci.*, 241:408–411, 1975.

38. Lishner, M.; R. Lang; I. Kedar; and M. Ravid. "Treatment of diabetic perforating ulcers (mal perforant) with local dimethylsulfoxide," *Journal of the American Geriatrics Society*, 33(1):41–43, January 1985.

39. Ludwig, C.U.; H.R. Stoll; R. Obrist; and J.P. Obrecht. "Prevention of cytotoxic drug induced skin ulcers with dimethyl sulfoxide (DMSO) and alpha tocopherol," *European Journal of Cancer & Clinical Oncology*, 23(3):327–329, March 1987.

40. Gordon, D.M. *Ann. N.Y. Acad. Sci.*, 141:551, 1967.

41. Hill, R.V. "Dimethyl sulfoxide in the treatment of retinal disease," *Ann. N.Y. Acad. Sci.*, 245:485–493, 1975.

42. Venegas, H. "Dimethyl sulfoxide therapy in sterility due to tubal obstruction," *Ann. N.Y. Acad. Sci.*, 245:494–496, 1975.

43. Kryzywicki, J. *J. Czas. Stomat.*, 11:1007, 1969.

44. Varshavski, A.I., and T.A. Guberskaia, "Use of dimethyl sulfoxide in the combined treatment of the exacerbation of chronic parenchymatous parotitis," *Stomatologiia*, 67(6):12–14, November-December 1988.

45. Kolomiets, L.I. "Effectiveness of ectericide, dimethyl sulfoxide and oxacillin in treating acute, odontogentic inflammatory jaw diseases," *Stomatologiia*, 60(4):33–35, 1981.

46. Scherbel, A.L.; L.J. McCormack; and M.J. Poppo. "Alteration of collagen in generalized scleroderma (progressive systemic sclerosi) after treatment with dimethyl sulfoxide," *Cleveland Clinic Quarterly*, 32–47, 1965.

Chapter 5
The Toxicity and Side Effects of DMSO

1. Leake, C.D. *Science*, 152:1646:9, 1966

2. Smith, E.R.; Z. Hadidian; and M.M. Mason. *Ann. N.Y. Acad. Sci.*, 141:96, 1967.

3. Smith, E.R.; Z. Hadidian; and M.M. Mason. *J. Clin. Pharmacol*, September-October 1968, pp.315–321.

4. Smith, Hadidian, and Brown, op. cit.

5. Brown, J.H. *Ann. N.Y. Acad. Sci.*, 141, 496, 1976.

6. John, H., and G. Laudahn. *Ann. N.Y. Acad. Sci.*, 141, 506, 1967.
7. Kligman, A.M. *J. Amer. Med. Assoc.*, 193, 796, 923, 1965.
8. Demos, C.H.; G.L. Beckloff; M.N. Donin; and P.M. Oliver. *Ann. N.Y. Acad. Sci.*, 141, 517, 1967.
9. Elfbaum, S.G., and K. Laden. *J. Soc. Cosmetic Chemists*, 19, 841–847, 1968; C.A. 71, 11478d.
10. Uranuma, T., Igaku. *Kenkyu*, 30:2235, 1960.
11. Block, L.H. *Drug & Cosmetic Ind.*, 95(3), 342–346, 1964.
12. Feinman, H.; M. Ben; and R. Levin. *Pharmacol.*, 6, 188, 1964.
13. Melville, K.I.; B. Klingner; and H.E. Shister. *Arch. Pharmacodyn.*, 174(2), 277–293, 1968.
14. Peterson, C.G., and R.D. Robertson. *Ann. N.Y. Acad. Sci.*, 141, 273, 1967.
15. Anon., *Munchener Med. Wschr.*, 108, 21, 1966.
16. Caujolle, F.; D. Caujolle; S. Cros; M. Calvet; and Y. Tollon. *Compt. Rend.*, 260(1), 327–330, 1965; C.A. 62, 13724c.
17. Ferm, J.H., and J. Embryol. *Exp. Morph.*, 16(1), 49–54, 1966.
18. David, N.A. *Annual Review of Pharmacol.*, 12, 353–373, 1972.
19. Ayre, J.E., and J. LeGuerrier. *Ann. N.Y. Acad. Sci.*, 141, 414, 1967.
20. Lohs, Von K.; W. Damerau; and T. Schramm. *Arch. Fur Geschwulstforschung*, 37(1), 1–3, 1971.
21. Hegre, A.M., and R.E. Smith. AMLC-TR-67-4 Aerospace Med. Lab. Lackland AFB Texas.
22. Kligman, A.M. *J. Invest. Dermat.*, 47, 375–392, 1966.
23. Sulzberger, M.B.; T.A. Cortese, Jr.; L. Fishman; H.S. Wiley; and P.S. Peyakovich. *Ann. N.Y. Acad. Sci.*, 141,437,1967.

24. McDermot, H.L.; A.J. Finkbeiner; and B. Zanette. *Can. J. Physicol. and Pharmacol.*, 45, 475, 1967.
25. Williams, K.I.H.; K.S. Whittmore; T.N. Mellin; and D.S. Layne. *Science*, 149, 203–204, 1965.
26. Hucker, H.B.; J.K. Miller; A.B. Hochberg; R. Brobyn; F.H. Riordon; and B. Calesnick. *J. Pharmacol. Exp. Ther.*, 155, 309–317, 1967.
27. Gerhards, E., and H. Gibian. *Ann. N.Y. Acad. Sci.*, 141, 65–76, 1967.
28. Borgstedt, H.H., and V. DiStefano. *Toxicol. & Appl. Pharmacol.*, 10, 523–528, 1967.
29. DiStefano, V., and H. Borgstedt. *Science*, 144(3622), 1137–1138, 1964; C.A. 61, 4868c.
30. *Bull. AT. Sci.*, 25(1):8–14, January 1969.
31. Caldwell, A.D.S.; P.G.T. Bye; and M.H. Briggs. *Nature*, 215, 1168, 1967.
32. Brobyn, R. *Medical Tribune*, October 3, 1968.
33. Jenkins, B.H. *Invest. Ophthalmol.*, 5(3), 329, 1966.
34. Jacob, S.W., and D.C. Wood. *Current Therap. Res.*, 9(4), 229–233, 1967.
35. Hull, F.W.; D.C. Wood; and R.D. Brobyn. *Northwest Medicine*, 68(1), 39–41, 1969.
36. Gordon, D.M. *Ann. N.Y. Acad. Sci.*, 141, 392, 1967.
37. Gordon, D.M., and K.E. Kleberger. *Arch. Ophthal.*, 79, 423, 1968.
38. Kleberger, K.E., and D.M. Gordon. *Forthschr. Med.*, 85(5), 171–174, 1967; C.A. 67, 52318n.
39. Sanders, M. *Ann. N.Y. Acad. Sci.*, 141, 649, 1967.
40. Wood, D.C.; F.S. Weber; and M.A. Palmquist. *J. Pharmacol. Exp. Therap.*, 177(3), 520–527, 1971.
41. Ibid., 528–535, 1971.

42. Brobyn, R.D. "The human toxicology of dimethyl sulfoxide," *Ann. N.Y. Acad. Sci.*, 243:497–506, 1975.
43. Wood, D.C.; D. Sweet; J. Van Dolah; J.C. Smith II; and I. Contaxis. *Ann. N.Y. Acad. Sci.*, 141, 346–380, 1967; C.A. 67, 460h.
44. Mueller, F.O.; P. O'Neill; and P.D. Trevor-Roper. *Brit. J. Ophthal.*, 51, 227, 1967.
45. Ibid., 13–30.
46. Kleberger, K.E. *Graefes Arch. Klin. Exp. Ophthal.*, 173, 269–281, 1967.
47. Rubin, L.F., and K.C. Barnett. *Ann. N.Y. Acad. Sci.*, 141, 333, 1967.
48. Barnett, K.C., and P.R.B. Noel. *Nature*, 214, 1115–1116, 1967.
49. Kleberger and Gordon. *Forthsch. Med.*, 85(5), 171–174, 1967; C.A. 67, 52318n.
50. Smith, E.R.; M.M. Mason; and E.E. Epstein. *Ann. N.Y. Acad. Sci.*, 141, 386, 1967.
51. Kleberger. *Ann. N.Y. Acad. Sci.*, 141, 381, 1967.
52. Kleberger. *Graefes Arch. Klin. Exp. Ophthal.*, 173, 269–281, 1967.
53. Ibid.
54. Ibid.
55. Wood, D.C.; D. Sweet; J. Van Dolah; J.C. Smith II; and J. Contaxis. *Ann. N.Y. Acad. Sci.*, 141, 346–380, 1967, C.A. 67, 460h.
56. Wood, D.C. *Science*, 155, 404, 1967.
57. Rubin, L.F., and P.A. Mattis. *Science*, 153, 83–84, 1966.
58. Caldwell, A.D.S.; P.G.T. Bye; and M.H. Briggs. *Nature*, 215, 1168, 1967.
59. Vogin, E.E.; S. Carson; G. Cannon; C.R. Linegar; and L.F. Rubin. *Toxicol. and Appl. Pharmacol.*, 16, 606–612, 1970.
60. Smith, E.R.; M.M. Mason; and E.E. Epstein. *J. Pharmacol. Exp. Ther.*, 170–172, 1969; C.A. 72, 30143c.
61. Gordon, D.M., and K.E. Kleberger, *Arch. Ophthal.*, 79, 423, 1968.

Chapter 6
The Potent Potion for Sports Injuries

1. Lang, J. "Potent potion for bum arm; Denehy ready now," *The Sporting News*, March 13, 1971.
2. Percy, E.C., and J.D. Carson. "The use of DMSO in tennis elbow and rotator cuff tendonitis: a double-blind study," *Medicine and Science in Sports and Exercise*, 13(4):215–219, 1981.
3. "DMSO: New Hope for Arthritis?" Select Committee on Aging, House of Representatives, Ninety-Sixth Congress. Washington, D.C.: U.S. Government Printing Office, Comm. Pub. No. 96-232, March 24, 1980, p. 136.

Chapter 7
Arthritis Therapy With DMSO and Diet

1. Morassi, P.; F. Massa; E. Mesensnel; D. Magris; and B. D'Angnolo. "Treatment of amyloidosis with dimethyl sulfoxide (DMSO)," *Minerva Medica*, 80(1):65–70, January 1989.
2. Akimova, T.F.; T.M. Novoselova; and A.P. Aliab'eva. "Current methods of treating acute gouty arthritis," *Terapevticheskii Arkhiv*, 53(7):127–129, 1981.
3. Yoshimitsu, K.; N. Koga; Y. Kitamura; K. Fukuda; E. Kittaka; N. Horino; N. Sakura; T. Tanaka; Y. Nishi; T. Sakano; et al. "Favorable effect of dimethyl

sulfoxide on secondary amyloidosis in juvenile rheumatoid arthritis," *Pediatric Pharmacology,* 4(3):177–181, 1984.

4. Murav'ev, I.V., and A.P. Aliab'eva. "Dimethyl sulfoxide in the treatment of amyloidosis in rheumatoid arthritis (case report)," *Terapevticheskii Arkhiv,* (11):38–39, 1981.

5. Tareev, E.M.; O.M. Vinogradova; L.N. Kochube; and T.V. Chegaeva. "Approaches to the treatment of amyloidosis," *Urologiia I Nefrologiia,* 6:56–63, November-December 1983.

6. Takahashi, A.; J. Matsumoto; S. Nishimura; N. Tanada; S. Imura; T. Isobe; and T. Shimoyama. "Improvement of endoscopic and histologic findings of AA-type gastrointestinal amyloidosis by treatment with dimethyl sulfoxide and prednisolone," *Gastroenterologia Japonica,* 20(2):143–147, April 1985.

Chapter 9
Using DMSO in Head and Spinal Cord Injuries

1. De la Torre, J.C.; J.W. Surgeon; P.K. Hill; and T. Khan. "DMSO in the treatment of brain infection: basic considerations," *Arterial Air Embolism and Acute Stroke* (eds. J.M. Hallenbeck and L.J. Greenbaum), Undersea Medical Society Report No. 11-15-77:138–161, 1977.

2. De la Torre, J.C., and P.K. Hill, "Ultrastructural studies on formation of edema and its treatment following experimental brain infarction in monkeys," *Dynamics of Brain Edema* (eds. H. Pappius and W. Feindel), Berlin: Springer, 1976, pp. 306–314.

3. De la Torre, J.C., and J.W. Surgeon. "Dexamethasone and DMSO in experimental transorbital cerebral infarction," *Stroke,* 7:577–583, 1976.

4. Deutsch, E. "Beeinflussung de blutgerinnung durch DMSO und kombinationen mit heparin," *DMSO Symposium, Vienna,* Berlin: Saladruck, 1966, p. 144.

5. White, R.P. ,Prostaglandin F_2 Alpha and experimental cerebral vasospasm in dogs," *Pharmacologist,* 13:292, 1972.

6. Weeks, J.R. "The prostaglandins: biologically active lipids with implications in circulatory physiology," *Circ. Res.,* 24:1223–1229, 1969.

7. LaHann, T.R., and A. Horita. "Effects of dimethyl sulfoxide (DMSO) on prostaglandin synthetase," *Proc. West. Pharmacol. Soc.,* 18:81–82, 1975.

8. Coceani, F. "Prostaglandins and the central nervous system," *Arch. Intern. Med.,* 133:119–129, 1974.

9. Bergstrom, S. "Prostaglandins: members of a new hormonal system," *Science,* 157:382–391, 1967.

10. Dujovny, M.; P.J. Barrionuevo; R.K. Laha; S. De Castro; and J.C. Maroon. "Experimental middle cerebral artery microsurgical embolectomy," *Surg. Forum,* 37:495–596, 1976.

11. Dujovny, M.; P.J. Barrionuevo; R.D. Laha; G. Solis; J. Maroon; and R.H. Hellstrom. "The role of DMSO and methylprednisolone in canine middle cerebral artery microsurgical embolectomy," *Stroke,* 8:6–7, 1977.

12. De la Torre, Surgeon, Hill, and Kahn, op. cit.
13. Kajihara, K.; H. Kawanaga; J.C. de la Torre; and S. Mullan. "Dimethyl sulfoxide in the treatment of experimental acute spinal cord injury," *Surgical Neurology*, 1:16–22, 1973.
14. De la Torre, J.C.; D.W. Rowed; H.M. Kawanaga; and S. Mullan. "Dimethyl sulfoxide in the treatment of experimental brain compression," *J. Neurosurg.*, 38:345–354, March 1973.
15. Schmeck, H.M., Jr. "Scientists seek to test controversial solvent on disease of muscles," *The New York Times*, January 15, 1981, p. A21.
16. Marshall, L.F.; P.E. Camp; and S.A. Bowers. "Dimethyl sulfoxide for the treatment of intracranial hypertension: a preliminary trial," *Neurosurgery*, 14(6):659–663, June 1984.
17. Zingerman, L.I. "Dimexide (dimethyl sulfoxide) in the treatment of multiple sclerosis," *Zhurnal Neuropatologii I Psikhiatrii Imeni S. S. Korsakova*, 84(9): 1330–1333, 1984.

Chapter 10
DMSO Therapy for Mental Disabilities

1. Gesell, A. *Developmental Diagnosis*, New York: Paul Hoeber, 1946.
2. Aspillaga, M.J.; C. Morizon; I. Avendano; M. Sanchez; and L. Capdeville. "Dimethyl sulfoxide therapy in severe retardation in mongoloid children," *Ann. N.Y. Acad. Sci.*, 243:421–431, 1975.
3. Giller, A. and M.E.M. de Bernadou. "Dimethyl sulfoxide therapy in nonmongoloid infantile oligophrenia," *Ann. N.Y. Acad. Sci.*, 243:432–448, 1975.
4. Givovich, L.; M. Colombo; and Y. Lacassie. "Present treatment of Down's syndrome," *Revista Chilena De Pediatria*, 53(5):496–502, September-October, 1982.
5. Hoffer, A. and M. Walker. *Smart Nutrients*. Garden City Park, N.Y.: Avery Publishing Group, 1993.

Chapter 11
The DMSO-Cancer Connection

1. Tucker, E.J. and A. Carrizo. "Hematoxylon dissolved in dimethyl sulfoxide used in recurrent neoplasms," *International Surgery*, 49:516–527, June 1968.
2. Volden, G.; E. Thorud; and O.H. Iversen. "Inhibition of methylcholanthrene-induced skin carcinogenesis in hairless mice by membrane-labilizing agent DMSO," *British Journal of Dermatology*, 109 Suppl. 25: 133–136, July 1983.
3. Unpublished treatise by Thomas D. Rogers, Northwestern State University, "Light and electron microscope studies of the chemotherapeutic effect of a combination of dimethyl sulfoxide and hematoxylon on a transplantable lymphosarcoma," January 1979.

Chapter 12
Infectious Diseases Respond to DMSO

1. "Antiviral drug, DMSO teamed

against shingles," *Drug Topics,* February 15, 1971.

2. Zuniga, A.; R. Burdach; and S. Rubio. "Dimethyl sulfoxide therapy in bronchiolitis," *Ann. N.Y. Acad. Sci.,* 243:460–467.

3. Zuniga, A. "Dimethyl sulfoxide therapy in subjective tinnitus of unknown origin," *Ann. N.Y. Acad. Sci.,* 243:468–474.

4. Zimmerman, S.J.; M.B. Maude; and M. Moldawer. "Freezing and storage of human semen in 50 healthy medical students. A comparative study of glycerol and dimethylsulfoxide as a preservative," *Fertility Sterility,* 15:505, 1964.

5. Smith, G.C. "Observations in treating Cutaneous Larva Migrans," *J.S. Carolina Med. Assoc.,* 62:265, 1966.

6. Katz, R. and R.W. Hood. "Topical thiabendazole for creeping eruption," *Arch. Dermatol.,* 94:643, 1966.

7. Bogoiavlenski, I.F.; I.O. Zaks; and S.I. Ivanov. "Dimexide therapy of septic complications in critical status," *Ruesteziologiia I Reanimatologiia,* (4):38–40, July-August 1984.

8. Scheinberg, M.A.; J.C. Permambuco; and M.D. Benson. "DMSO and colchicine therapy in amyloid disease," *Annals of the Rheumatic Diseases,* 43(3): 421–423, June 1984.

9. Pravata, G.; G. Pinto; M. Bosco; G. Noto; and M. Arico. "Unusual localization of lichen amyloidosus. Topical treatment with dimethyl sulfoxide," *Acta Dermato-Venereologia,* 69(3):259–260, 1989.

10. Fil, I.; A.D. Zhenchenko; A. Ukh-

ov; and N.P. Popovich. "Prevention of suppurative complications of surgical wounds at a polyclinic," *Klinicheskaia Khirurgiia,* (1):58–59, 1988.

11. Sachek, M.G.; D.K. Novikov; and V.P. Bulakin. "Basis of immunocorrective therapy among patients with chronic osteomyelitis," *Vestnik Khirurgii Imeni I.I. Grekova,* 136(3):51–53, March 1986.

12. Glozman, V.N. "Clinico-diagnostic aspects of the use of proteases and dimexide in ochiepididymitis," *Urologia I Nefrologia,* (6):50–52, 1986.

Chapter 13
Misreporting of DMSO for Scleroderma and Interstitial Cystitis

1. Becker, D.P.; H.F. Young; F.E. Nulsen; et al. "Physiological effects of dimethyl sulfoxide on peripheral nerves: possible role in pain relief," *Exp. Neurol,* 24:272–276, 1969.

2. Engel, M.F. "Dimethyl sulfoxide in the treatment of scleroderma," *Southern Medical Journal,* 65:71–73, January 1972.

3. Heise, H., and P. Skierlo. "Circumscribed scleroderma—local treatment with dexamethasone-dimethyl sulfoxide preparation," *Dermatologische Monatsschrift,* 172(1):29–32, 1986.

4. Sergeev, V.P. "Mechanism of the therapeutic efficacy of dimexide in patients with circumscribed scleroderma," *Vestnik Dermatologii I Venerologii,* (7):64–66, July 1983.

5. Scherbel, A.L. "The effect of per-

cutaneous dimethyl sulfoxide on cutaneous manifestations of systemic sclerosis," *Ann. N.Y. Acad. Sci.*, 411:120–130, 1983.

6. Williams, H.J.; D.E. Furst; S.L. Dahl; V.D. Steen; C. Marks; E.J. Alpert; A.M. Henderson; C.O. Samuelson, Jr.; J.N. Dreyfus; A. Weinstein; et al. "Double-blind, multicenter controlled trial comparing topical dimethyl sulfoxide and normal saline for treatment of hand ulcers in patients with systemic sclerosis," *Arthritis and Rheumatism*, 28(3):308–314, March 1985.

7. Perez-Marrero, R.; L.E. Emerson; and J.T. Feltis. "A controlled study of dimethyl sulfoxide in interstitial cystitis," *Journal of Urology*, 140(1):36–39, July 1988.

8. Conejero Sugra-ness, J.; G. Llamazares Cach; J. Avila Padilla; F. Sarrias Lorenz; L. Sabin; and P. Zamora. "Treatment of the complex irritative bladder syndrome with dimethyl sulfoxide," *Actas Urologicas Espanolas*, 9(6):527–530, November-December 1985.

9. Okamura, K.; M. Mizunaga; S. Arima; S. Tokunaka; F. Inada; T. Takamura; and S. Yachiku. "The use of dimethyl sulfoxide in the treatment of intractable urinary frequency," *Hinyokika Kiyo-Acta Urologica Japonica*, 31(4):627–631, April 1985.

10. Tereszkiewicz, J. and T. Spruch. "Urethral syndrome in women and its treatment with dimethyl sulfoxide," *Ginekologia Polska*, 58(7):473–477, 1987.

11. Osanai, H.; K. Yamauchi; M. Morikawa; Y. Nakata; S. Tokunaka; F. Inada; and S. Yachiku.

"A case of bladder amyloidosis," *Hinyokika Kiyo-Acta Urologica Japonica*, 32(2):261–267, February 1986.

Appendix I

1. Kito, S.; E. Itoga; M. Inokawa; M. Hironaka; T. Kishida; and T. Shinoda. "Studies on biological actions of dimethyl sulfoxide in familial amyloidosis," *Ann. N.Y. Acad. Sci.*, 411:52–66, 1983.

2. Sabatelli, M.; C. Casali; C. Scoppetta; A. Frustaci; and P. Tonali. "Familial amyloid polyneuropathy. Description of two cases treated with dimethyl sulfoxide," *Rivista Di Neurobiologia*, 30(2-3):261–267, April-September 1984.

3. Monfrecola, G.; R. Iandoli; G. Bruno; and D. Martellotta. "Lichen amyloidosus: a new therapeutic approach," *Acta Dermato-Venereologica*, 65(5):453–455, 1985.

4. Hsieh, S.D.; R. Yamamoto; K. Saito; Y. Iwamoto; T. Kuzuya; S. Ohba; S. Kobori; and K. Saito. "Amyloidosis presented with whitening and loss of hair which improved after dimethyl sulfoxide treatment," *Japanese Journal of Medicine*, 26(3):393–395, August 1987.

5. Wang, W.J.; C.S. Lin; and C.K. Wong. "Response of systemic amyloidosis to dimethyl sulfoxide," *Journal of the American Academy of Dermatology*, 15(2 part 2):402–405, August 1986.

6. Ravid, M.; J. Shapira; R. Lang; and I. Kedar. "Prolonged dimethyl sulphoxide treatment in 13 patients with systemic amy-

loidosis," *Annals of the Rheumatic Diseases*, 41(6):587–592, 1982.

7. Gruys, E.; R.J. Sijens; and W.J. Biewenga. "Dubious effect of dimethyl sulphoxide therapy on amyloid deposits and amyloidosis," *Veterinary Research Communications*, 5(1) 21–32, September 1981.

8. Yachiku, S. "Experience with dimethyl sulfoxide treatment for primary localized amyloidosis of the bladder," *Journal of Urology*, 135(3):580–582, March 1986.

9. Dai, K.Y.; J.C. Montet; X.M. Zhao; J. Amic; and R. Choux. "Dissolving agents of human mixed cholesterol stones," *Gastroenterologie Clinique Et Biologique*, 12(4):312–319, April 1988.

10. Asakawa, S.; H. Igimi; and H. Shimura. "A new direct solubilizer for bilirubinate calcium stones," *Nippon Geka Gakkai Zasshi–Journal of the Japanese Surgical Society*, 84(10):1072–1083, October 1983.

11. Sotolong, J.R., Jr.; F. Swerdlow; H.I. Schiff; and H.E. Schapira. "Successful treatment of lupus erythematosus cystitis with DMSO," *Urology*, 23(2):125–127, February 1984.

12. Kolomiets, L.I. "Effectiveness of ectericide, dimethyl sulfoxide, and oxacillin in treating acute, odontogenic inflammatory jaw diseases," *Stomatologiia*, 60(4):33–35, 1981.

13. Kavli, G.; K. Midelfart; G. Volden; and H. Krokan. "Photochemical reactions of Heracleum Iaciniatum. Influence of dimethyl sulphoxide and corticosteroids," *British Journal of Dermatology*, 109 Suppl 25:137–140, July 1983.

Bibliography

Albert, H.M., "Effects of DMSO on the Healing of Wounds," *Presse Med.*, 75, 20, 1967.

Annals New York Academy of Sciences, "Biological Actions of Dimethyl Sulfoxide (DMSO)," Vol. 141, 1–671:1967.

Arno, I.C., Wapner, P.M., and Brownstein, I.E., "Experiences With DMSO in Relief of Postpartum Episiotomy Pain," *Annals New York Academy of Sciences*, 141, 403, 1967.

Ayre, J.E., and Leguerrier, J., "Some (Regressive) Effects of DMSO Dexamethasone Upon Cervical Cells in Cervical Dysplasia and Carcinoma in Situ," *Annals New York Academy of Sciences*, 141, 414, 1967.

Bernath, Z., Chacon, E., Bennett, N., and Riveros, A., "Experiencia Clinica en Tratamiento del Sindrome Asmatico con una Combinacion de DMSO 1.3 Dimetixantina-Etilendiamina, Clorfeniramina y un Anti-Inflamatorio," *Rev. Medica de Valparaiso*. Dic. 1969.

Berrios De La Luz, R., Pfister, H., Junemann, C., and Perales, L., "Terapia Para Artrosis y Artritis con Artrotin un Preparado a Base de DMSO, Gama-Cetofenibutazona y Dexametazona," *Boletin de la Soc. Chilena de Reumatologia, Vol. IX, No. 1*, Abril 1971; Santiago, Chile.

Bien, K., "Particular Properties of Dimethyl Sulfoxide (DMSO) in the Light of Current Clinical Investigations," *Polski Tygod. Lekar.*, 21, 688, 1966.

Blum, E.O., "Erfahrungen mit Dolicur bei Chirurgischen Erkrankungen Unter Besonderer Beruecksichtigung der Vertraeglichkeit," *DMSO Symposium*, Herausgegeben von Priv.—Doz. Laudahn, G., Saladruck, Berlin, 1965, p. 102.

Bottomly, D.R., Shimazaki, Y., and Bachman, D.M., "Controlled Study of Dimethyl Sulfoxide Effects in Patients with Connective Tissue Diseases," *Arthritis Rheumato.*, 7, 294, 1964.

Brown, J.H., "Treatment of Aerotits and Aerosinusitis With Topical DMSO," *Aerospace Medicine*, 38, 629, 1967.

Brucher, E., Munizaga, G., and Torres, P., "Accion Terapeutica de Merinex en Diversas Afecciones Organica-Cerebrales," *Rev. Hosp. Psiquiatrico, Vol. 1*, Enero 1970, Santiago, Chile.

Cerimele, D., and Pisanu, G., "Rapporto fra Aziones dei Corisonici ed Aggiunta Dimetilsulfossido (Importanza delia Concentrazione)," *Redaziones il.*, 21, VII, 1966.

Chan, J.C., and Gadebusch, H.H., "Virucidal Properties of Dimethyl Sulfoxide," *Applied Microbiology*, 16, 1625, 1968.

Cors, J., "Anti-Inflammatory Effects of DMSO," *Bull Trav. Soc. Pharm. Lyon*, 9, 213, 1965.

Day, P.L., "Final Evaluation of One Thousand Cases Treated in Orthopaedic Practice With DMSO," *DMSO Symposium*, Vienna. Herausgageben von Priv.—Doz. Daudhan, G., and Gertich, K. (eds.), 1966, p. 107.

Escobar, E., and Cornejo, J., "Una Neuva Quimioterapia Antiblastica, Potenciada e Hipotoxica, Ciclofosfamido-Sulfoxidanta (DMSO)," *Rev. de Hosp. San Fco. de Borja*, Vol. 6 No. 3, Septbre, 1971, Stgo., Chile.

Finney, J.W., and Urschel, H. and Co., "Protection of the Ischemic Heart With DMSO Alone or DMSO With Hydrogen Peroxide," *Annals New York Academy of Sciences*, Vol. 141, 1, 231–241, 1967.

Frommhold, W., and Bublitz, G., "Untersuchungen uber Unterhautifibrosen nach Telekobalttherapie und ihre Behandlungsmoeglichkeiten mit Dimethylsulfoxyd (DMSO)," *Strahlentherapie*, 133, 529, 1967.

Gerhards, E., "Uber Stoffwechsel und Stoffwechselwirkungen von Dimethylsulfoxyd," *DMSO Symposium*, 1965, Laudahn, G. (ed.), Saladruck, Berlin, 1965, p. 18.

Grismali, J., and y Varela, L., "Uso de Ipran en Neurologia," *Rev. Hosp. San Fco. De Borja*, Vol. 5, No. 4, Dic. 1970, Santiago, Chile.

Grismali, J., and y Varela, L., "Terapia con Merinex en Neurosis Depresiva de Angustia e Histerica," *Rev. Hosp. San Fco. de Borja*, Vol. 5, No. 2, Junio 1970, Santiago, Chile.

Herschler, R.J., and Jacob, S.W., "DMSO-Therapy in Peripheral Vascular Disease," U.S. Patent Pending, 1964 (Patent royalties assigned to University of Oregon Medical School).

Herschler, R.J., and Jacob, S.W., "DMSO-Therapy in Burns," U.S. Patent Pending, 1964 (Patent royalties assigned to University of Oregon Medical School).

Herschler, R.J., and Jacob, S.W., "DMSO: A New Drug from Lignin," *TAPPI* 48:43A–46A, 1965.

Jacob, S.W., "Dimethyl Sulfoxide (DMSO), Its Basic Pharmacology and Usefulness in the Therapy of Headache," *Headache*, 5:78–81, October, 1965.

Jacob, S.W., "Dimethyl Sulfoxide (DMSO)," *McGraw-Hill Yearbook of Science and Technology*, 1966, McGraw-Hill Book Company

Jacob, S.W., "DMSO: Potential Usefulness in Physical Therapy," *Physical Therapy*, 49:470, 1969.

Jacob, S.W., "Dimethyl Sulfoxide (DMSO): Current Concepts in Toxicology, Pharmacology, and Clinical Usefulness in Surgery," *American Surgeon*, 35:564, 1969.

Jacob, S.W., Bischell, M., Eberlec, G., and Herschler, R.J., "The Influence of Dimethyl Sulfoxide on the Transport of Insulin Across a Biologic Membrane," *Federation Proceedings* 23:410, 1964.

Jacob, S.W., Bischel, M., and Herschler, R.J., "Dimethyl Sulfoxide (DMSO): A New Concept in Pharmacotherapy," *Current Therapeutic Research* 6: 134–135, 1964.

Jacob, S.W., Bischel, M., and Herschler, R.J., "Dimethyl Sulfoxide (DMSO): Effects on the Permeability of Biologic Membranes (Preliminary Report)," *Current Therapeutic Research* 6:193–198, 1964.

Jacob, S.W., Herschler, R.J., and Rosenbaum, E.E., "Dimethyl Sulfoxide (DMSO): Laboratory and Clinical Evaluation," *Journal of the American Veterinary Medical Association*, 147, 12:1350–1359, December 15, 1965.

Jacob, S.W., and Rosenbaum, E.E., "The Toxicology of Dimethyl Sulfoxide (DMSO)," *Headache*, 6:127–135, October, 1966.

Jacob, S.W., and Rosenbaum, E.E., "Dimethyl Sulfoxide (DMSO), An Evaluation After Two Years of Clinical Experience," *DMSO Symposium,* 1966, Vienna, p. 83, Saladruck, Berlin, 1966.

Jacob, S.W., and Wood, D.C., "Notes on Dimethyl Sulfoxide (DMSO)," Symposium: Vienna, Austria, November 8–9, 1966. *Current Therapeutic Research* 9:229–233, 1967.

Jacob, S.W., and Wood, D.C., "Summary of Dimethyl Sulfoxide Symposium," *Arznei-For* 17: 1086, 1967.

Jacob, S.W., and Wood, D.C., "Dimethyl Sulfoxide (DMSO) Toxicology, Pharmacology and Clinical Experience," *Amer. Your. Surg.* 114:414–427, 1967.

Jacob, S.W., Wood, D.C., and Brown, J.H., "Therapeutic Potential of Diemthyl Sulfoxide (DMSO)," *Aerospace Medicine,* Aerospace Med. 40, 75, 1969.

Kajihara, K., Kawanaga, H., de La Torre, J.C., and Mullan, Sean, "Dimethyl Sulfoxide in the Treatment of Experimental Acute Spinal Cord Injury," *Surgical Neurology,* 1973, Vol. 1 No. 1, pg. 16–22.

Kaminsky, A., "Dimethyl Sulfoxide: Its Possibilities in Dermatology," *Rev. Assoc. Med. Arg.,* 79, 556, 1965.

Kamiya, S., Wakao, T., and Nishioka, K., "Studies on Improvement of Eye Drops. 3. Bacteriological Consideration of DMSO," *Rinsho Ganka (Japanese Journal of Clinical Opthalmology),* 20, 143, 1966.

Kocsis, J.J., Harkaway, S., Vogel, W.H., Brink, J.J., and Stein, D.G., "Dimethyl Sulfoxide Breakdown of Blood-Brain Barrier," *Science,* 160, 1471, 1968.

Lau, H., Limberger, J., and Muller, H., "Treatment of Mastopathies With Dimethyl Sulfoxide," *Deut. Med. Wochschr.,* 93, 2102, 1968.

MacCallum, F.O., and Juel-Jensen, B.E., "Herpes Simplex Virus Skin Infection in Man Treated with Idoxuridine in Dimethyl Sulfoxide, Results of Double Blind Controlled Trial," *Brit. Med. J.,* 2, 805, 1966.

Matsumoto, J., "Clinical Trials of Dimethyl Sulfoxide in Rheumatoid Arthritis Patients in Japan," *Annals New York Academy of Sciences,* 141, 560, 1967.

Munizaga, G., "Decaimiento Psico-Organico y Consideraciones

Terapeuticas," *Rev. Hosp. San Fco. Borja,* Vol. 5, No. 3, Septbre. 1970. Santiago, Chile.

Narula, P.N., and Jacob, S.W., "The Cryoprotective Effect of Dimethyl Sulfoxide and Glycerol on Cell Cultures at Various Temperatures," *Cryobiology* 2:32, 1965.

Narula, P.N., and Jacob, S.W., "The Cryoprotective Effect of Methyl Cellulose (Methacel) With Dimethyl Sulfoxide and Glycerol on Cell Cultures," *Cryobiology* 2:32, 1965.

Nassar, C., "Experiencia Clinica con Merinex en Ninos con Deficit Mental y Dificultades de Aprendizaje Basico," *Rev. Med. de Valparaiso,* Vol. XXII, Dic. 1969.

Paul, M.M., "Comparison of DMSO and Conventional Methods of Therapy in the Treatment of Soft Tissue Athletic Injuries," *DMSO Symposium,* Vienna, 1966, Laudahn, G. (ed.), Saladruck, Berlin, 1966, p. 101.

Paulin, H.J., Murphy, J.B., and Larson, R.E., "Determination of Dimethyl Sulfoxide in Plasma and Cerebrospinal Fluid by Gas-Liquid Chromatography," *Anal. Chem.* 38, 651, 1966.

Penrod, D.S., Bacharach, B., and Templeton, J.Y., "III. Dimethyl Sulfoxide for Incisional Pain After Thoracotomy: Preliminary Report," *Annals New York Academy of Sciences,* 141, 493, 1967.

Perce, H.L., "Dimethyl Sulfoxide (DMSO) the Wonder Drug," *Current Pediatry,* 13, 7, 1964.

Perlman, F., and Wolfe, H.F., "Dimethyl-Sulfoxide as a Penetrant Carrier of Allergens Through Intact Human," *J. Allergy,* 38, 299, 1966.

Persky, L., and Stewart, B.H., "The Use of Dimethyl Sulfoxide in the Treatment of Genitourinary Disorders," *Annals New York Academy of Sciences,* 141, 551, 1967.

Rosenbaum, E.E., Herschler, R.J., and Jacob, S.W., "Dimethyl Sulfoxide (DMSO) in Musculoskeletal Disorders," *JAMA* 192:309–313, 1965.

Rosenbaum, E.E., and Jacob, S.W., "Dimethyl Sulfoxide (DMSO) in the Treatment of Musculoskeletal Injuries and Inflammations, II. The Treatment of Rheumatoid Arthritis, Degenerative Arthritis, and Gouty Arthritis, a Preliminary Report," *Northwest Medicine* 63:227–229, 1964.

Rosenbaum, E.E., and Jacob, S.W., "Dimethyl Sulfoxide (DMSO) in the

Treatment of Acute Musculoskeletal Injuries and Inflammations, I. Dimethyl Sulfoxide in Acute Subdeltoid Bursitis," *Northwest Medicine* 63:167–168, 1964.

Rosenbaum, E.E., and Jacob, S.W., "The Use of Dimethyl Sulfoxide (DMSO) for the Treatment of Intractable Pain in Surgical Patients," *Surgery* 58:258–266, 1965.

Sabah, D., "Tratamiento Combinado con Gamma-Cetofenibutazona, Dexametasona y DMSO en Artritis Reumatoidea y Otras Colagenopatias," Boletin Soc. Chilena de Reumatologia, Vol. VII, No. 12, Septbre. 1970, Stgo., Chile.

Solano-Aguilar, E., "Dimethyl Sulfoxide con Triamcinolona en Varias Dermatosis," *Rev. Med. Costa Rica*, 33, 231, 1966.

Steimberg, A., "Clinical Applications of Dimethyl Sulfoxide in Collagenous and Musculoskeletal Diseases," *DMSO Symposium*, Vienna, 1966, Laudahn, G. (ed.), Saladruck, Berlin, 1966, p. 20.

Steimberg, A., "The Employment of Dimethyl Sulfoxide as an Anti-Inflammatory Agent and Steroid-Transporter in Diversified Clinical Diseases," *Annals New York Academy of Sciences*, 141, 532, 1967.

Stein, D.G., and Brink, J.J., "Prevention of Retrograde Amnesia by Injection of Magnesium Pemoline," *Dimethylsulfoxide-Psychopharmacology*, 14, 240, 1969.

Stelzer, J.M., Colaizzi, J.L., and Wurdack, P.J., "Influence of Dimethyl Sulfoxide (DMSO) on Percutaneous Absorption of Salicylic Acid and Sodium Salcylate From Ointments," *J. Pharm. Sci.*, 57, 1732, 1968.

Stewart, B.H., "Dimethyl Sulfoxide (DMSO) in the Treatment of Troublesome Genitourinary Disorders: A Preliminary Report," *Cleveland Clinic Quarterly*, 33, 81, 1966.

Stewart, B.H., Versky, L., and Kiser, W.S., "Use of Dimethyl Sulfoxide (DMSO) in Treatment of Interstitial Cystitis," *J. Urol.* 98, 671, 1967.

Stewart, G., and Jacob, S.W., "Use of Dimethyl Sulfoxide (DMSO) in the Treatment of Post Amputation Pain," *American Surgeon* 31:460–462, 1965.

Stoughton, R.B., and Fritsh, W., "Influence of Dimethyl Sulfoxide (DMSO) on Human Percutaneous Absorption," *Arch. Dermatol.*, 90, 512, 1964.

Stringer, H., and Engel, G.B., "Dimethyl Sulfoxide for Nail Infection," *Lancet*, 7441, 825, 1966.

Tellex, A., "Experiencia Terapeutica con Ipran en Psiquiatria de la Edad Avanzada," *Rev. Hospital Psiquiatrico*, Vol 1. No. 2, Junio 1970, Santiago, Chile.

Torre de la, J.C., Rowed, D.W., Kawanaga, H.M., and Mullan, S., "Dimethyl Sulfoxide in the Treatment of Experimental Brain Compression," *Journal of Neurosurgery*, Volume 38, March 1973.

Tucker, E.J., and Carrizo, A., "Hematoxylon Dissolved in Dimethylsulfoxide Used in Recurrent Neoplasms," *Intern. Surg.*, 49, 516, 1968.

Venerando, A., "On Therapeutic Action of Dimethyl Sulphoxide (RE 421) in Sport Trauma and in Osteoarticular Atlas Diseases," *Gaz. Intern. Med. Chir.*, 70, 1605, 1965, in Italian.

Vishwkarma, S.K., "Dimethyl Sulfoxide in Tympanoplasty. A Preliminary Report," *Plastic Reconstructive Surgery*, 42, 15, 1968.

Weitgasser, H., "Dermatological Investigations with Dimethylsulfoxide (DMSO)," *Z. Haut-Geschlechts Krankh.*, 21, 749, 1967.

Weitgasser, H., "Die Lokalbehandlung von Chronischen Paronychien mit Einer Kombination von Triamcinolon-Acetonid und Dimetilsulfoxide," *Z. Haut-Geschlechts Krankh.*, 44, 27, 1969.

Wodniansky, P., "Dupuytrem und Sklerodermie," *DMSO Symposium*, Vienna, 1966, Laudahn, G. (ed.), Saladruck, Berlin, 1966, p. 158.

Yeats, R.O., Preliminary Test Using DMSO as a Vehicle for Drugs in Leprosy," *Annals New York Academy of Sciences*, 141, 668, 1967.

Ziv-Silberman, G., "DMSO in the Treatment of Chronic Mastitis," *Veterinary Record*, 81, 527, 1967.

Zuckner, J., and Uddin, J., "Local Applications of Dimethyl Sulfoxide (DMSO) and DMSO Combined With Trincinolone Acetonide in Rheumatoid Arthritis," *Nature*, 1389, 55, 1965.

Index